Janna L. Morrison and Timothy R.H. Regnault
(Eds.)

Nutrition in Pregnancy

Volume II

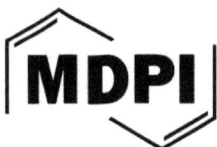

This book is a reprint of the Special Issue that appeared in the online, open access journal, *Nutrients* (ISSN 2072-6643) from 2014–2016, available at:

http://www.mdpi.com/journal/nutrients/special_issues/nutrition-pregnancy

Guest Editors
Janna L. Morrison
Professor, School of Pharmacy and Medical Sciences
University of South Australia
Australia

Timothy R.H. Regnault
Associate Professor, Departments of Obstetrics and Gynaecology/Physiology and Pharmacology
Scientist, Children's Health Research Institute
Western University
Canada

Editorial Office
MDPI AG
St. Alban-Anlage 66
Basel, Switzerland

| *Publisher* | *Assistant Editor* |
| Shu-Kun Lin | Xiaocen Zhang |

1. Edition 2017

MDPI • Basel • Beijing • Wuhan • Barcelona • Belgrade

ISBN 978-3-03842-368-3 (Hbk) Vol. 2   ISBN 978-3-03842-308-9 (Hbk) Vol. 1-2
ISBN 978-3-03842-369-0 (PDF) Vol. 2   ISBN 978-3-03842-309-6 (PDF) Vol. 1-2

Table of Contents

Section 1: Micronutrients and Diet Composition during Pregnancy

Section 2: New Studies of Vitamin D and Its Role in Fetal Development

List of Contributors

Antonysunil Adaikalakoteswari Warwick Medical School, University of Warwick, Coventry CV2 2DX, UK.

Neil Anderson Academic department of Diabetes and Metabolism, George Eliot Hospital, Nuneaton CV10 7DJ, UK.

Euclides Avila Department of Reproductive Biology, National Institute of Medical Sciences and Nutrition Salvador Zubirán, Vasco de Quiroga No. 15, Tlalpan 14000, Mexico City, Mexico.

Cynthia Barrera Department of Nutrition, Faculty of Medicine, University of Chile, Av. Independencia 1027, Independencia, Santiago 8380453, Chile.

Karla A. Bascuñán Department of Nutrition, Faculty of Medicine, University of Chile, Av. Independencia 1027, Independencia, Santiago 8380453, Chile.

Michelle L. Blumfield School of Health Sciences, and Priority Research Centre in Physical Activity and Nutrition, Faculty of Health and Medicine, University of Newcastle, Callaghan, New South Wales 2308, Australia.

Francis G. Bowling Mater Research Institute, Level 4, Translational Research Institute, University of Queensland, 37 Kent St, TRI, Woolloongabba, QLD 4102, Australia; Mater Children's Hospital, Mater Health Services, South Brisbane, QLD 4101, Australia.

Rodrigo Chamorro Department of Nutrition, Faculty of Medicine, University of Chile, Av. Independencia 1027, Independencia, Santiago 8380453, Chile.

Karen Charlton School of Medicine, University of Wollongong, NSW 2522, Australia.

Xuemei Chen Laboratory of Reproductive Biology, School of Public Health, Chongqing Medical University, Chongqing 400016, China.

Yoon Young Cho Division of Endocrinology and Metabolism, Department of Medicine, Thyroid Center, Samsung Medical Center, Sungkyunkwan University School of Medicine, 81 Irwon-Ro, Gangnam-Gu, Seoul 135-710, Korea.

Rihwa Choi Department of Laboratory Medicine and Genetics, Samsung Medical Center, Sungkyunkwan University School of Medicine, 81 Irwon-Ro, Gangnam-Gu, Seoul 135-710, Korea.

Jae Hoon Chung Division of Endocrinology and Metabolism, Department of Medicine, Thyroid Center, Samsung Medical Center, Sungkyunkwan University School of Medicine, 81 Irwon-Ro, Gangnam-Gu, Seoul 135-710, Korea.

Vicki L. Clifton Robinson Research Institute, School of Paediatrics and Reproductive Health, Adelaide University, Lyell McEwin Hospital, Haydown Road, Elizabeth Vale, SA 5112, Australia.

Marta Cuervo Department of Nutrition, Food Sciences and Physiology, Center for Nutritional Research, University of Navarra, Pamplona 31008, Spain; CIBERobn Physiopathology of Obesity and Nutrition, Institute of Health Carlos III (ISCIII), Madrid 28029, Spain.

Ian Darnton-Hill The Boden Institute of Obesity, Nutrition, Exercise & Eating Disorders, University of Sydney, NSW 2006, Australia; The Friedman School of Nutrition Science and Policy, Tufts University, Medford, MA 021111, USA.

Barbara Davidson Global Health Center, Perinatal Institute and Division of Biostatistics and Epidemiology, Cincinnati Children's Hospital Medical Center, 3333 Burnet Avenue, Cincinnati, OH 45229, USA.

Adekunle Dawodu Global Health Center, Perinatal Institute and Division of Biostatistics and Epidemiology, Cincinnati Children's Hospital Medical Center, 3333 Burnet Avenue, Cincinnati, OH 45229, USA.

Paul A. Dawson Mater Research Institute, Level 4, Translational Research Institute, University of Queensland, 37 Kent St, TRI, Woolloongabba, QLD 4102, Australia.

Lorenza Díaz Department of Reproductive Biology, National Institute of Medical Sciences and Nutrition Salvador Zubirán, Vasco de Quiroga No. 15, Tlalpan 14000, Mexico City, Mexico.

Yubin Ding Laboratory of Reproductive Biology, School of Public Health, Chongqing Medical University, Chongqing 400016, China.

Kristyn Dunlop Department of Physiology and Pharmacology, Western University, London, ON N6A-5C1, Canada.

Marta Durand-Carbajal Department of Reproductive Biology, National Institute of Medical Sciences and Nutrition Salvador Zubirán, Vasco de Quiroga No. 15, Tlalpan 14000, Mexico City, Mexico.

Aoife Elliott Mater Research Institute, Level 4, Translational Research Institute, University of Queensland, 37 Kent St, TRI, Woolloongabba, QLD 4102, Australia; Mater Children's Hospital, Mater Health Services, South Brisbane, QLD 4101, Australia.

Rufei Gao Laboratory of Reproductive Biology, School of Public Health, Chongqing Medical University, Chongqing 400016, China.

Yanqing Geng Laboratory of Reproductive Biology, School of Public Health, Chongqing Medical University, Chongqing 400016, China.

Jessica A. Grieger Robinson Research Institute, School of Paediatrics and Reproductive Health, Adelaide University, Lyell McEwin Hospital, Haydown Road, Elizabeth Vale, SA 5112, Australia.

Maria de Lourdes Guerrero National Institute of Medical Sciences and Nutrition, Vasco de Quiroga No. 15, Tlalpan, Mexico City 14000, Mexico.

Junlin He Laboratory of Reproductive Biology, School of Public Health, Chongqing Medical University, Chongqing 400016, China.

Lisu Huang MOE-Shanghai Key Lab of Children's Environmental Health, Xinhua Hospital affiliated to Shanghai Jiao Tong University School of Medicine, Shanghai 200092, China.

Seonwoo Kim Biostatistics Team, Samsung Biomedical Research Institute, 81 Irwon-Ro, Gangnam-Gu, Seoul 135-710, Korea.

Sun Wook Kim Division of Endocrinology and Metabolism, Department of Medicine, Thyroid Center, Samsung Medical Center, Sungkyunkwan University School of Medicine, 81 Irwon-Ro, Gangnam-Gu, Seoul 135-710, Korea.

Alexander Lawson Department of Pathology, Heartlands Hospital, Birmingham B9 5SS, UK.

Soo-Youn Lee Department of Laboratory Medicine and Genetics, Samsung Medical Center, Sungkyunkwan University School of Medicine, 81 Irwon-Ro, Gangnam-Gu, Seoul 135-710, Korea.

Yanli Li Laboratory of Reproductive Biology, School of Public Health, Chongqing Medical University, Chongqing 400016, China.

Xinggui Liao Laboratory of Reproductive Biology, School of Public Health, Chongqing Medical University, Chongqing 400016, China.

Xueqing Liu Laboratory of Reproductive Biology, School of Public Health, Chongqing Medical University, Chongqing 400016, China.

Catherine Lucas School of Medicine, University of Wollongong, NSW 2522, Australia.

Jose Alfredo Martínez Department of Nutrition, Food Sciences and Physiology, Center for Nutritional Research, University of Navarra, Pamplona 31008, Spain; CIBERobn Physiopathology of Obesity and Nutrition, Institute of Health Carlos III (ISCIII), Madrid 28029, Spain.

Anne T. McMahon School of Medicine, University of Wollongong, NSW 2522, Australia.

Philip G. McTernan Warwick Medical School, University of Warwick, Coventry CV2 2DX, UK.

Uzonna C. Mkparu Columbia University Medical Center, Institute of Human Nutrition, New York, NY 10027, USA.

Janna L. Morrison Early Origins of Adult Health Research Group, School of Pharmacy and Medical Sciences, Sansom Institute for Health Research, University of South Australia, Adelaide, SA 5001, Australia.

Ardythe L. Morrow Global Health Center, Perinatal Institute and Division of Biostatistics and Epidemiology, Cincinnati Children's Hospital Medical Center, 3333 Burnet Avenue, Cincinnati, OH 45229, USA.

Soo-young Oh Department of Obstetrics and Gynecology, Samsung Medical Center, Sungkyunkwan University School of Medicine, 81 Irwon-Ro, Gangnam-Gu, Seoul 135-710, Seoul, Korea.

Andrea Olmos-Ortiz Department of Reproductive Biology, National Institute of Medical Sciences and Nutrition Salvador Zubirán, Vasco de Quiroga No. 15, Tlalpan 14000, Mexico City, Mexico.

Fengxiu Ouyang MOE-Shanghai Key Lab of Children's Environmental Health, Xinhua Hospital affiliated to Shanghai Jiao Tong University School of Medicine, Shanghai 200092, China.

Yong-Mei Peng Children's Hospital of Fudan University, 399 Wanyuan Road, Shanghai 20102, China.

Claudia Puigrredon Obstetrics and Gynecology Department, Clinical Hospital of the University of Chile, Av. Santos Dumont 999, Independencia, Santiago 8380453, Chile.

Timothy R.H. Regnault Departments of Physiology and Biochemistry, Department of Physiology and Pharmacology, and Department of Obstetrics and Gynecology, Western University, London, ON N6H-5W9, Canada; Children's Health Research Institute, London, ON N6C-2V5, Canada; Lawson Health Research Institute, London, ON N6C-2R5, Canada.

Jorge Sandoval Obstetrics and Gynecology Department, Clinical Hospital of the University of Chile, Av. Santos Dumont 999, Independencia, Santiago 8380453, Chile.

Susana Santiago Department of Nutrition, Food Sciences and Physiology, Center for Nutritional Research, University of Navarra, Pamplona 31008, Spain.

Ponnusamy Saravanan WISDEM Centre, University Hospital Coventry and Warwickshire, Coventry CV2 2DX, UK; Warwick Medical School, University of Warwick, Coventry CV2 2DX, UK; Academic department of Diabetes and Metabolism, George Eliot Hospital, Nuneaton CV10 7DJ, UK.

Carmen Sayon-Orea Department of Preventive Medicine and Public Health, University of Navarra, Pamplona 31008, Spain.

Kavitha Sivakumar Warwick Medical School, University of Warwick, Coventry CV2 2DX, UK.

Phoebe Starling School of Medicine, University of Wollongong, NSW 2522, Australia.

Gyanendra Tripathi Warwick Medical School, University of Warwick, Coventry CV2 2DX, UK.

Alejandra Valencia Department of Nutrition, Faculty of Medicine, University of Chile, Av. Independencia 1027, Independencia, Santiago 8380453, Chile.

Alfonso Valenzuela Lipid Center, Institute of Nutrition and Food Technology (INTA), University of Chile, Av. El Líbano 5524, Macul, Santiago 8380453, Chile.

Rodrigo Valenzuela Department of Nutrition, Faculty of Medicine, University of Chile, Av. Independencia 1027, Independencia, Santiago 8380453, Chile.

Manu Vatish Nuffield Department of Obstetrics & Gynaecology, University of Oxford, Oxford OX3 9DU, UK.

Meng Wang Department of Epidemiology and Health Statistics, School of Public Health, Shandong University, 44 WenhuaXilu Road, Jinan 250012, Shandong, China; Zhejiang Provincial Center for Disease Control and Prevention, 3399 Binsheng Road, Hangzhou 310051, Zhejiang, China.

Weiye Wang MOE-Shanghai Key Lab of Children's Environmental Health, Xinhua Hospital affiliated to Shanghai Jiao Tong University School of Medicine, Shanghai 200092, China.

Xia Wang MOE-Shanghai Key Lab of Children's Environmental Health, Xinhua Hospital affiliated to Shanghai Jiao Tong University School of Medicine, Shanghai 200092, China.

Yingxiong Wang Laboratory of Reproductive Biology, School of Public Health, Chongqing Medical University, Chongqing 400016, China.

Zhi-Ping Wang Department of Epidemiology and Health Statistics, School of Public Health, Shandong University, 44 WenhuaXilu Road, Jinan 250012, Shandong, China.

Craig Webster Department of Pathology, Heartlands Hospital, Birmingham B9 5SS, UK.

Zhenzhen Wei MOE-Shanghai Key Lab of Children's Environmental Health, Xinhua Hospital affiliated to Shanghai Jiao Tong University School of Medicine, Shanghai 200092, China.

Jessica G. Woo Global Health Center, Perinatal Institute and Division of Biostatistics and Epidemiology, Cincinnati Children's Hospital Medical Center, 3333 Burnet Avenue, Cincinnati, OH 45229, USA.

Catherine Wood Academic department of Diabetes and Metabolism, George Eliot Hospital, Nuneaton CV10 7DJ, UK.

Chittaranjan S. Yajnik Diabetes Research Centre, KEM Hospital, Pune 411011, India.

Hui Yang Department of Epidemiology and Health Statistics, School of Public Health, Shandong University, 44 WenhuaXilu Road, Jinan 250012, Shandong, China.

Heejin Yoo Biostatistics and Clinical Epidemiology Center, Samsung Medical Center, 81 Irwon-Ro, Gangnam-Gu, Seoul 135-710, Korea.

Xiaodan Yu MOE-Shanghai Key Lab of Children's Environmental Health, Xinhua Hospital affiliated to Shanghai Jiao Tong University School of Medicine, Shanghai 200092, China.

Huijuan Zhang Departments of Pathology and Bio-Bank, the International Peace Maternity and Child Health Hospital, Shanghai Jiao Tong University, Shanghai 200030, China.

Jun Zhang MOE-Shanghai Key Lab of Children's Environmental Health, Xinhua Hospital affiliated to Shanghai Jiao Tong University School of Medicine, Shanghai 200092, China.

Zhong-Tang Zhao Department of Epidemiology and Health Statistics, School of Public Health, Shandong University, 44 WenhuaXilu Road, Jinan 250012, Shandong, China.

About the Guest Editors

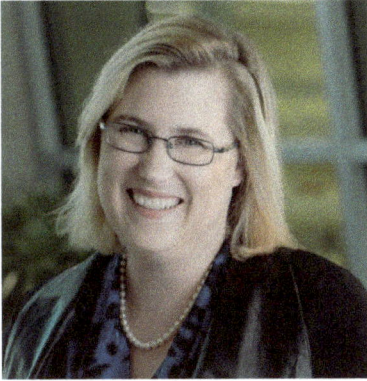

Janna Morrison, Prof., is Head of the Early Origins of the Adult Health Research Group in the Sansom Institute for Health Research at the University of South Australia. Prof Morrison held fellowships from the Heart Foundation 2004–2013 and is currently a NHMRC Career Development Fellow (2014–2017). Her current research focusses on how the fetal cardiovascular system responds to changes in nutrient supply before conception and during pregnancy. Initial work focused on understanding how the small baby maintains its blood pressure in utero and if these mechanisms might lead to an increased risk of hypertension in adult life. With the aid of an American Physiological Society Career Enhancement Award, she began investigating the effects of being small on heart development and has shown a role for upregulation of a hypertrophic signaling pathway. This is an important step in developing interventions to improve the heart health of babies born small. More recently, she has looked at the other end of the spectrum, the effects of maternal obesity on heart development. After completing her Ph.D. at the University of British Columbia, Janna held postdoctoral positions at the University of Toronto and the University of Adelaide before joining the Sansom Institute for Health Research in 2006. Janna received a South Australian Tall Poppy Science Award (2006) and is a fellow of the Cardiovascular section of the American Physiological Society (2015).

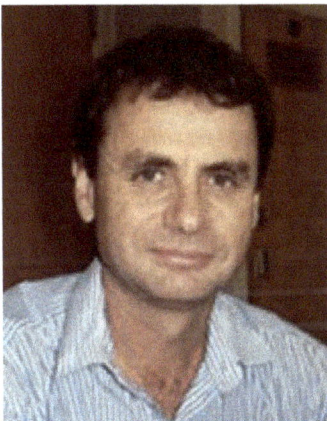

Timothy Regnault, Dr., is an Associate Professor in the Departments of Obstetrics and Gynaecology/ Physiology and Pharmacology at Western University, Canada. His research activities are focused around the *in utero* origins of adult metabolic disease. Through the use of cell-based and animal/human model systems, and technologies such as PET/CT and MRI, his laboratory investigates how stressors such as hypoxia, oxidative stress and infection and poor maternal diet during fetal life, impact placental, and fetal blood vessel, liver, adipose, kidney, heart and muscle development and function *in utero*, and how modifications to these systems *in utero* may underlie an increased adverse postnatal life metabolic disease risk. These studies aim to address what reprogramming events these stressors initiate in the womb and what the implications of these outcomes are for the onset and severity of childhood and adult diseases; such as insulin resistance and associated non-communicable diseases including obesity, cardiovascular disease and hypertension. More importantly, the research sets out to understand the degree of plasticity of these changes by investigating if they are locked after being reprogrammed, or are there windows of opportunity for intervention and rescue of some of these unfavorable *in utero*-induced changes.

Preface to "Nutrition in Pregnancy"

Maternal nutrition during pregnancy, and how this impacts placental and fetal growth and metabolism, is of considerable interest to women, their partners and their health care professionals. In developing countries, maternal undernutrition is a major factor contributing to adverse pregnancy outcomes and an increased adverse metabolic health risk in postnatal life. Conversely, with the increased prevalence of high calorie diets and resulting overweight and obesity issues in developed countries, the impact of overnutrition on pregnancy outcome is highlighted as a contributing factor for adverse metabolic outcomes in offspring later in life. Both epidemiological and animal studies now highlight that undernutrition, overnutrition, and diet composition negatively impact fetoplacental growth and metabolic patterns, having adverse later-life metabolic effects for the offspring. This Special Issue Book aims to highlight new research in a number of these abovementioned areas across the early life course.

A great deal of data now highlights the periconceptional period as a critical period upon which insults may generate later-life physiological and metabolic changes in the resulting offspring. In the review submitted by Padhee and colleagues, the procedures of ARTs are examined, specifically in terms of how common procedures associated with the handling and preparation of gametes and embryos may impact later-life metabolism, particularly impacting offspring cardiometabolic health. These later-life poor metabolic outcomes are also understood to be established during pregnancy. In surveying preconceptional women, pregnant and lactating women and women of reproductive age, Cuervo et al. report that these groups are not consuming appropriate foods for their physiological status, based upon the Spanish dietary guidelines and highlight a real need for improved education and community outreach programs to these groups of women to ensure adequate maternal and thus fetal nutrition.

Poor maternal nutritional intake after the periconceptional period during pregnancy can also negatively impact fetal growth trajectory and can result in fetal growth restriction. Vonnahme et al., describe the effects of maternal undernutrition on vascularity of nutrient transferring tissue during different stages of pregnancy. In addition to maternal nutrient supply, the effectiveness of the placenta in transporting nutrients and oxygen to the fetus is important in determining fetal growth. A range of adaptations to placental development occur when the fetus is growth-restricted and these are described by Zhang et al. Regardless of the cause of low birth weight, Zheng et al. show a relationship between the placental microbiome and fetal growth. Zohdi et al. describe the effects of maternal protein restriction during pregnancy on fetal development that increase the risk of cardiovascular disease later in life. Davis et al. illustrate the importance of the adrenal gland in the fetal adaptation to placental insufficiency, highlighting the important role of norepinephrine in regulating fetal growth but not pancreatic mass in the growth-restricted fetus. Wood-Bradley and team provide a review of the literature surrounding the potential mechanisms by which maternal nutrition (focusing on malnutrition due to protein restriction, micronutrient restriction and excessive fat intake) influences offspring kidney development and thereby function in later life. In the same light, Blumfield et al. detail evidence that a maternal diet during pregnancy that is low in protein is related to higher systolic blood pressure in childhood. Furthermore, Colon-Ramos and colleagues investigated the potential association between maternal dietary patterns during pregnancy and birth outcomes in a diverse population with a historically high burden of low birth weight and other adverse birth outcomes.

Experiences in the perinatal period also play a key role in defining how offspring respond to stress(es) in postnatal life. On this point, Tsuduki and colleagues report upon the impact of a high fat diet during mouse lactation, where it appears to increase the susceptibility of later-life obesity induced through postnatal social stress. This paper highlights the importance of understanding how an early life environment predisposes offspring to potential detrimental responses to postnatal adverse situations. In a review by Dunlop et al., the impact of fetal growth restriction on postnatal metabolism in skeletal muscle, but also the effect of a "second hit", such as a Western diet in postnatal life, is presented.

While meeting dietary guidelines is important, overall maternal health status also plays a pivotal role in determining fetal nutrient supply. In situations of maternal disease, such as infection with human immunodeficiency virus (HIV), the ability of the mother to consume sufficient substrates to maintain herself and meet fetal demands is often compromised. Also in situations of HIV, resting energy expenditure is increased and the disease may limit dietary intake and reduce nutrient absorption, in addition to influencing the progression of HIV disease as reported by Ramlal and colleagues. Their study described typical diets of HIV-infected, pregnant Malawian women and highlighted that poor quality maternal diets should be enhanced to meet demands of this particular group of pregnant women, vulnerable to both HIV and malnutrition.

While deficiencies in nutrition during pregnancy can result in adverse offspring outcomes, once pregnant, maternal weight gain during and after pregnancy are critical issues both for maternal and fetal health. In the pilot RCT report led by Martin et al., a cohort of women were recruited with the aim of reducing postpartum weight retention and improving breastfeeding outcomes. The findings indicate that the approach reported is feasible and acceptable to pregnant women and that the methodology, including the collection of blood for biomarker assessment, could be adapted based on qualitative feedback to a larger, adequately powered RCT. Assessing maternal body composition, as part of monitoring maternal well-being, prior to and during pregnancy is critical to

Preface to "Nutrition in Pregnancy"

Maternal nutrition during pregnancy, and how this impacts placental and fetal growth and metabolism, is of considerable interest to women, their partners and their health care professionals. In developing countries, maternal undernutrition is a major factor contributing to adverse pregnancy outcomes and an increased adverse metabolic health risk in postnatal life. Conversely, with the increased prevalence of high calorie diets and resulting overweight and obesity issues in developed countries, the impact of overnutrition on pregnancy outcome is highlighted as a contributing factor for adverse metabolic outcomes in offspring later in life. Both epidemiological and animal studies now highlight that undernutrition, overnutrition, and diet composition negatively impact fetoplacental growth and metabolic patterns, having adverse later-life metabolic effects for the offspring. This Special Issue Book aims to highlight new research in a number of these abovementioned areas across the early life course.

A great deal of data now highlights the periconceptional period as a critical period upon which insults may generate later-life physiological and metabolic changes in the resulting offspring. In the review submitted by Padhee and colleagues, the procedures of ARTs are examined, specifically in terms of how common procedures associated with the handling and preparation of gametes and embryos may impact later-life metabolism, particularly impacting offspring cardiometabolic health. These later-life poor metabolic outcomes are also understood to be established during pregnancy. In surveying preconceptional women, pregnant and lactating women and women of reproductive age, Cuervo et al. report that these groups are not consuming appropriate foods for their physiological status, based upon the Spanish dietary guidelines and highlight a real need for improved education and community outreach programs to these groups of women to ensure adequate maternal and thus fetal nutrition.

Poor maternal nutritional intake after the periconceptional period during pregnancy can also negatively impact fetal growth trajectory and can result in fetal growth restriction. Vonnahme et al., describe the effects of maternal undernutrition on vascularity of nutrient transferring tissue during different stages of pregnancy. In addition to maternal nutrient supply, the effectiveness of the placenta in transporting nutrients and oxygen to the fetus is important in determining fetal growth. A range of adaptations to placental development occur when the fetus is growth-restricted and these are described by Zhang et al. Regardless of the cause of low birth weight, Zheng et al. show a relationship between the placental microbiome and fetal growth. Zohdi et al. describe the effects of maternal protein restriction during pregnancy on fetal development that increase the risk of cardiovascular disease later in life. Davis et al. illustrate the importance of the adrenal gland in the fetal adaptation to placental insufficiency, estimate the requirements for dietary energy during gestation and when investigating relationships between maternal nutritional status and offspring development. Forsum and co-workers investigate the possibility of estimating body density and the use of a two-component model (2CM) to calculate total body fat, concluding it may present a new clinically appropriate methodology.

Many nutritional studies in pregnancy have focused on the impact of changes in total or macronutrient intake. This current issue features several studies that expand our knowledge regarding nutrient uptake during pregnancy, but have focused on changes in micronutrients during pregnancy. Grieger and Clifton, provide updated evidence from epidemiological and RCTs on the impact of dietary and supplemental intakes of omega-3 long-chain polyunsaturated fatty acids, zinc, folate, iron, calcium, and vitamin D, as well as dietary patterns, on infant birth weight. Additionally, in studying maternal intakes of polyunsaturated fatty acids (PUFAs), Bascuñán et al. report a Chilean study that highlights the need for new strategies to improve n-3 PUFA intake throughout pregnancy and breastfeeding periods and the need to develop dietary interventions to improve the quality of consumed foods with particular emphasis on n-3 PUFA for adequate fetal development. Fish intake during pregnancy is recognized as an important source of PUFAs. Starling and co-workers present a systematic review of fish intake during pregnancy and fetal neurodevelopment. The review covers approximately a 14 year period of publications between January 2000 and March 2014 involving over 270 papers, of which only eight were selected for a qualitative comparison of study findings.

Deficiencies in a range of micronutrients in low vs. middle income countries that may act through epigenetic mechanisms to influence fetal development and risk of chronic disease in adult life are identified by Darnton-Hill et al. They also discuss supplementation programs. One particular micronutrient that is important for sulphonation of steroids and hormones is sulphate. Dawson et al. describe the requirements for sulphate during pregnancy, the consequences of reduced sulphonation capacity and the use of animal models to adequately understand the role of sulphate in human pregnancy. Folic acid and Vitamin B12, are crucial factors for metabolic pathways, and have been extensively studied and demonstrated to play important roles in preventing the development of neural tube defects (NTDs). Wang et al. present data that in a local Chinese population consumption of non-staple foods such as milk, fresh fruits, and nuts were associated with decreasing NTDs risk in offspring. Further independent roles for folate and Vitamin B12 deficiency amongst pregnant women are presented in this Issue. The relationship between maternal Vitamin B12 and neonatal HDL is presented by Adaikalakotwewari et al. Further, folate deficiency resulting in birth defects is highlighted by Li et al., who present a mouse model to provide evidence that folate deficiency can impair decidual angiogenesis.

The importance of adequate Vitamin D in women of reproductive age and its role in fetal development is of great interest and importance. A review of calcitrol biosynthesis during pregnancy, particularly in the placenta is presented by Olmos-Ortiz et al. Additionally, Choi et al. describe the high prevalence of Vitamin D deficiency in Korean women during pregnancy, particularly in the winter, while Yu et al. report the cord blood Vitamin D in babies born in Shanghai. Finally regarding Vitamin D, the impact of sun exposure and Vitamin D supplementation on achieving appropriate Vitamin D status in women whom are breastfeeding is explored by Dawodu and colleagues.

In this Special Issue Book, several new studies highlighted the importance of diet intake and composition upon maternal and fetal well-being parameters in human population and animal studies. Many of these studies show that deficiencies in consumption/delivery of components (e.g., protein, vitamins, PUFAs) of a diet can lead to adverse fetal/offspring development and detail how consumption of certain foods may have beneficial effects on fetal/offspring growth and development. We hope that the articles contained within this Special Issue Book, and the material they reference and describe, are of interest to women, their partners and their health care professionals in promoting continual and informed dialogue about nutrition in pregnancy.

Janna L. Morrison and Timothy R.H. Regnault
Guest Editors

Section 1:

Micronutrients and Diet Composition during Pregnancy

A Review of the Impact of Dietary Intakes in Human Pregnancy on Infant Birthweight

Jessica A. Grieger and Vicki L. Clifton

Abstract: Studies assessing maternal dietary intakes and the relationship with birthweight are inconsistent, thus attempting to draw inferences on the role of maternal nutrition in determining the fetal growth trajectory is difficult. The aim of this review is to provide updated evidence from epidemiological and randomized controlled trials on the impact of dietary and supplemental intakes of omega-3 long-chain polyunsaturated fatty acids, zinc, folate, iron, calcium, and vitamin D, as well as dietary patterns, on infant birthweight. A comprehensive review of the literature was undertaken via the electronic databases Pubmed, Cochrane Library, and Medline. Included articles were those published in English, in scholarly journals, and which provided information about diet and nutrition during pregnancy and infant birthweight. There is insufficient evidence for omega-3 fatty acid supplements' ability to reduce risk of low birthweight (LBW), and more robust evidence from studies supplementing with zinc, calcium, and/or vitamin D needs to be established. Iron supplementation appears to increase birthweight, particularly when there are increases in maternal hemoglobin concentrations in the third trimester. There is limited evidence supporting the use of folic acid supplements to reduce the risk for LBW; however, supplementation may increase birthweight by ~130 g. Consumption of whole foods such as fruit, vegetables, low-fat dairy, and lean meats throughout pregnancy appears beneficial for appropriate birthweight. Intervention studies with an understanding of optimal dietary patterns may provide promising results for both maternal and perinatal health. Outcomes from these studies will help determine what sort of dietary advice could be promoted to women during pregnancy in order to promote the best health for themselves and their baby.

Reprinted from *Nutrients*. Cite as: Grieger, J.A.; Clifton, V.L. A Review of the Impact of Dietary Intakes in Human Pregnancy on Infant Birthweight. *Nutrients* **2015**, *7*, 153–178.

1. Introduction

Optimal nutrition supply to the developing fetus is paramount in achieving appropriate fetal growth and development. During pregnancy, dietary energy and nutrient requirements are generally increased to support increased maternal metabolism, blood volume and red cell mass expansion, and the delivery of nutrients to the fetus [1,2]. In a recent systematic review and meta-analysis of 90 dietary studies among pregnant women in developed countries (n = 126,242), compared to dietary recommendations in the specific countries, energy and fiber intakes were generally lower, total fat and saturated fat intakes were higher, and carbohydrate intake was borderline or lower than recommendations [3]. Key nutrients including folate, iron, zinc, calcium, vitamin D, and essential fatty acids function to promote red blood cell production, enzyme activity, bone development, and brain development. Current evidence indicates, however, that micronutrient intake during pregnancy is less than optimal [4]. This is of concern given the current consensus that maternal nutrition is relevant to both the short- and long-term health of the infant.

Human studies assessing maternal dietary intakes on birth outcomes date back to the early 1940s, when the appropriate energy and protein intakes to achieve a full-term infant ($\geq$2500 g) were uncertain [5–8]. However, the available evidence at the time suggested that mothers with insufficient weight gain during pregnancy had higher rates of premature birth than mothers with appropriate pregnancy weight gain [9,10]. Undernutrition, then, was seen to markedly affect pregnancy outcome, potentially through inadequate energy availability to the developing fetus. Comparatively, the recent surge in the prevalence of overweight and obesity worldwide has been identified as another significant complication of pregnancy [11–13], potentially via fetal exposure to excess energy availability. The long-term detrimental influence of maternal obesity and excess maternal nutrition on the risk of disease in childhood and beyond has been described [14–16].

Unfortunately, there has been no single comprehensive review examining infant birthweight related to important maternal nutrients that may play a role in fetal birthweight. Therefore, this review will provide updated information from epidemiological studies and the latest evidence from systematic reviews/meta-analyses on the impact of long chain omega 3 polyunsaturated fatty acids (LC $n3$ PUFA), zinc, iron, folate, calcium, and vitamin D on fetal birthweight. These nutrients were chosen due to their nutritional importance in pregnancy and the potential mechanisms relevant to birthweight. A distinction will be made between studies conducted in developed and developing countries due to differences in dietary intakes and prevalence of infants with low birthweight (LBW). Maternal nutrient deficiencies can occur in women who are of normal weight, obese, or underweight, and thus the impact of nutrient deficiencies will be discussed in the context of pregnancy undernutrition and overnutrition. The impact of whole dietary patterns on birthweight will also be discussed in order to highlight diet quality as a global holistic marker of nutritional intake.

2. Methods

A comprehensive review of the literature was undertaken via the electronic databases PubMed, Cochrane Library, and Medline. The most recent systematic reviews and meta-analyses were used to capture information from epidemiological and RCTs, with any subsequent studies published after the systematic reviews also included. Reviews were initially searched for using the search keywords "omega 3 fatty acids birthweight small for gestational age pregnancy"; "zinc birthweight small for gestational age pregnancy"; "iron birthweight small for gestational age pregnancy"; "folate birthweight small for gestational age pregnancy"; "calcium birthweight small for gestational age pregnancy"; "vitamin D birthweight small for gestational age pregnancy"; and "diet birthweight small for gestational age pregnancy". Articles were limited to human studies published in English, and articles were included where they provided information about diet and nutrition during pregnancy and the birthweight outcomes of the fetus. Outcomes focussed on low birth weight (LBW: <2500 g) and small for gestational age (SGA: <10th percentile for gestational age), but also included intrauterine growth restriction (IUGR: <3rd percentile for gestational age) and large for gestational age (LGA: >90th percentile for gestational age); and macrosomia (>4000 g at birth). Key mechanistic studies were included to highlight the importance of different nutrients during pregnancy and transfer through the placenta. Supporting animal studies were included where there was a lack of human studies on the effects of maternal under- and overnutrition.

3. Review

3.1. Undernutrition and Fetal Growth

The major determinant of intrauterine fetal growth is the placental supply of nutrients to the fetus, which is dependent upon placental size, morphology, and blood supply [17]. Several animal studies have shown direct relationships between placental size and birthweight [18,19]. Experimental restriction of placental growth [20–22], food restriction [23], and isocaloric low protein diets [24,25] resulted in reduced placental weight and altered placental efficiency, leading to reduced birthweight and IUGR. The timing of delivery of nutrients through the placenta is also important [26]. In pregnant sheep, severe undernutrition during the peri-conceptual period led to preterm delivery [17]; global undernutrition in early pregnancy reduced the placental:fetal weight ratio [27]; global undernutrition in early to mid-gestation increased placental size [28,29]; and global undernutrition in late gestation reduced fetal growth [30]. In rats, a low protein diet in early pregnancy increased placental growth [31], whereas in late pregnancy there was reduced fetal weight [32]. A recent review has neatly summarized the animal models, demonstrating how dietary manipulation impacts perinatal programming [33]. It can be summarized that following maternal reduced nutrition (*i.e.*, a low protein isocaloric diet, or global food restriction at 20%–70% calorie intake), offspring exhibited structural disorganization and impaired programming of the appetite-regulating system located in the hypothalamus. Due to changes in orexigenic pathways and increased white adipose tissue, the potential increased risk of obesity later in life is inevitable.

Maternal undernutrition during critical periods in humans may also influence fetal adipocyte metabolism and fat mass, leading to obesity in later life [34]. Thus, alterations in fetal nutritional supply can drive developmental adaptations influencing growth and metabolism. These alterations affect not only postnatal outcomes but also contribute to increased susceptibility to disease in later life.

In a systematic review and meta-analysis of 78 studies ($n = 1,025,794$ women), risk of preterm birth was increased in the cohort studies of underweight women by 29%, and a 64% increased risk for LBW [35]. Low birthweight is a proxy for maternal undernutrition [36]. It is associated with reduced fat mass and lean mass [37,38], poor cognition in childhood [39], and increased risk for type 2 diabetes [40] and high blood pressure [41,42] in adulthood. These studies support a link between maternal nutrition, infant birthweight, and the short- and long-term consequences. However, there are limited epidemiological studies suggesting the optimal maternal dietary intakes for optimal infant birthweight.

3.2. Epidemiological Studies and Randomized Controlled Trials Assessing Birthweight

3.2.1. Long chain omega-3 Polyunsaturated Fatty Acids

Fatty acids are among the essential nutrients for intrauterine growth [43]. Among the long chain omega-3 polyunsaturated fatty acids (LC *n3* PUFA), docosahexanoic acid (DHA) plays a critical role in fetal growth and central nervous system development. It has been estimated that the average complete DHA accretion rate *in utero* is 43 mg/kg/day [44]. As the fetus does not accumulate appreciable amounts of fat until the last trimester of gestation, if adequate DHA is not available during this critical window of development, the deleterious effect on the brain dopaminergic and serotonergic systems is irreversible [45]. There has been much recent investigation into the importance of LC *n3* PUFA in pregnancy [46–48] and associations between LC *n3* PUFA intakes and birth outcomes is emerging.

The most recent review that included 14 epidemiological studies assessing fish/seafood intake on birth outcomes revealed a positive association in 6 of the studies; 4 studies showed an inverse association, and the remaining studies revealed no association [49]. Overall in these studies, daily intake of fish ranged from 3.4 g to 47 g, or 8–12 fish meals per month. It is noted that 11 of the studies collected dietary data during pregnancy, while 3 studies collected dietary information following delivery [49].

There is emerging research, particularly in developed countries on *n3* fatty acid supplementation and birthweight. The most recent meta-analysis of 15 RCTs reported that birthweight was slightly higher among infants born to women in the

LC *n*-3 PUFA supplemented group compared to placebo (RR 42.2; 95% CI: 14.8, 69.7); however, risk of LBW was not significantly different (RR 0.92; 95% CI: 0.83, 1.02) [49] (Table 1). In a further phase 3 double blind RCT with smaller sample size (*n* = 303), supplementation with 600 mg/day DHA from <20 week gestation to birth led to a 172 g greater birthweight [50]. Interestingly, it was reported that only 78% of the capsules were consumed, thus mean daily intakes of DHA was lower than anticipated (469 mg/day). The conflicting evidence of an increase in birthweight with LC *n3* PUFA supplementation and the lack of studies in developing countries suggest the need for further, high-quality studies to be replicated and confirmed. Moreover, the clinical significance of an increase in birthweight of 42 g and 172 g, identified by Imhoff-Kunsch *et al.* [49] and Carlson *et al.* [50], is unclear, particularly as supplementation only marginally affected LBW.

3.2.2. Zinc

Zinc is essential for normal fetal growth and development [51]. In the USA, dietary zinc intake is recommended to increase from 8 mg/day in non-pregnant women to 11 mg/day during gestation [52]. Most of the zinc gained is deposited in the fetus and in the uterine muscle. Several studies have identified that maternal zinc absorption is not significantly different throughout gestation or compared to the non-pregnant state [51,53,54], but does appear to increase during lactation [51,55]. Potential mechanisms for adjustment of zinc metabolism may include reduced endogenous gastrointestinal zinc excretion [51,56] or the release of maternal tissue zinc [57].

Zinc deficiency is thought to influence embryonic and fetal development through reduced cell proliferation, reduced protein synthesis, or reductions in rates of tubulin polymerization, rather than increased rates of cellular oxidative damage, increased rates of apoptosis, or reduced binding of hormones and transcription factors dependent on zinc-finger regions [58,59]. Studies in animals have identified that zinc deficiency is teratogenic, such that it can interfere with normal embryonic development. For instance, offspring of mother hens with zinc deficiency were born with several skeletal defects and abnormalities of the brain, with many deaths occurring within 4 days [60], and when rats were fed a zinc-deficient diet during pregnancy, fewer offspring were born and many were growth-retarded, with multiple anomalies [61]. The consideration that zinc deficiency is a teratogenic risk in humans may be supported by the correlation of low plasma zinc concentrations in the first and third trimesters of pregnancy with respective increases in risk for malformations [62] and LBW [63]. Other adverse consequences of maternal zinc deficiency include increased maternal mortality, prolonged labor, prematurity [64], and adverse fetal development [65].

In a review of 46 studies conducted in developed and developing countries, 23 studies reported a positive relationship between maternal zinc concentrations and birthweight [64]. Since publication of that review, 3 studies have reported on zinc and birthweight, all in developing countries: 2 studies reported no relationship between low maternal zinc status and LBW infants [66,67], whereas among pregnant women from Tanzania, increased odds of LBW were observed with low maternal zinc concentrations [68]. Only a few studies assessing maternal dietary intakes of zinc were found, of which a study among women from New Jersey ($n = 818$) reported those with intakes of ≤ 6 mg/day had a two-fold increased risk of LBW compared to intakes >6.1 mg/day [69]; however, dietary intakes of zinc between 8 and 11 mg/day were not associated with LBW [70,71]. Currently there is insufficient evidence to presume that maternal zinc deficiency is teratogenic or that maternal zinc deficiency is related to neonatal birthweight. Further studies are required assessing mechanistic pathways between maternal zinc status and infant birthweight.

In the most recent Cochrane review of 20 RCTs, compared to placebo (or other micronutrient supplementation combinations), zinc supplementation (5–44 mg/day) had no effect on reducing risk for LBW or SGA [72] (Table 1). Similarly, in a systematic review and meta-analysis of 20 trials that was published in the same year, maternal zinc supplementation (between 5 and 50 mg/day) had no effect on LBW or SGA [73] (Table 1). In that review, however, only 6 trials were deemed to be of high quality, and the overall quality of evidence for LBW or SGA was very low. More robust evidence from supplementation studies needs to be established, and appropriate biomarkers to assess zinc status may need to be developed to support increasing dietary zinc intakes during pregnancy for infant birthweight.

3.2.3. Iron

Dietary iron requirements during pregnancy increase due to the expansion of red cell mass to accommodate fetal and placental growth, and to allow for the blood loss that occurs at delivery. Increased dietary iron requirements are difficult to achieve through diet alone, and beginning pregnancy with already low intakes increases the likelihood of outcomes such as preterm birth and LBW [74,75]. Thus, the prevalence of iron deficiency (with and without anemia) is reported to increase during each trimester [76,77].

Only 1 study was located assessing dietary iron intakes on fetal body weight. In this study among 1274 pregnant women aged 18–45 years from the UK, it was found that for every 10 mg increase in dietary iron intake, fetal birthweight was predicted to increase by 70 g (95% CI: 10, 130; $p = 0.02$); however, when adjusting for maternal age, cotinine levels, alcohol intake, maternal weight, height, parity, ethnicity, gestational age, and fetal sex, the change of 34 g was not significant [78].

There is considerably more information on maternal iron status and birthweight. A recent review of 25 observational studies revealed anemia (defined as Hb < 110 g/L) during pregnancy increased the risk for LBW (OR 1.25; 95% CI: 1.08, 1.25) compared to non-anemic women (Hb ≥ 110 g/L); however, when including only the nine studies with adjusted estimates, this was no longer significant (aOR 1.13; 95% CI: 0.94, 1.35) [79]. Interestingly, there was a 30% increased risk for LBW when anemia occurred during the first two trimesters of pregnancy compared to the final trimester. Maternal anemia was not associated with birthweight or SGA, and there was no significant difference in birthweight between high- and low-income countries [79].

Some studies have also assessed ferritin concentration, which is an indicator of iron stores. Both low ferritin (<12 g/L, indicating depleted iron stores) and high ferritin (≥60 g/L) levels were significantly associated with lower birthweight (106 g and 123 g, respectively) compared with women with intermediate ferritin concentrations [74]. In a sample of 580 black women from Alabama, USA, plasma ferritin levels in the highest quartile at 19 weeks (95.8 μg/L), 26 weeks (55.4 μg/L), and 36 weeks (41.4 μg/L) were associated with a lower mean birthweight than those in the lower three quartiles, by 142–226 g [80], whereas infants of mothers with depleted iron stores ($n = 51$, serum ferritin <10.0 μg/L) had a lower birth weight by ~336 g compared to infants of mothers with adequate serum ferritin >20.0 μg/L ($n = 20$) [81]. A final study reported serum ferritin <12 μg/L was associated with 192 g lower birthweight [82].

In the same review described above [79], a meta-analysis on 16 RCTs was carried out that assessed iron supplementation compared to control supplementation on birthweight (Table 1). Iron-only supplementation led to a mean difference in birthweight of 40.8 g (0.97 to 80.6) and reduced LBW (RR 0.81; 95% CI: 0.71, 0.91), but not SGA. Although duration of iron supplementation was not associated with birthweight, it was found that for every 10 mg increase in daily iron intake, birth weight increased by 15.1 (6.0 to 24.2) g, and for every 10 g/L increase in mean Hb concentration in the third trimester or at delivery, birthweight increased by 143 (95% CI: 68, 218) g [79].

Table 1. Summary of supplementation studies and relative risk for low birthweight.

Study Population	Supplementation Intervention	RR (95% CI)
	Long chain omega-3 polyunsaturated fatty acids	
Meta-analysis of 15 RCTs [49]	80 mg/day–2.2 g/day (8 trials, n = 3247)	0.92 (0.83, 1.02)
	Zinc	
Cochrane review of 20 RCTs (n > 15,000 women) [72]	5–44 mg/day (14 trials, n = 5643)	0.93 (0.78, 1.12)
	5–44 mg/day (8 trials, n = 4252)	1.02 (0.94, 1.11) [a]
Systematic review and meta-analysis of 20 RCTs (n = 6209) [73]	15–50 mg/day (n = 11 trials, n = 937/5416 LBW babies)	1.06 (0.91, 1.23)
	25–45 mg/day (5 trials, n = 1155/3441 SGA babies)	1.03 (0.91, 1.23) [a]
	Iron	
Meta-analysis of 48 RCTs (n = 17,793) [79]	10–140 mg/day (n = 10 trials)	0.81 (0.71, 0.91)
		0.84 (0.66, 1.07) [a]
	Folate	
Cochrane review of 31 trials (n = 17,771) [83]	Dose range not reported (4 studies, n = 3113 on LBW)	0.83 (0.66, 1.04)
	Calcium	
Cochrane review of 21 trials (n = 16,602) [84]	≥1000 mg/day (5 trials, n = 13,638, mainly calcium carbonate)	0.83 (0.63, 1.09)
	≥600 mg/day (5 trials, n = 1177, mainly calcium carbonate)	0.86 (0.61, 1.22) [b]
	Vitamin D	
Cochrane review of 6 trials on various maternal and infant outcomes (n = 623) [85]	1000 IU/day; 600,000 IU at month 7 and 8; 1 dose of 200,000 IU in third trimester (3 trials, n = 463)	0.48 (0.23, 1.01) [b]

[a] small for gestational age; [b] intrauterine growth restriction.

Mechanisms linking iron status to birthweight are not established. An early study identified an inverse relationship between hemoglobin levels and placenta weight [86], in which further possible roles of the placenta in the regulation of iron transfer and the transport proteins involved have been implicated [87–89]. Additional mechanistic studies are needed to better understand the link between iron status and birthweight, as multiple studies have reported positive effects.

3.2.4. Folate

Folate requirements are increased during pregnancy due to the demand of fetal growth [90]. It has long been established that folic acid at or around the time of conception reduces the risk for neural tube defects [91–93], and it is currently recommended that a 400 µg/day folic acid supplementation is taken three months before and early on in pregnancy [52,94,95]. However, the effect of routine folic acid supplementation on birth outcomes is not currently known.

Maternal folate status is largely determined by folate supplement use and though a number of other factors such as dietary folate intake and genetic variations in genes [90]. Red blood cell folate (RBC) is a biomarker of long-term folate status reflecting the previous 2–4 months, while serum and plasma folate represent short-term folate status and are therefore commonly used to reflect current folate supplement use [96].

No systematic reviews were located that reported on folate status and birth outcomes. However, in the most recent review of the literature assessing folate status and birth outcomes [97], maternal RBC folate status appeared to be associated with birthweight ($n = 5$ studies), and there was an increased risk for SGA with low or decreasing RBC folate (125–300 nmol/L) in two of four studies. However the majority of these studies were of poor quality, folate status was collected at different time points during gestation, and some of the studies were underpowered and thus were unable to identify a meaningful outcome. Comparatively, a number of high-quality studies were identified that assessed serum or plasma folate on birth outcomes. Only 2 of 15 studies reported significant associations between high or increasing serum or plasma folate during pregnancy and increased birthweight, while 1 study showed a significantly decreased risk of LBW with increasing folate levels in the second trimester. Folic acid supplement use was identified in 18 studies, of which 5 reported positive outcomes with supplement use in the second and third trimesters; and there was mixed evidence reporting folic acid supplement use and LBW or SGA. Although the majority of these studies were of high quality, some studies reported pre-conception folate intake and some RCTs were also summarized in the results. Thus, the ability to draw appropriate conclusions about the effect of dietary folate intake and folate status on birth outcomes is difficult. No further studies have been carried out since that review, further limiting the ability to understand the impact of maternal folate intake on birth outcomes, and at what time point during gestation folate should be measured.

In a Cochrane review assessing folic acid alone or with other micronutrients *versus* no folic acid (Table 1), the mean difference in birthweight was significantly greater in the folic acid supplement groups compared to no folic acid supplement (mean difference 135.75 g; 95% CI: 47.85, 223.68), but not LBW (RR 0.83; 95% CI: 0.66, 1.04; 4 studies, n = 3113 participants) [83]. In that review, it was revealed that supplementation typically took place from the 8th week of pregnancy until three days postpartum. The indication that most studies were also conducted 30–45 years ago suggests the need for current, well-designed clinical trials to assess the effectiveness of folic acid supplement use on birthweight parameters, given that current folic supplement use is recommended to assist other neonatal outcomes, namely neural tube defects.

3.2.5. Calcium

Calcium absorption and urinary calcium excretion are approximately two-fold higher during pregnancy compared to pre-conception or after delivery [98–100]. These changes are evidenced at the end of the first trimester and available for the peak fetal demands in the third trimester. Calcium is transported across the placenta by an active transport process, being important in many developmental functions and critical for skeletal development [101]. There does not appear to be an additional need for calcium in pregnancy [102].

Few studies have reported on associations between calcium intake and birthweight. Studies in developing countries have reported higher calcium intakes (≥1200 mg/day *vs.* <800 mg/day) were associated with higher birthweight (~3400 g *vs.* 3000 g) [71], particularly when calcium intakes reached dietary recommendations [103,104]. It is to be noted, however, that birthweight of 3000 g with lower daily calcium intake of 800 mg is not considered an inappropriate birthweight.

In a recent Cochrane review of 21 trials, no effect of calcium supplementation was found for LBW or IUGR, despite all 5 trials providing high dose supplementation (≥1000 mg/day) [84] (Table 1). Comparatively, higher birthweights were apparent following calcium supplementation compared to placebo (mean difference 64.66 g; 95% CI: 15.75, 113.58) in 19 trials with 8287 women [84]; however, the clinical importance of an increase of 64 g is unknown.

3.2.6. Vitamin D

The major circulating form of vitamin D is 25-hydroxyvitamin D (25(OH)D) and the most biological potent form is calcitriol (1,25-dihydroxyvitamin D_3) (1,25(OH)$_2$D$_3$)). 25(OH)D readily crosses experimentally perfused placentas in humans [105,106] and rodents [107], such that cord blood 25(OH)D levels at term are typically three-quarters that of maternal values [108]. In comparison, $1,25(OH)_2D_3$ does not appear to cross the placenta, with lower levels detected in cord blood [109]. Although there is no recommended increase in vitamin D intake during pregnancy [95,110], it is apparent that neonates born to vitamin D-deficient mothers will also be deficient [111,112]. There is mixed evidence regarding the effect of maternal 25(OH)D on bone health at birth; however, studies assessing skeletal health in childhood suggest 25(OH)D levels during pregnancy may have more impact at this later stage [113].

Currently, the estimated average requirement for calcium and vitamin D during pregnancy according to the Institute of Medicine (IOM) is 800 mg/day and 400 IU/day (10 µg/day), respectively [110]. The recommendation for calcium is similar to that reported by the National Health and Medical Research Council (NHMRC) in Australia (840 mg/day); however, the requirement for vitamin D is half (5 µg/day, 200 IU/day) [95].

The most recent meta-analysis revealed that 25(OH)D insufficiency (<37.5 nmol/L) during pregnancy was associated with increased risk for small SGA (OR 1.85; 95% CI 1.52, 2.26, 6 studies) compared to higher 25(OH)D levels [114]. Importantly, even adjusting for confounders such as 25(OH)D concentration cut-offs (<37.5 and <80 nmol/L), gestational age (<16 and >16 weeks), and study design (case-control and other), the association remained significant. In the same review that included 4 studies on LBW, mothers with 25(OH)D concentrations <37.5 nmol/L during pregnancy had infants with lower birth weight (random weighted mean difference −130.92; 95% CI 186.69, 75.14 g) compared to infants of mothers with levels greater than this [114].

A Cochrane review of 3 RCTs identified vitamin D treatment alone as borderline significant in reducing risk for SGA compared to no supplements/placebo (Table 1) [85]. Currently, there is insufficient evidence to promote the use of a vitamin D supplement (with or without calcium) during pregnancy to reduce the risk of LBW babies. The NHMRC in Australia recommends consuming 5 µg/day vitamin D [95] whereas the IOM advocates 10 µg/day for those in the USA or Canada [110]. In Australia, it has also been suggested that pregnant women who receive regular exposure to sunlight do not require supplementation; however, for those who have little access to sunlight, a vitamin D supplement of 10 µg/day would not be excessive [95]. Although various vitamin D supplements are currently on the market in doses ranging from 5 to10 µg, further studies are required to assess whether supplemental vitamin D can improve infant health outcomes.

3.3. Dietary Pattern Studies

Assessment of single nutrients on various study outcomes such as birthweight presents several caveats as a result of the highly interrelated nature of dietary exposures. Thus it is difficult to separate out the specific effects of nutrients or foods in relation to infant birthweight, disease risk, or other health outcomes. Studies assessing whole foods rather than specific nutrients may provide valuable information on optimal nutrition during pregnancy, and therefore dietary pattern analysis aims to overcome some of the difficulties that are often lost in nutrient-based analyses. Higher consumption of food groups within each identified dietary pattern indicates higher scores/adherence to this type of pattern.

Among women participating in the Auckland Birthweight Collaborative study ($n = 1714$), higher scores on the *traditional* food pattern (characterized by fruit, vegetables, yogurt, and lean meat) in early pregnancy was associated with reduced odds for SGA (OR 0.86; 95% CI: 0.75, 0.99) [115]. Similarly, compared to the *Western* dietary pattern ($n = 7619$) characterized by a high intake of high-fat dairy, refined grains, processed meat, beer, and sweets, 26%–32% reduced odds for SGA were found for both the *health conscious* dietary pattern ($n = 7479$), characterized by a higher intake of fruits, vegetables, poultry, and breakfast cereals, and for the *intermediate* dietary pattern ($n = 29,514$), characterized by low fat dairy and fruit but also including some red meat, dairy, and vegetables [116]. Among women from Spain, higher scores on the Alternate-Healthy Eating Index in the first trimester were associated with reduced risk of fetal growth restriction compared to women with the lowest score [117]. Among women participating in the Osaka Maternal and Child Health Study in Japan, those in the wheat products pattern (bread, confectionery, and soft drinks, $n = 303$) had infants with lower birthweight, and compared with women in the rice, fish, and vegetables pattern, women in the *wheat products* pattern had higher odds of an infant being born SGA (OR 5.2; 95% CI: 1.1, 24.4) [118].

In pregnant women from the Generation R study in the Netherlands, both low and medium adherence to the Mediterranean diet in the first trimester was associated with lower birthweight [119]. In two population-based cohort studies from Spain, higher intakes of fish, legumes, and dairy products were associated with higher infant birthweight and reduced risk for IUGR, while intake of cereal, fruits, and nuts had no relationship with birthweight [120]. Similarly, in women from the Danish National Birth Cohort ($n = 35,530$), higher intake of Mediterranean foods reduced the odds for preterm birth [121].

The first dietary pattern analysis to assess *pre-conception* diet on perinatal outcomes was carried out in a sample of 309 pregnant women from an area of low socioeconomic status in Australia [122]. The study revealed no association between any of the dietary patterns identified with LBW or SGA; however, there was an approximate 50% reduced risk for preterm delivery following the high protein

14

and fruit pattern, and there was a 50% increased risk for preterm delivery following a high fat, sugar, and takeaway pattern [122].

There is emerging data on dietary pattern assessment and fetal growth. Generally, these studies were reported in large prospective cohorts, thus capturing a large sample size, which improves the generalizability to other populations. The single study that assessed pre-conception diet and perinatal outcomes warrants further investigation, as improving diet pre-conception presents an ideal opportunity to modify dietary intake prior to pregnancy in order to optimize birth outcomes. Nevertheless, these studies suggest that consumption of whole foods such as fruit, vegetables, low-fat dairy, and lean meats throughout pregnancy appears beneficial in reducing risk for LBW babies, but it is unclear if healthier food choices in a certain trimester are optimal. Assessing quantities of the different foods relevant to national food consumption guidelines would also be a valuable component to dietary pattern analyses.

3.4. Summary

According to the reviewed epidemiological studies, there does not appear to be any consistent or conclusive evidence regarding the optimal intake for maternal dietary LCPUFA, zinc, calcium, or vitamin D for optimal birthweight. Larger studies are needed that assess LCPUFA intakes and blood concentrations over the course of pregnancy, and to determine at what time point and at what level is most important in determining optimal birth outcomes. There is insufficient evidence to presume that maternal zinc deficiency is teratogenic or that maternal zinc deficiency is related to neonatal birthweight; therefore, further studies are required assessing mechanistic pathways between maternal zinc status and infant birthweight. Iron supplementation increases infant birthweight and the magnitude that was identified with higher Hb concentrations (*i.e.*, for each 10 g/L increase in mean Hb concentration in late pregnancy or at delivery, birthweight increased by 143 g), could be critical for the survival of neonates born with lower birthweight. There is limited evidence supporting the use of folic acid supplements to reduce the risk for LBW; however, supplementation may increase birthweight by ~130 g. Further trials assessing calcium supplementation need to be undertaken, particularly among women with low baseline calcium intakes, to support the few epidemiology studies identifying higher calcium intakes with higher birthweight. Serum 25(OH)D levels of at least 37.5 nmol/L appear optimal in reducing the risk for SGA and increasing birthweight; however, clarification as to what defines a normal 25(OH)D level is required, in addition to high-quality study designs. Currently there is not enough evidence to support the use of fish oil supplements to reduce the risk of LBW in low-risk or high-risk pregnancies, and more robust evidence from studies supplementing with zinc, calcium, and/or vitamin D needs to be established.

Attempting to draw inferences on the role of maternal nutrition in determining the fetal growth trajectory is difficult. Dietary pattern studies appear to show positive associations between healthier dietary patterns and infant birthweight. In particular, foods such as lean meat, vegetables, fruit, whole grains, and low-fat dairy all contain beneficial nutrients such as protein, fiber, iron, zinc, calcium, and folate. Intervention studies assessing whole foods rather than specific nutrients may provide valuable information on optimal nutrition during pregnancy, and how certain dietary patterns improve maternal and perinatal outcomes. Outcomes from these studies will help determine what sort of dietary advice could be promoted to women during pregnancy in order to promote the best health for themselves and their babies.

3.5. Overnutrition and Fetal Growth

The global increase in overweight and obesity [11–13] indicates that more women entering pregnancy are overweight/obese [11,123]. Maternal BMI is a proxy measure of nutritional status [12,124–129]. Epidemiological studies have reported that maternal overweight (*i.e.*, BMI ≥ 25 kg/m^2) increases the risk for LGA and fetal macrosomia (Table 2). In a sample of women from Canada, class 3 obesity (BMI ≥ 40 kg/m^2, $n = 249$) was protective against LBW (aOR 0.07; 95% CI: 0.01, 0.36), but not SGA, compared to women with normal BMI (18.5–24.9 kg/m^2, $n = 446$); but class 3 obesity was also associated with LGA (aOR 4.29; 95% CI: 2.67, 6.89); birthweight > 4000 g (aOR 3.70; 95% CI: 2.22, 6.16) and birthweight > 4500 g (aOR 5.78; 95% CI: 2.11, 15.86) [124]. In contrast, recent data from a retrospective 12-year cohort study of 75,432 women in Australia identified obesity as an independent risk factor for SGA compared to normal weight (adjusted OR 1.22; 95% CI: 1.14, 1.31) [130], similar to the 24% increased risk for SGA with maternal obesity in a multi-ethnic New Zealand population (adjusted OR 1.24; CI: 1.11, 1.39) [131].

16

Table 2. Odds ratios for adverse perinatal outcomes according to different pre-pregnancy/maternal body mass index.

Study Population	n	BMI (kg/m²)	Perinatal Outcome OR (95% CI)	
			LGA	SGA
Retrospective case-control study (n = 100), UK [a] [132]	Not reported	≥40.0	3.11 (1.25, 7.79) *	-
Retrospective population-based cohort study of 5047 singleton nulliparous pregnancies, China [b] [133]	579	<18.5		1.67 (1.07, 2.61) †
	926	24.0–27.9	1.46 (1.02, 2.08) †	
	342	≥28	1.91 (1.17, 3.10) †	
South Australian Pregnancy Outcome Unit, with singleton pregnancies (n = 19, 672), [c] [12]	364	<18.5	0.38 (0.22, 0.67)	2.12 (1.58, 2.85)
	2943	25.0–29.9	1.59 (1.41, 1.81)	0.75 (0.61, 0.92)
	1528	30.0–34.9	1.60 (1.37, 1.85)	0.77 (0.59, 0.99)
	684	35.0–39.9	1.91 (1.58, 2.30)	1.12 (0.82, 1.52)
	453	≥40.0	2.17 (1.76, 2.68)	0.56 (0.34, 0.94)
Birth cohort study. Queensland, Australia [d] [126]	211	≥30.0	2.73 (1.49, 5.01)	-
Singleton fetuses at the University of California (1981 through 2001). Weight measured on first pre-natal visit [e] [128]	Not reported	>29.0	3.04 (1.86, 4.98) White	-
			0.33 (0.04, 2.85) African American	-
			2.93 (1.00, 8.58) Latina	-
			3.55 (1.39, 9.07) Asian	-
Retrospective cohort study of women who had received prenatal care in the whole urban prenatal care centers of Kazerun, Iran [f] [129]	816	<19.8	0.48 (0.30, 0.77)	-
	682	26.0–29.9	1.27 (0.87, 1.86)	-
	186	≥29.0	1.21 (0.61, 2.41)	-
Prospective study in Thai women, at <28 weeks' gestation [g] [125]	200	≥27.5	1.4 (0.5, 4.3)	-
Danish cohort of women carrying singleton births [h] [127]	116	<18.5	0.32 (0.27, 0.38)	-
	3160	25.0–29.9	1.70 (1.60, 1.78)	-
	1898	30.0–34.9	2.20 (2.08, 2.33)	-
	1363	≥35.0	2.73 (2.55, 2.94)	-
Retrospective cohort study among women and infants from the Better Outcomes Registry and Network dataset, Canada [i] [124]	249	≥40.0	3.70 (2.22, 6.16)	0.75 (0.38, 1.45)

* Fetal macrosomia (≥4000 g) † Relative Risk; [a] Reference BMI category: 20.0–25.0 kg/m². [b] Analysis adjusted for maternal age, maternal education, and gestational weight gain. Reference BMI category: 18.5–24.9 kg/m² (n = 3200). [c] Analysis adjusted for maternal age, parity, smoking status, and hospital status. Reference BMI category: 18.5–24.9 kg/m² (n = 5,261). [d] Analysis adjusted for pre-pregnancy obesity, previous pregnancy, marital status, education level, and maternal smoking. Reference BMI category: <30 kg/m². [e] Analysis adjusted for maternal age, parity, educational level, insurance status, gestational diabetes, gestational age, birthweight, induction of labor, use of epidural anesthesia, length of labor, and weight gain. Reference BMI category: 19.8–26.0 kg/m². [f] Analysis adjusted for pre-pregnancy BMI and gestational weight gain, and additionally adjusted for maternal age, education level, occupation, family history of hypertension, family history of diabetes, and parity. Reference BMI category: 19.8–26.0 kg/m². [g] Relative risk. Reference BMI category: 18.5–23.0 kg/m². [h] Analysis adjusted for maternal age, parity, smoking during pregnancy, gestational age, birthweight, GDM, sex, and calendar year. BMI reference category: 18.5–24.0 kg/m². [i] Analysis adjusted for maternal smoking, education quartile, and family income quartile. Reference BMI category: 18.5–24.9 kg/m².

Several obesogenic models in animals have identified short-term consequences of maternal high fat feeding. In rats, exposure to maternal overnutrition or obesity during pregnancy was associated with obese offspring [134–138], with additive effects occurring when pups consumed a high fat diet post-weaning [139]. Overfeeding sheep from conception to mid-gestation to induce overweight and obesity also led to fetal overgrowth [140]. Other animal studies have investigated the long-term effects of excess maternal nutrition. One of the earliest was in the baboon, where overfeeding in the pre-weaning period permanently increased adiposity through larger fat cells; this was particularly evident in females [141]. Rats who were overfed to become obese prior to conception, were fed normally during pregnancy, and whose offspring were fed a normal diet, were more frequently obese as adults compared to controls [138]. Longer term high-fat feeding in rats also has been associated with insufficient placental function, reduced pup survival, and fetal death [142], suggesting that uterine stress as a result of maternal obesity alters proper development of the placental vasculature, leading to poor fetal development.

Obesity and pregnancy also individually contribute to a state of chronic inflammation. Maternal high fat consumption programs the appetite-regulating system of offspring towards orexigenic pathways, leptin resistance, and adiposity [33]. Mechanisms underpinning the relationship between maternal obesity and adverse perinatal outcomes have been reported; however, a biologic pathway has not been established. Pro-inflammatory cytokines are elevated in obese compared to normal pregnancies [143], which can ultimately impact the maternal–fetal interface, leading to a higher risk of fetal infection and fetal complications [144]. Maternal obesity also can result in placental oxidative stress [145]. The increase in oxidative stress may impair placentation and establishment of sufficient blood supply, potentially impacting fetal metabolism [146]. The placenta is involved with the delivery of nutrients, oxygen, and hormones to the fetus, thus is ultimately responsible for the growth trajectory of the fetus [147].

Increasing pre-pregnancy BMI has been associated with increased placental weight and placental size, which were associated with adverse perinatal outcomes [148]; and maternal obesity was also associated with placenta insufficiency and increased placental lesions [149]. Moreover, IUGR is associated with placental insufficiency [150]. As maternal obesity can also be associated with undernutrition in the mother as well as the fetus (reviewed in [151]), neonatal consequences include IUGR but also altered epigenetic programming, which has been linked to later life disease in the offspring (reviewed in [152]). It is difficult to identify whether fetal programming with maternal overweight/obesity shares the same mechanisms of maternal undernutrition; the mechanisms underlying the way in which fetal systems cope with excess fuels during intrauterine development remain relatively unexplored. These findings provide evidence that excess BMI plays a significant role in altered *in utero* environment, which can have significant adverse effects on the fetus both in the short and longer term.

Gestational Weight Gain

The effects of maternal obesity on maternal and infant outcomes are further confounded by pre-pregnancy BMI [153,154] as well as excess gestational weight gain [155–158]. In two recent systematic reviews and meta-analyses, high gestational weight gain was associated with lower risk of LBW (RR 0.64; 95% CI: 0.53, 0.78) [159], whereas low total gestational weight gain (<12.5 kg to <7 kg depending on pre-pregnancy BMI category) was associated with increased risk of LBW (RR 1.85; 95% CI: 1.72, 2.00) [160]. However, in a population-based cohort study of 3536 women with class 3 obesity, those who lost weight during pregnancy had increased risk for SGA babies (aOR 2.34; 95% CI: 1.15, 4.76) [161]. Subsequent meta-analysis on interventions aimed at reducing gestational weight gain revealed there were no significant differences in birthweight between the dietary/physical activity intervention and control groups [162,163]. The IOM has recently revised gestational weight gain recommendations according to different BMI categories which attempt to improve the short- and long-term health of the mother and the child [164].

3.6. Summary

The effects of maternal BMI on infant birthweight are important given the increasing prevalence of overweight and obesity in women of childbearing age. The strong evidence of association between childhood obesity and other metabolic abnormalities such as hypertension, diabetes, and cardiovascular disease signifies the importance of modifying body weight to an appropriate level prior to conception, to improve infant and adult outcomes. Although this is ideal, it is far from practical and is unlikely in a real-world situation. Dietary modification should be at the forefront of efforts to improve maternal health, regardless of BMI, in an effort to positively impact perinatal health. Further larger and more robust studies are required to identify the importance of limiting weight gain during pregnancy, and to follow up on longer term health outcomes in the mother, infant, and child.

4. Conclusions

This review summarizes comprehensive data from epidemiological studies and the latest evidence from RCTs on maternal dietary intakes and infant birthweight. Research to date has not identified an effective supplementation strategy to combat the adverse perinatal effects associated with suboptimal maternal diet; indeed, supplementation strategies may only be beneficial when a deficiency is observed. Thus, a complete understanding of the underlying dietary profile is warranted to avoid needless supplementation where no deficiency exists. In many cases, the mean birthweight of the study population was >3000 g, suggesting that any increases in birthweight that were identified may not be of clinical benefit. Suboptimal dietary intakes (intakes below recommended levels) occur not only in developing countries, but also in developed countries, irrespective of BMI. The global obesity epidemic brings new challenges in understanding, managing, and treating obesity in pregnancy, to improve both short- and long-term child health outcomes. Successful weight gain modifications show promise in reducing the risk of LGA babies but do not appear to modify rates of SGA. To date, the most promising results come from dietary pattern analyses, in which consumption of whole foods including fruit, vegetables, whole grains, low-fat dairy, and lean meats might be beneficial toward producing an infant of appropriate birthweight.

This review has highlighted the inconsistencies between studies and the limited success of dietary interventions studies to improve infant outcomes. We have identified the need for further RCTs that are carefully implemented and targeted to women with clear dietary deficiencies, as well as the need to reduce the increasing prevalence of women entering pregnancy with an overweight BMI through dietary interventions. Understanding pre-conception diet also deserves attention as dietary intakes appear to change minimally prior to and during pregnancy [165,166]. Up to 50% of pregnancies are unplanned [167]; therefore, informing women prior to pregnancy on the importance of healthy eating should be encouraged so as to maintain a healthy diet during pregnancy.

Acknowledgments: Funding support was provided by the National Health and Medical Research Council Senior Fellowship (ID 510703 to VLC).

Author Contributions: Jessica A. Grieger compiled the review and wrote the manuscript. Vicki L. Clifton participated in the writing and critical review of the manuscript.

Conflicts of Interest: The authors declare no conflict of interest.

References

1. Australian Government Department of Health and Ageing. *National Health and Medical Research Council. Nutrient Reference Values for Australia and New Zealand Including Recommended Dietary Intakes*; Australian Government Department of Health and Ageing: Canberra, Australia, 2013.
2. Kaiser, L.L.; Allen, L. Position of the american dietetic association: Nutrition and lifestyle for a healthy pregnancy outcome. *J. Am. Diet. Assoc.* **2002**, *102*, 1479–1490.
3. Blumfield, M.L.; Hure, A.J.; Macdonald-Wicks, L.; Smith, R.; Collins, C.E. Systematic review and meta-analysis of energy and macronutrient intakes during pregnancy in developed countries. *Nutr. Rev.* **2012**, *70*, 322–336.

4.   Blumfield, M.L.; Hure, A.J.; Macdonald-Wicks, L.; Smith, R.; Collins, C.E. A systematic review and meta-analysis of micronutrient intakes during pregnancy in developed countries. *Nutr. Rev.* **2013**, *71*, 118–132.

5.   Klein, J. The relationship of maternal weight gain to the weight of the newborn infant. *Am. J. Obstet. Gynecol.* **1946**, *52*, 574–580.

6.   Schofield, C.P.; Wheildon, A.; McNaughton, J.; Beet, L. *Report of Committee of Inquiry into the Medical Aspects of the Decline of the Birth Rate, Including Reports of Special Investigations;* Special Report Series No. 4. P98; National Health and Medical Research Council: Canberra, Australia, 1948.

7.   Smith, C.A. Effects of maternal under nutrition upon the newborn infant in holland (1944–1945). *J. Pediatr.* **1947**, *30*, 229–243.

8.   Sontag, L.W.; Wines, J. Relation of mothers' diets to status of their infants at birth and in infancy. *Am. J. Obstet. Gynecol.* **1947**, *54*, 994–1003.

9.   Tompkins, W.T.; Wiehl, D.G. Nutritional deficiencies as a casual factor in toxemia and premature labor. *Am. J. Obstet. Gynecol.* **1951**, *62*, 898–919.

10. Venkatachalam, P.S. Maternal nutritional status and its effect on the newborn. *Bull. World Health Organ.* **1962**, *26*, 193–201.

11. Callaway, L.K.; Prins, J.B.; Chang, A.M.; McIntyre, H.D. The prevalence and impact of overweight and obesity in an australian obstetric population. *Med. J. Aust.* **2006**, *184*, 56–59.

12. Dodd, J.M.; Grivell, R.M.; Nguyen, A.M.; Chan, A.; Robinson, J.S. Maternal and perinatal health outcomes by body mass index category. *Aust. N. Z. J. Obstet. Gynaecol.* **2011**, *51*, 136–140.

13. Guelinckx, I.; Devlieger, R.; Beckers, K.; Vansant, G. Maternal obesity: Pregnancy complications, gestational weight gain and nutrition. *Obes. Rev.* **2008**, *9*, 140–150.

14. Catalano, P.M. Obesity and pregnancy—The propagation of a viscous cycle? *J. Clin. Endocrinol. Metab.* **2003**, *88*, 3505–3506.

15. Ehrenberg, H.M.; Mercer, B.M.; Catalano, P.M. The influence of obesity and diabetes on the prevalence of macrosomia. *Am. J. Obstet. Gynecol.* **2004**, *191*, 964–968.

16. Gillman, M.W.; Rifas-Shiman, S.L.; Kleinman, K.; Oken, E.; Rich-Edwards, J.W.; Taveras, E.M. Developmental origins of childhood overweight: Potential public health impact. *Obesity Silver Spring* **2008**, *16*, 1651–1656.

17. Fowden, A.L.; Forhead, A.J. Endocrine mechanisms of intrauterine programming. *Reproduction* **2004**, *127*, 515–526.

18. Baur, R. Morphometry of the placental exchange area. *Adv. Anat. Embryol. Cell Biol.* **1977**, *53*, 3–65.

19. Mellor, D.J. Nutritional and placental determinants of foetal growth rate in sheep and consequences for the newborn lamb. *Br. Vet. J.* **1983**, *139*, 307–324.

20. Owens, J.A.; Falconer, J.; Robinson, J.S. Glucose metabolism in pregnant sheep when placental growth is restricted. *Am. J. Physiol.* **1989**, *257*, R350–357.

21. Thureen, P.J.; Trembler, K.A.; Meschia, G.; Makowski, E.L.; Wilkening, R.B. Placental glucose transport in heat-induced fetal growth retardation. *Am. J. Physiol.* **1992**, *263*, R578–R585.

22. Vatnick, I.; Schoknecht, P.A.; Darrigrand, R.; Bell, A.W. Growth and metabolism of the placenta after unilateral fetectomy in twin pregnant ewes. *J. Dev. Physiol.* **1991**, *15*, 351–356.

23. Lederman, S.A.; Rosso, P. Effects of food restriction on fetal and placental growth and maternal body composition. *Growth* **1980**, *44*, 77–88.

24. Jansson, N.; Pettersson, J.; Haafiz, A.; Ericsson, A.; Palmberg, I.; Tranberg, M.; Ganapathy, V.; Powell, T.L.; Jansson, T. Down-regulation of placental transport of amino acids precedes the development of intrauterine growth restriction in rats fed a low protein diet. *J. Physiol.* **2006**, *576*, 935–946.

25. Rutland, C.S.; Latunde-Dada, A.O.; Thorpe, A.; Plant, R.; Langley-Evans, S.; Leach, L. Effect of gestational nutrition on vascular integrity in the murine placenta. *Placenta* **2007**, *28*, 734–742.

26. Belkacemi, L.; Nelson, D.M.; Desai, M.; Ross, M.G. Maternal undernutrition influences placental-fetal development. *Biol. Reprod.* **2010**, *83*, 325–331.

27. Heasman, L.; Clarke, L.; Firth, K.; Stephenson, T.; Symonds, M.E. Influence of restricted maternal nutrition in early to mid gestation on placental and fetal development at term in sheep. *Pediatr. Res.* **1998**, *44*, 546–551.

28. Faichney, G.J.; White, G.A. Effects of maternal nutritional status on fetal and placental growth and on fetal urea synthesis in sheep. *Aust. J. Biol. Sci.* **1987**, *40*, 365–377.

29. McCrabb, G.J.; Egan, A.R.; Hosking, B.J. Maternal undernutrition during mid-pregnancy in sheep. Placental size and its relationship to calcium transfer during late pregnancy. *Br. J. Nutr.* **1991**, *65*, 157–168.

30. Mellor, D.J.; Murray, L. Effects of placental weight and maternal nutrition on the growth rates of individual fetuses in single and twin bearing ewes during late pregnancy. *Res. Vet. Sci.* **1981**, *30*, 198–204.

31. Langley-Evans, S.C.; Welham, S.J.; Sherman, R.C.; Jackson, A.A. Weanling rats exposed to maternal low-protein diets during discrete periods of gestation exhibit differing severity of hypertension. *Clin. Sci. Lond.* **1996**, *91*, 607–615.

32. Langley-Evans, S.C.; Nwagwu, M. Impaired growth and increased glucocorticoid-sensitive enzyme activities in tissues of rat fetuses exposed to maternal low protein diets. *Life Sci.* **1998**, *63*, 605–615.

33. Breton, C. The hypothalamus-adipose axis is a key target of developmental programming by maternal nutritional manipulation. *J. Endocrinol.* **2013**, *216*, R19–R31.

34. Vickers, M.H.; Krechowec, S.O.; Breier, B.H. Is later obesity programmed *in utero*? *Curr. Drug Targets* **2007**, *8*, 923–934.

35. Han, Z.; Mulla, S.; Beyene, J.; Liao, G.; McDonald, S.D.; Knowledge Synthesis, G. Maternal underweight and the risk of preterm birth and low birth weight: A systematic review and meta-analyses. *Int. J. Epidemiol.* **2011**, *40*, 65–101.

36. Thame, M.; Wilks, R.J.; McFarlane-Anderson, N.; Bennett, F.I.; Forrester, T.E. Relationship between maternal nutritional status and infant's weight and body proportions at birth. *Eur. J. Clin. Nutr.* **1997**, *51*, 134–138.

37. Lapillonne, A.; Braillon, P.; Claris, O.; Chatelain, P.G.; Delmas, P.D.; Salle, B.L. Body composition in appropriate and in small for gestational age infants. *Acta Paediatr.* **1997**, *86*, 196–200.

38. Padoan, A.; Rigano, S.; Ferrazzi, E.; Beaty, B.L.; Battaglia, F.C.; Galan, H.L. Differences in fat and lean mass proportions in normal and growth-restricted fetuses. *Am. J. Obstet. Gynecol.* **2004**, *191*, 1459–1464.

39. Emond, A.; Drewett, R.; Blair, P.; Emmett, P. Postnatal factors associated with failure to thrive in term infants in the avon longitudinal study of parents and children. *Arch. Dis. Child.* **2007**, *92*, 115–119.

40. Newsome, C.A.; Shiell, A.W.; Fall, C.H.; Phillips, D.I.; Shier, R.; Law, C.M. Is birth weight related to later glucose and insulin metabolism?—A systematic review. *Diabet. Med.* **2003**, *20*, 339–348.

41. Campbell, D.M.; Hall, M.H.; Barker, D.J.; Cross, J.; Shiell, A.W.; Godfrey, K.M. Diet in pregnancy and the offspring's blood pressure 40 years later. *Br. J. Obstet. Gynaecol.* **1996**, *103*, 273–280.

42. Roseboom, T.J.; van der Meulen, J.H.; van Montfrans, G.A.; Ravelli, A.C.; Osmond, C.; Barker, D.J.; Bleker, O.P. Maternal nutrition during gestation and blood pressure in later life. *J. Hypertens.* **2001**, *19*, 29–34.

43. Cetin, I.; Alvino, G.; Cardellicchio, M. Long chain fatty acids and dietary fats in fetal nutrition. *J. Physiol.* **2009**, *587*, 3441–3451.

44. Lapillonne, A.; Groh-Wargo, S.; Gonzalez, C.H.; Uauy, R. Lipid needs of preterm infants: Updated recommendations. *J. Pediatr.* **2013**, *162*, S37–S47.

45. Carlson, S.E. Docosahexaenoic acid supplementation in pregnancy and lactation. *Am. J. Clin. Nutr.* **2009**, *89*, 678S–684S.

46. Allen, K.G.; Harris, M.A. The role of *n*-3 fatty acids in gestation and parturition. *Exp. Biol. Med. Maywood* **2001**, *226*, 498–506.

47. Fleith, M.; Clandinin, M.T. Dietary pufa for preterm and term infants: Review of clinical studies. *Crit. Rev. Food Sci. Nutr.* **2005**, *45*, 205–229.

48. Koletzko, B.; Lien, E.; Agostoni, C.; Bohles, H.; Campoy, C.; Cetin, I.; Decsi, T.; Dudenhausen, J.W.; Dupont, C.; Forsyth, S.; *et al.* The roles of long-chain polyunsaturated fatty acids in pregnancy, lactation and infancy: Review of current knowledge and consensus recommendations. *J. Perinat. Med.* **2008**, *36*, 5–14.

49. Imhoff-Kunsch, B.; Briggs, V.; Goldenberg, T.; Ramakrishnan, U. Effect of *n*-3 long-chain polyunsaturated fatty acid intake during pregnancy on maternal, infant, and child health outcomes: A systematic review. *Paediatr. Perinat. Epidemiol.* **2012**, *26* (Suppl. 1), 91–107.

50. Carlson, S.E.; Colombo, J.; Gajewski, B.J.; Gustafson, K.M.; Mundy, D.; Yeast, J.; Georgieff, M.K.; Markley, L.A.; Kerling, E.H.; Shaddy, D.J. DHA supplementation and pregnancy outcomes. *Am. J. Clin. Nutr.* **2013**, *97*, 808–815.

51. Fung, E.B.; Ritchie, L.D.; Woodhouse, L.R.; Roehl, R.; King, J.C. Zinc absorption in women during pregnancy and lactation: A longitudinal study. *Am. J. Clin. Nutr.* **1997**, *66*, 80–88.

52. Institute of Medicine. *Dietary Reference Intakes: Estimated Average Requirements*; The National Acadamies Press: Washington, DC, USA, 2011.

53. Swanson, C.A.; King, J.C. Zinc utilization in pregnant and nonpregnant women fed controlled diets providing the zinc rda. *J. Nutr.* **1982**, *112*, 697–707.

54. Swanson, C.A.; Turnlund, J.R.; King, J.C. Effect of dietary zinc sources and pregnancy on zinc utilization in adult women fed controlled diets. *J. Nutr.* **1983**, *113*, 2557–2567.

55. Moser-Veillon, P.B. Zinc needs and homeostasis during lactation. *Analyst* **1995**, *120*, 895–897.

56. Jackson, M.J.; Giugliano, R.; Giugliano, L.G.; Oliveira, E.F.; Shrimpton, R.; Swainbank, I.G. Stable isotope metabolic studies of zinc nutrition in slum-dwelling lactating women in the Amazon valley. *Br. J. Nutr.* **1988**, *59*, 193–203.

57. Masters, D.G.; Keen, C.L.; Lonnerdal, B.; Hurley, L.S. Release of zinc from maternal tissues during zinc deficiency or simultaneous zinc and calcium deficiency in the pregnant rat. *J. Nutr.* **1986**, *116*, 2148–2154.

58. Jankowski-Hennig, M.A.; Clegg, M.S.; Daston, G.P.; Rogers, J.M.; Keen, C.L. Zinc-deficient rat embryos have increased caspase 3-like activity and apoptosis. *Biochem. Biophys. Res. Commun.* **2000**, *271*, 250–256.

59. Mackenzie, G.G.; Zago, M.P.; Keen, C.L.; Oteiza, P.I. Low intracellular zinc impairs the translocation of activated nf-kappa b to the nuclei in human neuroblastoma imr-32 cells. *J. Biol. Chem.* **2002**, *277*, 34610–34617.

60. Kienholz, E.W.; Turk, D.E.; Sunde, M.L.; Hoekstra, W.G. Effects of zinc deficiency in the diets of hens'. *J. Nutr.* **1961**, *75*, 211–221.

61. Hurley, L.S.; Swenerton, H. Congenital malformations resulting from zinc deficiency in rats. *Proc. Soc. Exp. Biol. Med.* **1966**, *123*, 692–696.

62. Jameson, S. Effects of zinc deficiency in human reproduction. *Acta Med. Scand. Suppl.* **1976**, *593*, 1–89.

63. Wells, J.L.; James, D.K.; Luxton, R.; Pennock, C.A. Maternal leucocyte zinc deficiency at start of third trimester as a predictor of fetal growth retardation. *Br. Med. J.* **1987**, *294*, 1054–1056.

64. Shah, D.; Sachdev, H.P. Effect of gestational zinc deficiency on pregnancy outcomes: Summary of observation studies and zinc supplementation trials. *Br. J. Nutr.* **2001**, *85* (Suppl. 2), S101–S108.

65. Merialdi, M.; Caulfield, L.E.; Zavaleta, N.; Figueroa, A.; DiPietro, J.A. Adding zinc to prenatal iron and folate tablets improves fetal neurobehavioral development. *Am. J. Obstet. Gynecol.* **1999**, *180*, 483–490.

66. Badakhsh, M.H.; Khamseh, M.E.; Seifoddin, M.; Kashanian, M.; Malek, M.; Shafiee, G.; Baradaran, H.R. Impact of maternal zinc status on fetal growth in an Iranian pregnant population. *Gynecol. Endocrinol.* **2011**, *27*, 1074–1076.

67. Samimi, M.; Asemi, Z.; Taghizadeh, M.; Azarbad, Z.; Rahimi-Foroushani, A.; Sarahroodi, S. Concentrations of serum zinc, hemoglobin and ferritin among pregnant women and their effects on birth outcomes in Kashan, Iran. *Oman Med. J.* **2012**, *27*, 40–45.

68. Rwebembera, A.A.; Munubhi, E.K.; Manji, K.P.; Mpembeni, R.; Philip, J. Relationship between infant birth weight </=2000 g and maternal zinc levels at Muhimbili National Hospital, Dar Es Salaam, Tanzania. *J. Trop. Pediatr.* **2006**, *52*, 118–125.

69. Scholl, T.O.; Hediger, M.L.; Schall, J.I.; Fischer, R.L.; Khoo, C.S. Low zinc intake during pregnancy: Its association with preterm and very preterm delivery. *Am. J. Epidemiol.* **1993**, *137*, 1115–1124.

70. Bawadi, H.A.; Al-Kuran, O.; Al-Bastoni, L.A.; Tayyem, R.F.; Jaradat, A.; Tuuri, G.; Al-Beitawi, S.N.; Al-Mehaisen, L.M. Gestational nutrition improves outcomes of vaginal deliveries in Jordan: An epidemiologic screening. *Nutr. Res.* **2010**, *30*, 110–117.

71. Khoushabi, F.; Saraswathi, G. Impact of nutritional status on birth weight of neonates in Zahedan City, Iran. *Nutr. Res. Pract.* **2010**, *4*, 339–344.

72. Mori, R.; Ota, E.; Middleton, P.; Tobe-Gai, R.; Mahomed, K.; Bhutta, Z.A. Zinc supplementation for improving pregnancy and infant outcome. *Cochrane Database Syst. Rev.* **2012**, *7*, CD000230.

73. Chaffee, B.W.; King, J.C. Effect of zinc supplementation on pregnancy and infant outcomes: A systematic review. *Paediatr. Perinat. Epidemiol.* **2012**, *26* (Suppl. 1), 118–137.

74. Ronnenberg, A.G.; Wood, R.J.; Wang, X.; Xing, H.; Chen, C.; Chen, D.; Guang, W.; Huang, A.; Wang, L.; Xu, X. Preconception hemoglobin and ferritin concentrations are associated with pregnancy outcome in a prospective cohort of chinese women. *J. Nutr.* **2004**, *134*, 2586–2591.

75. Scholl, T.O.; Hediger, M.L. Anemia and iron-deficiency anemia: Compilation of data on pregnancy outcome. *Am. J. Clin. Nutr.* **1994**, *59*, 492S–500S.

76. Scholl, T.O. Maternal iron status: Relation to fetal growth, length of gestation, and iron endowment of the neonate. *Nutr. Rev.* **2011**, *69* (Suppl. 1), S23–S29.

77. Zhou, L.M.; Yang, W.W.; Hua, J.Z.; Deng, C.Q.; Tao, X.; Stoltzfus, R.J. Relation of hemoglobin measured at different times in pregnancy to preterm birth and low birth weight in Shanghai, China. *Am. J. Epidemiol.* **1998**, *148*, 998–1006.

78. Alwan, N.A.; Greenwood, D.C.; Simpson, N.A.; McArdle, H.J.; Godfrey, K.M.; Cade, J.E. Dietary iron intake during early pregnancy and birth outcomes in a cohort of british women. *Hum. Reprod.* **2011**, *26*, 911–919.

79. Haider, B.A.; Olofin, I.; Wang, M.; Spiegelman, D.; Ezzati, M.; Fawzi, W.W. Anaemia, prenatal iron use, and risk of adverse pregnancy outcomes: Systematic review and meta-analysis. *BMJ* **2013**, *346*, f3443.

80. Goldenberg, R.L.; Tamura, T.; DuBard, M.; Johnston, K.E.; Copper, R.L.; Neggers, Y. Plasma ferritin and pregnancy outcome. *Am. J. Obstet. Gynecol.* **1996**, *175*, 1356–1359.

81. Singla, P.N.; Tyagi, M.; Kumar, A.; Dash, D.; Shankar, R. Fetal growth in maternal anaemia. *J. Trop. Pediatr.* **1997**, *43*, 89–92.

82. Ribot, B.; Aranda, N.; Viteri, F.; Hernandez-Martinez, C.; Canals, J.; Arija, V. Depleted iron stores without anaemia early in pregnancy carries increased risk of lower birthweight even when supplemented daily with moderate iron. *Hum. Reprod.* **2012**, *27*, 1260–1266.

83. Lassi, Z.S.; Salam, R.A.; Haider, B.A.; Bhutta, Z.A. Folic acid supplementation during pregnancy for maternal health and pregnancy outcomes. *Cochrane Database Syst. Rev.* **2013**, *3*, CD006896.

84. Buppasiri, P.; Lumbiganon, P.; Thinkhamrop, J.; Ngamjarus, C.; Laopaiboon, M. Calcium supplementation (other than for preventing or treating hypertension) for improving pregnancy and infant outcomes. *Cochrane Database Syst. Rev.* **2011**, CD007079.

85. De-Regil, L.M.; Palacios, C.; Ansary, A.; Kulier, R.; Pena-Rosas, J.P. Vitamin D supplementation for women during pregnancy. *Cochrane Database Syst. Rev.* **2012**, *2*, CD008873.

86. Godfrey, K.M.; Redman, C.W.; Barker, D.J.; Osmond, C. The effect of maternal anaemia and iron deficiency on the ratio of fetal weight to placental weight. *Br. J. Obstet. Gynaecol.* **1991**, *98*, 886–891.

87. Bastin, J.; Drakesmith, H.; Rees, M.; Sargent, I.; Townsend, A. Localisation of proteins of iron metabolism in the human placenta and liver. *Br. J. Haematol.* **2006**, *134*, 532–543.

88. Lipinski, P.; Stys, A.; Starzynski, R.R. Molecular insights into the regulation of iron metabolism during the prenatal and early postnatal periods. *Cell. Mol. Life Sci.* **2013**, *70*, 23–38.

89. McArdle, H.J.; Lang, C.; Hayes, H.; Gambling, L. Role of the placenta in regulation of fetal iron status. *Nutr. Rev.* **2011**, *69* (Suppl. 1), S17–S22.

90. Greenberg, J.A.; Bell, S.J.; Guan, Y.; Yu, Y.H. Folic acid supplementation and pregnancy: More than just neural tube defect prevention. *Rev. Obstet. Gynecol.* **2011**, *4*, 52–59.

91. MRC vitamin study research group. Prevention of neural tube defects: Results of the medical research council vitamin study. *Lancet* **1991**, *338*, 131–137.

92. De-Regil, L.M.; Fernandez-Gaxiola, A.C.; Dowswell, T.; Pena-Rosas, J.P. Effects and safety of periconceptional folate supplementation for preventing birth defects. *Cochrane Database Syst. Rev.* **2010**, CD007950.

93. Rieder, M.J. Prevention of neural tube defects with periconceptional folic acid. *Clin. Perinatol.* **1994**, *21*, 483–503.

94. Czeizel, A.E.; Dudas, I. Prevention of the first occurrence of neural-tube defects by periconceptional vitamin supplementation. *N. Engl. J. Med.* **1992**, *327*, 1832–1835.

95. National Health and Medical Research Council. *Nutrient Reference Values for Australia and New Zealand Including Recommended Dietary Intakes*; National Health and Medical Research Council: Canberra, Australia, 2005.

96. Shane, B. Folate status assessment history: Implications for measurement of biomarkers in nhanes. *Am. J. Clin. Nutr.* **2011**, *94*, 337S–342S.

97. Van Uitert, E.M.; Steegers-Theunissen, R.P. Influence of maternal folate status on human fetal growth parameters. *Mol. Nutr. Food Res.* **2013**, *57*, 582–595.

98. Cross, N.A.; Hillman, L.S.; Allen, S.H.; Krause, G.F.; Vieira, N.E. Calcium homeostasis and bone metabolism during pregnancy, lactation, and postweaning: A longitudinal study. *Am. J. Clin. Nutr.* **1995**, *61*, 514–523.

99. Gertner, J.M.; Coustan, D.R.; Kliger, A.S.; Mallette, L.E.; Ravin, N.; Broadus, A.E. Pregnancy as state of physiologic absorptive hypercalciuria. *Am. J. Med.* **1986**, *81*, 451–456.

100. Heaney, R.P.; Skillman, T.G. Calcium metabolism in normal human pregnancy. *J. Clin. Endocrinol. Metab.* **1971**, *33*, 661–670.

101. Kovacs, C.S. Bone metabolism in the fetus and neonate. *Pediatr. Nephrol.* **2013**, *29*, 793–803.

102. Prentice, A. Micronutrients and the bone mineral content of the mother, fetus and newborn. *J. Nutr.* **2003**, *133*, 1693S–1699S.

103. Durrani, A.M.; Rani, A. Effect of maternal dietary intake on the weight of the newborn in Aligarh city, India. *Niger. Med. J.* **2011**, *52*, 177–181.

104. Sabour, H.; Hossein-Nezhad, A.; Maghbooli, Z.; Madani, F.; Mir, E.; Larijani, B. Relationship between pregnancy outcomes and maternal vitamin D and calcium intake: A cross-sectional study. *Gynecol. Endocrinol.* **2006**, *22*, 585–589.

105. Hillman, L.S.; Slatopolsky, E.; Haddad, J.G. Perinatal vitamin D metabolism. Iv. Maternal and cord serum 24,25-dihydroxyvitamin D concentrations. *J. Clin. Endocrinol. Metab.* **1978**, *47*, 1073–1077.

106. Wieland, P.; Fischer, J.A.; Trechsel, U.; Roth, H.R.; Vetter, K.; Schneider, H.; Huch, A. Perinatal parathyroid hormone, vitamin D metabolites, and calcitonin in man. *Am. J. Physiol.* **1980**, *239*, E385–E390.

107. Haddad, J.G., Jr.; Boisseau, V.; Avioli, L.V. Placental transfer of vitamin D3 and 25-hydroxycholecalciferol in the rat. *J. Lab. Clin. Med.* **1971**, *77*, 908–915.

108. Kovacs, C.S. Vitamin D in pregnancy and lactation: Maternal, fetal, and neonatal outcomes from human and animal studies. *Am. J. Clin. Nutr.* **2008**, *88*, 520S–528S.

109. Kovacs, C.S. Fetus, neonate and infant. In *Vitamin D*, 3rd ed.; Feldman, D., Ed.; Academic Press: New York, NY, USA, 2011; pp. 625–646.

110. Dietary Reference Intakes for Calcium and Vitamin D. Institute of Medicine: Washington, DC, USA, 2011. Available online: http://www.nal.usda.gov/fnic/DRI/DRI_Calcium_Vitamin_D/FullReport.pdf (accessed on 15 February 2014).

111. Aly, Y.F.; El Koumi, M.A.; Abd El Rahman, R.N. Impact of maternal vitamin D status during pregnancy on the prevalence of neonatal vitamin D deficiency. *Pediatr. Rep.* **2013**, *5*, e6.

112. Hashemipour, S.; Lalooha, F.; Zahir Mirdamadi, S.; Ziaee, A.; Dabaghi Ghaleh, T. Effect of vitamin D administration in vitamin D-deficient pregnant women on maternal and neonatal serum calcium and vitamin D concentrations: A randomised clinical trial. *Br. J. Nutr.* **2013**, *110*, 1611–1616.

113. Javaid, M.K.; Crozier, S.R.; Harvey, N.C.; Gale, C.R.; Dennison, E.M.; Boucher, B.J.; Arden, N.K.; Godfrey, K.M.; Cooper, C.; Princess Anne Hospital Study Group. Maternal vitamin D status during pregnancy and childhood bone mass at age 9 years: A longitudinal study. *Lancet* **2006**, *367*, 36–43.

114. Aghajafari, F.; Nagulesapillai, T.; Ronksley, P.E.; Tough, S.C.; O'Beirne, M.; Rabi, D.M. Association between maternal serum 25-hydroxyvitamin D level and pregnancy and neonatal outcomes: Systematic review and meta-analysis of observational studies. *BMJ* **2013**, *346*, f1169.

115. Thompson, J.M.; Wall, C.; Becroft, D.M.; Robinson, E.; Wild, C.J.; Mitchell, E.A. Maternal dietary patterns in pregnancy and the association with small-for-gestational-age infants. *Br. J. Nutr.* **2010**, *103*, 1665–1673.

116. Knudsen, V.K.; Orozova-Bekkevold, I.M.; Mikkelsen, T.B.; Wolff, S.; Olsen, S.F. Major dietary patterns in pregnancy and fetal growth. *Eur. J. Clin. Nutr.* **2008**, *62*, 463–470.

117. Rodriguez-Bernal, C.L.; Rebagliato, M.; Iniguez, C.; Vioque, J.; Navarrete-Munoz, E.M.; Murcia, M.; Bolumar, F.; Marco, A.; Ballester, F. Diet quality in early pregnancy and its effects on fetal growth outcomes: The infancia y medio ambiente (childhood and environment) mother and child cohort study in Spain. *Am. J. Clin. Nutr.* **2010**, *91*, 1659–1666.

118. Okubo, H.; Miyake, Y.; Sasaki, S.; Tanaka, K.; Murakami, K.; Hirota, Y.; Osaka, M.; Child Health Study, G.; Kanzaki, H.; Kitada, M.; *et al.* Maternal dietary patterns in pregnancy and fetal growth in japan: The osaka maternal and child health study. *Br. J. Nutr.* **2012**, *107*, 1526–1533.

119. Timmermans, S.; Steegers-Theunissen, R.P.; Vujkovic, M.; den Breeijen, H.; Russcher, H.; Lindemans, J.; Mackenbach, J.; Hofman, A.; Lesaffre, E.E.; Jaddoe, V.V.; *et al.* The mediterranean diet and fetal size parameters: The generation r study. *Br. J. Nutr.* **2012**, *108*, 1–11.

120. Chatzi, L.; Mendez, M.; Garcia, R.; Roumeliotaki, T.; Ibarluzea, J.; Tardon, A.; Amiano, P.; Lertxundi, A.; Iniguez, C.; Vioque, J.; *et al.* Mediterranean diet adherence during pregnancy and fetal growth: Inma (spain) and rhea (greece) mother-child cohort studies. *Br. J. Nutr.* **2012**, *107*, 135–145.

121. Mikkelsen, T.B.; Osterdal, M.L.; Knudsen, V.K.; Haugen, M.; Meltzer, H.M.; Bakketeig, L.; Olsen, S.F. Association between a mediterranean-type diet and risk of preterm birth among danish women: A prospective cohort study. *Acta Obstet. Gynecol. Scand.* **2008**, *87*, 325–330.

122. Grieger, J.A.; Grzeskowiak, L.E.; Clifton, V.L. Preconception dietary patterns in human pregnancies are associated with preterm delivery. *J. Nutr.* **2014**, *144*, 1075–1080.

123. Athukorala, C.; Rumbold, A.R.; Willson, K.J.; Crowther, C.A. The risk of adverse pregnancy outcomes in women who are overweight or obese. *BMC Pregnancy Childbirth* **2010**, *10*, 56.

124. Gaudet, L.; Tu, X.; Fell, D.; El-Chaar, D.; Wu Wen, S.; Walker, M. The effect of maternal class iii obesity on neonatal outcomes: A retrospective matched cohort study. *J. Matern. Fetal Neonatal Med.* **2012**, *25*, 2281–2286.

125. Kongubol, A.; Phupong, V. Prepregnancy obesity and the risk of gestational diabetes mellitus. *BMC Pregnancy Childbirth* **2011**, *11*, 59.

126. Ng, S.K.; Olog, A.; Spinks, A.B.; Cameron, C.M.; Searle, J.; McClure, R.J. Risk factors and obstetric complications of large for gestational age births with adjustments for community effects: Results from a new cohort study. *BMC Public Health* **2010**, *10*, 460.

127. Ovesen, P.; Rasmussen, S.; Kesmodel, U. Effect of prepregnancy maternal overweight and obesity on pregnancy outcome. *Obstet. Gynecol.* **2011**, *118*, 305–312.

128. Ramos, G.A.; Caughey, A.B. The interrelationship between ethnicity and obesity on obstetric outcomes. *Am. J. Obstet. Gynecol.* **2005**, *193*, 1089–1093.

129. Tabatabaei, M. Gestational weight gain, prepregnancy body mass index related to pregnancy outcomes in Kazerun, fars, Iran. *J. Prenat. Med.* **2011**, *5*, 35–40.

130. McIntyre, H.D.; Gibbons, K.S.; Flenady, V.J.; Callaway, L.K. Overweight and obesity in Australian mothers: Epidemic or endemic? *Med. J. Aust.* **2012**, *196*, 184–188.

131. Anderson, N.H.; Sadler, L.C.; Stewart, A.W.; Fyfe, E.M.; McCowan, L.M. Independent risk factors for infants who are small for gestational age by customised birthweight centiles in a multi-ethnic New Zealand population. *Aust. N. Z. J. Obstet. Gynaecol.* **2013**, *53*, 136–142.

132. Vinayagam, D.; Chandraharan, E. The adverse impact of maternal obesity on intrapartum and perinatal outcomes. *ISRN Obstet. Gynecol.* **2012**, *2012*, 939762.

133. Liu, X.; Du, J.; Wang, G.; Chen, Z.; Wang, W.; Xi, Q. Effect of pre-pregnancy body mass index on adverse pregnancy outcome in north of china. *Arch. Gynecol. Obstet.* **2011**, *283*, 65–70.

134. Chen, H.; Simar, D.; Lambert, K.; Mercier, J.; Morris, M.J. Maternal and postnatal overnutrition differentially impact appetite regulators and fuel metabolism. *Endocrinology* **2008**, *149*, 5348–5356.

135. Guo, F.; Jen, K.L. High-fat feeding during pregnancy and lactation affects offspring metabolism in rats. *Physiol. Behav.* **1995**, *57*, 681–686.

136. Levin, B.E.; Govek, E. Gestational obesity accentuates obesity in obesity-prone progeny. *Am. J. Physiol.* **1998**, *275*, R1374–R1379.

137. Nivoit, P.; Morens, C.; van Assche, F.A.; Jansen, E.; Poston, L.; Remacle, C.; Reusens, B. Established diet-induced obesity in female rats leads to offspring hyperphagia, adiposity and insulin resistance. *Diabetologia* **2009**, *52*, 1133–1142.

138. Shankar, K.; Harrell, A.; Liu, X.; Gilchrist, J.M.; Ronis, M.J.; Badger, T.M. Maternal obesity at conception programs obesity in the offspring. *Am. J. Physiol. Regul. Integr. Comp. Physiol.* **2008**, *294*, R528–R538.

139. Rajia, S.; Chen, H.; Morris, M.J. Maternal overnutrition impacts offspring adiposity and brain appetite markers-modulation by postweaning diet. *J. Neuroendocrinol.* **2010**, *22*, 905–914.

140. George, L.A.; Uthlaut, A.B.; Long, N.M.; Zhang, L.; Ma, Y.; Smith, D.T.; Nathanielsz, P.W.; Ford, S.P. Different levels of overnutrition and weight gain during pregnancy have differential effects on fetal growth and organ development. *Reprod. Biol. Endocrinol.* **2010**, *8*, 75.

141. Lewis, D.S.; Bertrand, H.A.; McMahan, C.A.; McGill, H.C., Jr.; Carey, K.D.; Masoro, E.J. Preweaning food intake influences the adiposity of young adult baboons. *J. Clin. Investig.* **1986**, *78*, 899–905.

142. Hayes, E.K.; Lechowicz, A.; Petrik, J.J.; Storozhuk, Y.; Paez-Parent, S.; Dai, Q.; Samjoo, I.A.; Mansell, M.; Gruslin, A.; Holloway, A.C.; *et al.* Adverse fetal and neonatal outcomes associated with a life-long high fat diet: Role of altered development of the placental vasculature. *PLoS One* **2012**, *7*, e33370.

143. Rizzo, G.S.; Sen, S. Maternal obesity and immune dysregulation in mother and infant: A review of the evidence. *Paediatr. Respir. Rev.* **2014**.

144. Sen, S.; Iyer, C.; Klebenov, D.; Histed, A.; Aviles, J.A.; Meydani, S.N. Obesity impairs cell-mediated immunity during the second trimester of pregnancy. *Am. J. Obstet. Gynecol.* **2013**, *208*, e131–e138.

145. Alanis, M.C.; Steadman, E.M.; Manevich, Y.; Danyelle, M.; Townsend, D.M.; Goetzl, L.M. Maternal obesity and placental oxidative stress in the first trimester. *Obes. Weight Loss Ther.* **2012**, *2*.

146. Schmatz, M.; Madan, J.; Marino, T.; Davis, J. Maternal obesity: The interplay between inflammation, mother and fetus. *J. Perinatol.* **2010**, *30*, 441–446.

147. Wallace, J.M. Adaptive maternal, placental and fetal responses to nutritional extremes in the pregnant adolescent: Lessons from sheep. In *Cambridge Studies in Biological and Evolutionary Anthropology (No. 59)*; Cambridge University Press: Cambridge, UK, 2011.

148. Wallace, J.M.; Horgan, G.W.; Bhattacharya, S. Placental weight and efficiency in relation to maternal body mass index and the risk of pregnancy complications in women delivering singleton babies. *Placenta* **2012**, *33*, 611–618.

149. Huang, L.; Liu, J.; Feng, L.; Chen, Y.; Zhang, J.; Wang, W. Maternal prepregnancy obesity is associated with higher risk of placental pathological lesions. *Placenta* **2014**, *35*, 563–569.

150. Kingdom, J.; Huppertz, B.; Seaward, G.; Kaufmann, P. Development of the placental villous tree and its consequences for fetal growth. *Eur. J. Obstet. Gynecol. Reprod. Biol.* **2000**, *92*, 35–43.

151. Correia-Branco, A.; Keating, E.; Martel, F. Maternal undernutrition and fetal developmental programming of obesity: The glucocorticoid connection. *Reprod. Sci.* **2014**.

152. Hochberg, Z.; Feil, R.; Constancia, M.; Fraga, M.; Junien, C.; Carel, J.C.; Boileau, P.; Le Bouc, Y.; Deal, C.L.; Lillycrop, K.; *et al.* Child health, developmental plasticity, and epigenetic programming. *Endocr. Rev.* **2011**, *32*, 159–224.

153. El-Chaar, D.; Finkelstein, S.A.; Tu, X.; Fell, D.B.; Gaudet, L.; Sylvain, J.; Tawagi, G.; Wen, S.W.; Walker, M. The impact of increasing obesity class on obstetrical outcomes. *J. Obstet. Gynaecol. Can.* **2013**, *35*, 224–233.

154. Magann, E.F.; Doherty, D.A.; Sandlin, A.T.; Chauhan, S.P.; Morrison, J.C. The effects of an increasing gradient of maternal obesity on pregnancy outcomes. *Aust. N. Z. J. Obstet. Gynaecol.* **2013**, *53*, 250–257.

155. Cedergren, M.I. Optimal gestational weight gain for body mass index categories. *Obstet. Gynecol.* **2007**, *110*, 759–764.

156. Chung, J.G.; Taylor, R.S.; Thompson, J.M.; Anderson, N.H.; Dekker, G.A.; Kenny, L.C.; McCowan, L.M.; Consortium, S. Gestational weight gain and adverse pregnancy outcomes in a nulliparous cohort. *Eur. J. Obstet. Gynecol. Reprod. Biol.* **2013**, *167*, 149–153.

157. Crane, J.M.; White, J.; Murphy, P.; Burrage, L.; Hutchens, D. The effect of gestational weight gain by body mass index on maternal and neonatal outcomes. *J. Obstet. Gynaecol. Can.* **2009**, *31*, 28–35.

158. Scott-Pillai, R.; Spence, D.; Cardwell, C.; Hunter, A.; Holmes, V. The impact of body mass index on maternal and neonatal outcomes: A retrospective study in a UK obstetric population, 2004–2011. *BJOG* **2013**, *120*, 932–939.

159. McDonald, S.D.; Han, Z.; Mulla, S.; Lutsiv, O.; Lee, T.; Beyene, J.; Knowledge Synthesis, G. High gestational weight gain and the risk of preterm birth and low birth weight: A systematic review and meta-analysis. *J. Obstet. Gynaecol. Can.* **2011**, *33*, 1223–1233.

160. Han, Z.; Lutsiv, O.; Mulla, S.; Rosen, A.; Beyene, J.; McDonald, S.D.; Knowledge Synthesis, G. Low gestational weight gain and the risk of preterm birth and low birthweight: A systematic review and meta-analyses. *Acta Obstet. Gynecol. Scand.* **2011**, *90*, 935–954.

161. Blomberg, M. Maternal and neonatal outcomes among obese women with weight gain below the new institute of medicine recommendations. *Obstet. Gynecol.* **2011**, *117*, 1065–1070.

162. Oteng-Ntim, E.; Varma, R.; Croker, H.; Poston, L.; Doyle, P. Lifestyle interventions for overweight and obese pregnant women to improve pregnancy outcome: Systematic review and meta-analysis. *BMC Med.* **2012**, *10*, 47.

163. Thangaratinam, S.; Rogozinska, E.; Jolly, K.; Glinkowski, S.; Roseboom, T.; Tomlinson, J.W.; Kunz, R.; Mol, B.W.; Coomarasamy, A.; Khan, K.S. Effects of interventions in pregnancy on maternal weight and obstetric outcomes: Meta-analysis of randomised evidence. *BMJ* **2012**, *344*, e2088.

164. Institute of Medicine and National Research Council of the National Academies. *Weight Gain during Pregnancy: Reexamining the Guidelines*; Institute of Medicine and National Research Council of the National Academies: Washington, DC, USA, 2009.

165. Crozier, S.R.; Robinson, S.M.; Godfrey, K.M.; Cooper, C.; Inskip, H.M. Women's dietary patterns change little from before to during pregnancy. *J. Nutr.* **2009**, *139*, 1956–1963.

166. Cuco, G.; Fernandez-Ballart, J.; Sala, J.; Viladrich, C.; Iranzo, R.; Vila, J.; Arija, V. Dietary patterns and associated lifestyles in preconception, pregnancy and postpartum. *Eur. J. Clin. Nutr.* **2006**, *60*, 364–371.

167. Finer, L.B.; Zolna, M.R. Unintended pregnancy in the united states: Incidence and disparities, 2006. *Contraception* **2011**, *84*, 478–485.

Polyunsaturated Fatty Acid Composition of Maternal Diet and Erythrocyte Phospholipid Status in Chilean Pregnant Women

Karla A. Bascuñán, Rodrigo Valenzuela, Rodrigo Chamorro, Alejandra Valencia, Cynthia Barrera, Claudia Puigrredon, Jorge Sandoval and Alfonso Valenzuela

Abstract: Chilean diets are characterized by a low supply of n-3 polyunsaturated fatty acids (n-3 PUFA), which are critical nutrients during pregnancy and lactation, because of their role in brain and visual development. DHA is the most relevant n-3 PUFA in this period. We evaluated the dietary n-3 PUFA intake and erythrocyte phospholipids n-3 PUFA in Chilean pregnant women. Eighty healthy pregnant women (20–36 years old) in the 3rd–6th month of pregnancy were included in the study. Dietary assessment was done applying a food frequency questionnaire, and data were analyzed through the Food Processor SQL® software. Fatty acids of erythrocyte phospholipids were assessed by gas-liquid chromatography. Diet composition was high in saturated fat, low in mono- and PUFA, high in n-6 PUFA (linoleic acid) and low in n-3 PUFA (alpha-linolenic acid and DHA), with imbalance in the n-6/n-3 PUFA ratio. Similar results were observed for fatty acids from erythrocyte phospholipids. The sample of Chilean pregnant women showed high consumption of saturated fat and low consumption of n-3 PUFA, which is reflected in the low DHA content of erythrocyte phospholipids. Imbalance between n-6/n-3 PUFA could negatively affect fetal development. New strategies are necessary to improve n-3 PUFA intake throughout pregnancy and breast feeding periods. Furthermore, it is necessary to develop dietary interventions to improve the quality of consumed foods with particular emphasis on n-3 PUFA.

Reprinted from *Nutrients*. Cite as: Bascuñán, K.A.; Valenzuela, R.; Chamorro, R.; Valencia, A.; Barrera, C.; Puigrredon, C.; Sandoval, J.; Valenzuela, A. Polyunsaturated Fatty Acid Composition of Maternal Diet and Erythrocyte Phospholipid Status in Chilean Pregnant Women. *Nutrients* **2014**, *6*, 4918–4934.

1. Introduction

During the last few decades, considerable scientific interest has been aroused about the beneficial effects of the adequate dietary intake of essential fatty acids. The early life period, *i.e.*, during pregnancy and early postpartum (perinatal period), has been one of the main research foci given that in this period, the composition of dietary fatty acids determines important effects on growth and development [1,2]. n-6 and n-3 polyunsaturated fatty acids (PUFA) are considered essential dietary nutrients, because mammals do not have the enzymatic capacity to insert a double-bond at the n-6 and n-3 position of saturated and/or n-9 precursors to form linoleic acid (LA, 18:2n-6) and alpha-linolenic acid (ALA, 18:3n-3), respectively [3,4].

LA and ALA are, in turn, the precursors of a family of fatty acids having a 20- or 22-carbon chain, such as arachidonic acid (AA, 20:4n-6) formed from LA and eicosapentaenoic acid (EPA, 20:5n-3) and docosahexaenoic acid (DHA, 22:6n-3) formed from ALA. AA and DHA are considered the most important metabolic products of LA and ALA, respectively [5,6]. AA and DHA are vital structural components of membrane phospholipids [7]. AA is widely distributed in all cell membrane phospholipids, while DHA is almost exclusively present in a high concentration in membrane phospholipids of cells from the central nervous system (neurons and glial cells) [8]. In humans, the higher rate of AA and DHA accretion occurs during the third trimester of pregnancy and the first two years after delivery [8–10]. In this context, both LA and ALA, as precursors of AA and DHA, are essential fatty acids and should be obligatory incorporated throughout the diet. LA is highly available in the Chilean diet, which is characterized as a Western diet. However, ALA is very restrictive, and preformed DHA is only scarcely consumed by our population, because of the low consumption of sea foods, which are the main primary source of this fatty acid [11].

Several studies have shown that pregnancy is a critical period for n-3 PUFA intake [12]. Maternal DHA supplementation during pregnancy results in higher scores on visual and neurocognitive tests in children at 12 months of age [13] and improves the early development of visual acuity and other neurodevelopmental indices [14]. Fetal metabolic demand of DHA increases during growth [15] in the last trimester of pregnancy, being the period where DHA accretion to the fetal brain and nervous system reaches its maximum speed [16]. Fetal supply of DHA is provided from maternal circulation at a rate, on average, of 67 mg of n-3 PUFA (primarily as DHA) per day [17]. On the other hand, maternal DHA requirements are increased in response to the expansion of red cell mass and placenta and for the accomplishment of the DHA needs of pregnant women [18].

The increased metabolic need of DHA during pregnancy can be compensated for by: (1) dietary intake; (2) increasing the capacity to metabolize ALA to DHA [19]; (3) preferential use of DHA reserves mobilized from adipose tissue [20]; and (4) saving DHA, because of amenorrhea during pregnancy [18,21]. Regarding diet, sources of n-3 PUFA are limited, and estimated intakes of EPA and DHA in various populations are below the recommended levels [22]; it is also known that DHA intake of women from industrialized countries is usually low. The average intake of DHA in Western countries is 70 to 200 mg/day [23–26], but in some cases, the intake is even lower (30–50 mg/day), resulting in women having less than the estimated daily accretion of DHA to the fetus in the third trimester [16]. These observations suggest a potential insufficient dietary intake of DHA for both mother and infant [27]. The assessment of the nutritional status of essential fatty acids during pregnancy is highly relevant, considering its effects on the offspring, infant development and the health of the mother [27].

The objective of this study was to evaluate the dietary supply of n-6 and n-3 PUFA and the nutritional PUFA status, through erythrocyte membrane phospholipid fatty acid measurement, in a group of healthy pregnant Chilean women. Furthermore, the nutrient intake of women was compared with the specific nutrient recommendations during pregnancy.

2. Material and Methods

2.1. Subjects

All women recruited to participate in the study were patients of the Obstetrics and Gynecology Department of the Clinical Hospital, University of Chile. Women (n = 80), between 20 and 35 years, being in the 3rd–6th month of pregnancy, with a history of previous successful breastfeeding (defined as having a previous child with breastfeeding up to six months) and an absence of any current pathology (hypertension, gestational diabetes, *etc.*) during pregnancy or congenital fetal malformation, were selected. Socioeconomic status was evaluated by the criteria proposed by the European Society for Opinion and Marketing Research (ESOMAR) [28], which includes the assessment of the educational level and current work activity of the individual with the highest income in the household. The study protocol was reviewed and approved by the Institutional Review Board of the Faculty of Medicine, University of Chile (Protocol 073-2011) and by the Ethic Committee of the Clinical Hospital, University of Chile (Protocol 507/11). All information regarding the study was given to each participant who voluntarily agreed to participate and signed the informed consent.

2.2. Food Analysis

Dietary evaluation was conducted by trained dietitians of the research group by the application of a food frequency questionnaire. To estimate nutritional composition (energy, macro- and micro-nutrients intake) of the habitual diet (between 3 and 6 months of gestation), mothers were extensively interviewed and asked for all groups of foods consumed during the previous month. In addition to the food frequency questionnaire, dietitians used a photographic "Atlas of Commonly Consumed Foods in Chile" [29], a validated graphic instrument that help to estimate the amount of each food consumed.

Dietary composition data from the food-frequency questionnaire was grouped into 9 food groups (cereals, fruits and vegetables, dairy, meats and eggs, legumes, fish and shellfish, high-lipid foods, oils and fats, sugars and processed foods). Cereals included all cereals and potatoes; fruits and vegetables included all kind of fruits, natural fruits juice and vegetables; dairy products included milk, cheese, fresh cheese and yogurts; meats and eggs included beef, chicken, pork and turkey meat and all their derived products, as well as eggs; fish and shellfish included hake, mackerel, tuna, salmon and shellfish (fresh and frozen); legumes included beans, chickpeas and lentils; high-lipid foods included olives, almonds, peanuts, walnuts, avocado, pistachios and hazelnuts; oils and fat included vegetable oils (mainly sunflower, soybean, canola, grape seed and olive oil) and fats (lard, butter, margarine, mayonnaise and cream); sugars and processed foods included sugar, honey, jam, delicacies, soft drinks, artificial juices, chocolates, cookies and sweet and savory snacks. Fatty acid intake from each food group was calculated as g per 100 g of consumed food, and then the average fatty acid intake was obtained.

Dietary data was analyzed using the software, Food Processor SQL® (ESHA Research, Salem, OR, USA), to calculate energy and nutrient intake. Diet composition was obtained using a database from the USDA National Nutrient Database for Standard Reference, which also contained information from locally-generated nutrient composition data.

2.3. Assessment of Nutritional Status

Participants were subjected to a clinical evaluation when incorporated into the study. A physician and a nurse assessed each participant regarding habitual health control under the standard clinical approach for pregnant women. Anthropometric data of weight (kg) and height (m) were assessed to determine body-mass index (BMI, kg/m^2). BMI was then used to establish maternal nutritional status according to gestational week following the national reference [30]. Energy and nutrient requirements were established according to WHO criteria [31] and recommended dietary intakes according to the American Institute of Medicine, 2001 [32].

2.4. Blood Samples

Blood was obtained at the first clinical evaluation at the beginning of the study (between 3 and 6 months of pregnancy) and stored in the presence of butylhydroxytoluene (BHT) as the antioxidant. Erythrocytes were then separated by centrifugation (3000 g × for 10 min at 20 °C) and frozen at −80 °C for further analyses.

2.5. Fatty Acid Analysis

2.5.1. Lipid Extraction from Erythrocyte Membranes

Quantitative extraction of total lipids from erythrocyte samples was carried out according to Bligh and Dyer [33], in the presence of BHT. Erythrocytes were homogenized in ice-cold chloroform/methanol (2:1 v/v) (containing magnesium chloride 0.5N and 0.01% (w/v) BHT) in an Ultraturrax homogenizer (Janke & Kunkel, Stufen, Germany). Lipids extracted from erythrocyte samples were separated by TLC (aluminum sheets 20 × 20 cm, silica gel 60 F-254, Merck, Santiago, Chile), using the solvent system, hexane/diethyl ether/acetic acid (80:20:1 v/v). After the development of plates and solvent evaporation, lipid spots were visualized by exposing the plates to a Camag UV (250 nm) lamp (Camag, Muttenz, Switzerland)) designed for TLC. The solvent system allows the separation of phospholipids, cholesterol, triacylglycerols and cholesterol esters according to their relative mobility. Spots of individual lipids were scraped from TLC plates and eluted with either diethyl ether or chloroform/methanol (2:1 v/v) [34].

2.5.2. Fatty Acid Methyl Ester (FAME) Synthesis

For fatty acid methyl ester (FAME) formation, phospholipids previously extracted from the silica gel spots with 15 mL of chloroform/methanol/water (10:10:1 v/v) and evaporated under nitrogen stream, were treated with methanolic boron trifluoride (12% methanolic solution) [35] and sodium hydroxide (0.5 N methanolic solution). FAME samples were cooled and extracted with 0.5 mL of hexane.

2.5.3. Gas Chromatography Analysis of FAME

FAME were separated and quantified by gas-liquid chromatography in Hewlett-Packard equipment (model 7890A, CA, USA) using a capillary column (Agilent HP-88, 100 m × 0.250 mm; I.D. 0.25 µm) and a flame ionization detector (FID). The injector temperature was set at 250 °C and the FID temperature at 300 °C. The oven temperature at injection was initially set at 120 °C and was programmed to increase until 220 °C at a rate of 5 °C per min. Hydrogen was utilized as the carrier gas at a flow rate of 35 cm per second in the column, and the inlet split ratio was set at 20:1. The identification and quantification of FAME were achieved by comparing the retention times and the peak area values (%) of the unknown samples to those of a commercial lipid standard (Nu-Chek Prep Inc., Elysian, MN, USA). C23:0 was used as the internal standard (Nu-Chek Prep Inc., Elysian, MN, USA.) using the Hewlett-Packard Chemstation (Palo Alto, CA, USA) data system.

2.6. Statistical Analyses

Dietary data were checked by contrasting the energy/nutrient intake data composition with dietary questionnaires, identifying potential outliers. In that case, a careful review of each food frequency questionnaire was done. A descriptive analysis was conducted, and the analysis of the variable's distribution was done using a Shapiro–Wilk test. Results are expressed as the mean $\pm$ SD (SE in Figure 1) or the median (interquartile range). To compare dietary nutrient intake with nutrient recommendations, a paired sample *t*-test was used. For all comparisons, statistical significance was set at α level ≤0.05. The statistical software used was SPSS v.15.0 (Chicago, IL, USA) and GraphPad Prism v.5.0 (GraphPad Software, San Diego, CA, USA) for figure processing.

3. Results

Table 1 shows the background and anthropometric data of the studied women. The sample was composed of young women (29.3 ± 5.9 years), mainly of medium socioeconomic status (70.9%). The gestational average was 22.6 ± 8.4 weeks. The distribution of nutritional status was 2.6% of women underweight, 51.2% normal weight, 29.5% overweight and 16.7% obese, indicating that over 50% of the sample presented a normal nutritional status.

Table 1. Background characteristics.

Variable	(*n* = 80) Mean ± SD
Age (Years)	29.3 ± 5.9
SES	
High (%)	13.9
Medium (%)	70.9
Low (%)	15.2
Preconception Weight (kg)	65.2 ± 10.9
Preconception BMI (kg/m²)	25.1 ± 3.6
Weight (kg) [a]	70.07 ± 10.7
Height (m) [a]	1.60 ± 0.04
BMI (kg/m²) [a]	26.9 ± 3.4
Gestational Age (Weeks)	22.6 ± 8.4
Nutritional Status	
Underweight (%)	2.6
Normal Weight (%)	51.2
Overweight (%)	29.5
Obese (%)	16.7

Data are expressed as the mean ± SD or as a percentage (%); SES, socioeconomic status; BMI, body mass index = kg/m²; [a] Anthropometric measures were taken at study enrollment.

3.1. Dietary Intake

The intake of women was analyzed according to energy intake and macro- and micro-nutrient dietary consumption. Daily nutrient dietary intake is shown in Table 2. Average energy was 2482 ± 670.5 kcal with 15.1%, 52.7% and 32.2% of energy coming from protein, lipids and carbohydrates, respectively. When intake data were compared with nutritional requirements, it was observed that the nutritional adequacy ((intake/requirement) × 100) of energy and macronutrients (carbohydrates, lipids and proteins) was all above the requirements. However, vitamins (folic, choline, thiamine, niacin and E) and minerals (iron, iodine, potassium, magnesium, zinc and copper) were under the recommended level. The intake of vitamins A, riboflavin, vitamins C and vitamins B12 and minerals (calcium, phosphorus and sodium) were above the recommended level (Table 2).

Table 2. Daily energy and nutrient dietary intake.

Energy/Nutrients	Intake	Requirement/RDA [a]	Adequacy (%) [b]	p-Value
Energy (kcal)	2482.0 ± 670.5	1835.8 ± 79.3	135	0.01
Protein (g)	94.0 ± 29.2	59.4 ± 3.4	158	0.001
Carbohydrate (g)	326.9 ± 106.4	238.3 ± 53.1	137	0.001
Fat (g)	88.8 ± 31.9	61.2 ± 2.6	145	0.001
Fiber (g)	30.5 ± 12.1	28	108	0.07
Cholesterol (mg) [c]	266.5 ± 104.4	-	-	-
Trans Fatty Acid (g) [c]	1.3 ± 1.5	-	-	-
Iron (mg)	14.4 ± 6.1	27	53	0.01
Folic Acid (μg) [d]	408.7 ± 261.9	600	68	0.01
Choline (mg)	217.2 ± 98.5	450	48	0.01
Iodine (μg) [e]	74.8 ± 67.2	220	33	0.01
Calcium (mg)	1111.9 ± 511.3	1000	119	0.05
Vitamin A (RAE) [f]	905 ± 513.5	770	117	0.02
Thiamin (mg)	1.2 ± 0.7	1.4	85	0.01
Riboflavin (mg)	1.5 ± 0.7	1.4	107	0.19
Niacin (mg)	11.6 ± 6.0	18	64	0.01
Vitamin C (mg)	196.0 ± 106.7	85	230	0.01
Vitamin E (α-tocopherol, mg)	5.8 ± 3.5	15	38	0.01
Vitamin B12 (μg)	4.3 ± 2.6	2.6	165	0.01
Phosphorus (mg)	985.1 ± 421.8	700	140	0.01
Sodium (g)	2.76 ± 1.9	1.5	164	0.01
Potassium (g)	2.9 ± 1.1	4.7	61	0.01
Magnesium (mg)	214.8 ± 101.8	350	61	0.01
Zinc (mg)	8.4 ± 4.63	11	76	0.01
Copper (μg)	914.4 ± 462.8	1000	91	0.10

Data are expressed as the mean ± SD; [a] RDA: Recommended Dietary Allowance, according to the Institute of Medicine, National Academies, USA [32]; [b] adequacy: (nutrient intake/nutrient daily recommendation) × 100; [c] for this nutrient, the proposed recommendation is "as low as possible while consuming a nutritionally adequate diet"; [d] folic acid intake does not include intake from fortified products (wheat flour); [e] iodine intake does not include intake from fortified products (salt); [f] RAE, retinol activity equivalent; 1 RAE = 1 mg retinol.

Daily fat and relevant n-6 and n-3 fatty acid intake are shown in Table 3. Total fat intake was over the recommendations. When saturated and unsaturated fat intakes were compared, it was observed that saturated fat was above the recommendations and total unsaturated fat (mono- and polyunsaturated) was under the recommendations. It is remarkable that the insufficient intake of ALA, EPA and DHA generated a high imbalance of the n-6/n-3 ratio (Table 3).

Fatty acid intake according to dietary food group is shown in Table 4. Fatty acid intake was analyzed and separated into nine dietary groups. Regarding total fat intake, higher fat consumption was obtained from oils and fats, followed by meats and eggs, cereals, high-lipid foods and dairy. Saturated fatty acid (SAFA) consumption was supplied by dairy, followed by meats and eggs and oils and fats. Monounsaturated fatty acids (MUFA) came from high-lipid foods, followed by oils and fats, meats and eggs, dairy and cereals. Regarding total PUFA intake, the higher supply came from oils and fats, followed by high-lipid foods, cereals, meats and eggs and dairy. The contribution of the different food groups to the dietary intake of n-6 and n-3 PUFA is shown in Figure 1A (LA and ALA) and Figure 1B (AA, EPA and DHA). It can be observed that the supply of LA was from high-lipid foods, followed by oils and fats and meats. ALA was notably less consumed than LA (Figure 1A). AA was provided mainly by meats, and EPA and DHA came almost exclusively from fish.

Table 3. Daily fat and relevant n-6 and n-3 fatty acid dietary intake.

Nutrients	Intake	RDA [a]	Adequacy (%) [b]	p-Value [c]
Total Fat (g)	88.8 ± 31.9	61.2 ± 2.6	145	0.001
Saturated Fat (g)	26.7 ± 11.7	15.6 ± 1.6	171	0.001
Monounsaturated Fat (g)	23.3 ± 10.5	29.0 ± 1.1	80	0.001
Polyunsaturated Fat (g)	16.3 ± 9.1	22.3 ± 0.8	73	0.001
LA (g) *	4.4 (2.8–6.7) [c]	13.0	45	0.001
ALA (g) *	0.6 (0.4–1.0) [c]	1.4	67	0.001
ARA (mg) *	60.0 (40–90) [c]	800	7.5	0.001
EPA (mg) *	10.0 (0–50) [c]	100	31	0.001
DHA (mg) *	40.0 (10–100) [c]	200	33	0.001
n-6/n-3 Ratio **	8.1 ± 6.1	-	-	-

Data are expressed as the mean ± SD, unless otherwise specified; [a] RDA: Recommended Dietary Allowance (RDA) according to the Institute of Medicine, National Academies, USA [32]; [b] adequacy: ((nutrient intake/nutrient daily recommendation) × 100); [c] for a comparison between mean intake and RDA proposed values; * Data expressed as the median (interquartile range); ** There is no RDA for this ratio; - no adequacy is shown; LA, linoleic acid; ALA, alpha-linolenic acid; ARA, arachidonic acid; EPA, eicosapentaenoic acid; DHA, docosahexaenoic acid.

Table 4. Fatty acid intake according to food groups.

Food Groups	Total Fat (g)	Total SAFA (g)	Total MUFA (g)	Total PUFA (g)
Cereals	9.7 (7.0–12.7)	1.7 (1.3–2.4)	1.0 (1.5–2.2)	1.2 (0.7–1.8)
Fruits and Vegetables	1.2 (0.7–1.6)	0.1 (0.07–0.17)	0.05 (0.02–0.07)	0.2 (0.1–0.3)
Dairy	8.4 (4.4–18.0)	4.9 (2.8–10.8)	1.9 (0.9–4.3)	0.2 (0.1–0.6)
Meats and Eggs	12.5 (8.3–20.4)	4.4 (2.8–6.7)	2.8 (1.8–5.7)	0.9 (0.5–1.2)
Fish and Seafood	0.7 (0.2–1.6)	0.17 (0.008–0.064)	0.2 (0.01–0.4)	0.1 (0.01–0.2)
Legumes	0.18 (0.4–0.39)	0.01 (0.006–0.04)	0.02 (0.007–0.06)	0.1 (0.02–0.2)
High-Lipid Foods	9.9 (3.7–14.4)	1.2 (0.5–1.8)	5.0 (2.5–7.6)	1.6 (0.6–3.7)
Oils and Fats	25 (4.9–36.2)	4.2 (2.2–6.4)	4.7 (3.2–9.1)	9.6 (3.9–15.0)
Sugar, Alcohol and Processed Foods	3.4 (0.84–8.1)	0.9 (0.2–3.0)	0.01 (0–0.02)	0.004 (0–0.09)

Data are expressed as the median (interquartile range); SAFA, saturated fatty acids; MUFA, monounsaturated fatty acids; PUFA, polyunsaturated fatty acids; Cereals, all cereals and potatoes; fruits and vegetables, fruits, natural fruits juice and vegetables; dairy products, milk, cheese, fresh cheese and yogurts; meats and eggs, beef, chicken, pork and turkey meat and all of their derived products, as well as eggs; fish and shellfish, hake, mackerel, tuna, salmon and shellfish (fresh and frozen); legumes, beans, chickpeas and lentils; high-lipid foods, olives, almonds, peanuts, walnuts, avocado, pistachios and hazelnuts; oils and fats, vegetable oils (mainly sunflower, soybean, canola, grape seed and olive oil) and fats (lard, butter, margarine, mayonnaise and creams); sugars and processed foods, sugar, honey, jam, delicacies, soft drinks, artificial juices, chocolates, cookies and sweet and savory snacks.

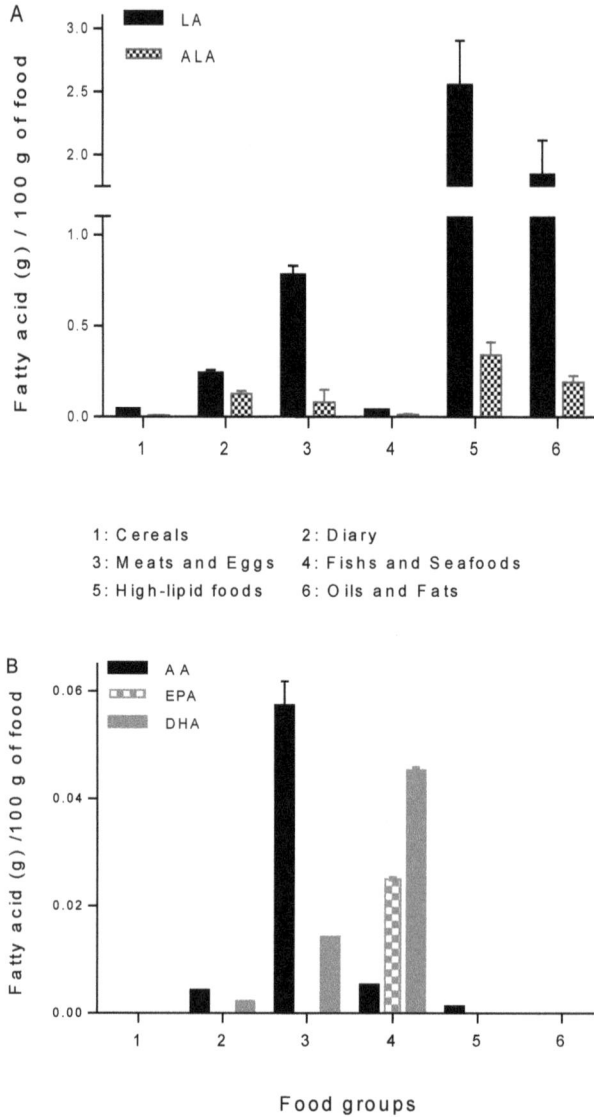

Figure 1. Data are expressed as the mean ± SE and represent the content of each fatty acid (g)/100g of food. Cereals, all cereals and potatoes; dairy products, milk, cheese, fresh cheese and yogurts; meats and eggs, beef, chicken, pork and turkey meat and all their derived products, as well as eggs; fish and shellfish, hake, mackerel, tuna, salmon and shellfish (fresh and frozen); high-lipid foods, olives, almonds, peanuts, walnuts, avocado, pistachios and hazelnuts; oils and fats, vegetable oils (mainly sunflower, soybean, canola, grape seed and olive oil) and fats (lard, butter, margarine, mayonnaise and creams).

3.2. Fatty Acid Composition of Erythrocyte Phospholipids

The fatty acid composition of phospholipids extracted from erythrocyte membranes is shown in Table 5. Total SAFA was the predominant fatty acid, followed by total PUFA and total MUFA. n-6 PUFA was almost four times the n-3 PUFA, LA and AA being the predominant fatty acids. DHA is the predominant n-3 PUFA, the values for ALA and EPA being closely similar. Table 5 also includes the results from the literature obtained for pregnant women of three different countries and continents (China, Belgium and the United States of America (USA)). The analysis of this information compared with our results is found in the Discussion section.

Table 5. Fatty acid composition of maternal erythrocyte membrane phospholipids

Fatty Acids [a]	Chilean Women [b]	Chinese Women [c]	Belgium Women [d]	USA Women [e]
Total SAFA	52.2 ± 2.8	46.4 (44.7–47.2)	46.0 ± 3.3	*
Total MUFA	13.3 ± 1.5	14.5 ± 3.5	12.7 ± 1.3	*
Total PUFA	35.4 ± 3.3	36.6 (34.1–38.7)	38.2 ± 3.5	*
Total n-6 PUFA	28.6 ± 3.6	26.5 (24.6–28.3)	*	27.91 ± 5.39
Total n-3 PUFA	6.8 ± 1.0	9.8 (8.6–11.8)	*	6.96 ± 2.27
18:2, n-6 (LA)	14.6 ± 3.4	15.0 ± 4.6	19.1 ± 3.2	9.0 ± 1.49
18:3, n-3 (ALA)	1.2 ± 0.4	*	0.22 ± 0.14	0.13 ± 0.06
20:4, n-6 (AA)	13.2 ± 1.8	7.3 (5.7–8.5)	8.4 ± 1.8	13.09 ± 3.3
20:5, n-3 (EPA)	1.6 ± 0.5	1.9 (1.7–2.2)	0.50 ± 0.31	0.30 ± 0.17
22:6, n-3 (DHA)	3.6 ± 0.6	5.6 (4.1–8.1)	4.8 ± 1.3	4.74 ± 1.68
n-6/n-3 PUFA Ratio	4.3 ± 1.0	2.6 (2.1–3.2)	*	4.71 ± 2.8

[a] Fatty acids are expressed as g per 100 g fatty acid methyl ester (FAME); [b] Data are expressed as the mean ± SD; SAFA, saturated fatty acids; MUFA, monounsaturated fatty acids; PUFA, polyunsaturated fatty acids; LA, linolenic acid; ALA, alpha-linolenic acid; AA, arachidonic acid; EPA, eicosapentaenoic acid; DHA, docosahexaenoic acid; SAFA includes: 6:0, 8:0, 10:0, 12:0, 14:0, 16:0, 18:0, 20:0, 22:0 and 24:0; MUFA includes 14:1 n-5, 16:1 n-7 and 18:1 n-9; PUFA includes 18:2 n-6, 18:3 n-3, 20:4 n-6, 20:5 n-3, 22:5 n-3 and 22:6 n-3; n-6/n-3 PUFA ratio: 20:4 n-6/(20:5 n-3 + 22:5 n-3 + 22:6 n-3); [c] Data from [22]; [d] Data from [36]; [e] Data from [37]; *: no data was available in this study.

4. Discussion

This study evaluated the dietary composition consumed by a sample of Chilean pregnant women with emphasis on their fatty acid intake and its association with the fatty acid profile of erythrocyte membrane phospholipids. Energy and macronutrient (carbohydrate, protein and fat) intake exceeded daily recommendations, but several vitamins and minerals were considerably under the recommended daily intake. The overconsumption of total fat and, especially, saturated fat in conjunction with an excessive intake of total n-6 PUFA (mainly LA) *versus* a lower intake of n-3 PUFA, particularly ALA, EPA and DHA, was observed. Considering these results, it is interesting to observe that LA (precursor of AA) intake is under the recommendation; however, this is not reflected in the AA content of erythrocyte membrane phospholipids (Table 5). ALA is also under the recommendation, and as a precursor of EPA and DHA, these n-3 PUFA show values far lower than the minimal recommendation. This suggest that the nutritional imbalance observed in the sample is due to either an efficient conversion of LA to AA (in spite of the low LA consumption), a very low conversion of ALA to DHA or to both effects [38]. This dietary imbalance is also observed in the fatty acid composition of erythrocyte phospholipids, which is considered the better marker for the nutritional fatty acid status [39].

The imbalance found between n-6 and n-3 PUFA (n-6/n-3 ratio) in the diet and in membrane phospholipids in pregnant women prompts a warning considering the effects of this imbalance in the human gestational period. During pregnancy, the rate of growth and development of the central nervous system is higher in the final stage (third trimester) and in the early postnatal period [17]. There is evidence demonstrating that the accumulation of DHA in the membrane of neuronal cells during pregnancy and early infancy reaches 50 mg/kg/month, whereas AA accumulates at a rate of 400 mg/kg/month, approximately [40–42]. Dietary intake of n-3 PUFA is associated with the enrichment of n-3 PUFA into the nervous system in pregnancy and the first month of extra-uterine life, strongly impacting infant neurodevelopment [43–46]. The low intake of DHA and the diminished status of this fatty acid in membrane phospholipids of maternal erythrocytes could determine a lower supply of the fatty acid to fetal tissues and, in turn, the depletion of maternal stores, as has been suggested [47]. Furthermore, the low intake of n-3 PUFA and the poor n-3 PUFA maternal status, particularly of DHA, could eventually determine lower neurocognitive development in infants [48].

The characterization of dietary fat intake of pregnant women based on the classification according to food groups (Tables 2 and 4) allowed us to determine the food source of total fat and the principal fatty acids in the diet. In relation to PUFA, the major food groups contributing to LA intake were the high-lipid foods, oils and fats and meats and eggs, whereas for ALA, these were high-lipids foods, oils and fats and dairy products. As expected, the highest proportion of EPA and DHA came from the group of fish and seafood, followed by the minimal contribution of meats and dairy products, only in the case of DHA. Regarding AA, the largest proportion came from meats, eggs and their derivatives, with a low contribution of other groups, such as dairy and seafood (Figure 1).

The high proportion of LA in the diet may be related to the high intake of vegetable oils, such as sunflower and soybean oils, and of fat from butter, margarine, meats and its derived products, all foods that are preferably consumed in the Chilean and occidental diet [49]. The low ALA intake came primarily from some oily seeds (walnuts, almonds) and vegetable oils (soybean and canola), with a lower proportion from dairy products. The low EPA and DHA intake observed in these pregnant women is a consequence of the low consumption of fish and shellfish, because this food group is the main and largest contributor to both fatty acids. The average daily intake of DHA was far below the recommended level, approximately allowing only 30% of the recommendation [50,51]. Results from other countries, included in Table 5, are very interesting. Regarding the comparison of fatty acid profile in membrane phospholipids with the other populations, the characteristics of our sample are similar to those reported in Belgium and USA pregnant women [37], pointing to a low n-3 PUFA and high n-6 PUFA content and, consequently, a higher n-6/n-3 ratio (compared only to USA women), contrary to what was reported in Chinese pregnant women [22]. Although these results are not strictly comparable, it is possible to establish that pregnant Chilean women have the lowest DHA concentration in the phospholipids of erythrocyte membranes.

The low intake of n-3 PUFA and the excessive intake of LA indicate that the average diet of Chilean pregnant woman has an imbalance towards the family of n-6 PUFA. Because of this reason, a complementary feeding program was available from 2009 in the country, consisting of a dry powdered milk product, which provides 90 mg of DHA per 200 mL [52], which is cost-free supplied to pregnant and lactating woman through the Chilean Primary Care Service system. The acceptability of the product was evaluated in pregnant women establishing that some modification of the milk product must be introduced [53]. It is also necessary to rethink the nutritional strategies to reduce saturated fat consumption, aiming to prevent chronically non-transmissible diseases [54] and to increase the n-3 PUFA consumption in this group and in the general population. The dietary imbalance observed in the intake of other important micronutrients during pregnancy, such as choline, iron, zinc and others vitamins or minerals, could negatively affect optimal infant development and maternal nutritional status [55,56], indicating that urgent dietary strategies in this group are needed.

Regarding fatty acids, although obviously the recommendation is to increase the consumption of seafood, the availability of these products is low, of high cost and concerns have arisen regarding contaminants [57]. The development of new food alternatives is essential to meet the daily recommendation of n-3 PUFA, specifically DHA, particularly in pregnant and lactating women. The traditional strategy to supplement DHA, such as fish oil capsules or emulsions, microalgae oil, *etc.*, has proven to be beneficial, particularly in improving neurological development [39]. The promotion of the consumption of vegetable oils with a high content of ALA (such as canola, chia, *Camelina*, flaxseed oil) [58,59] could be a new and interesting strategy to provide n-3 PUFA during this important physiological period [60]. It was demonstrated that consumption of canola oil (10% ALA) by Chilean women during pregnancy reduced the risk of premature delivery and improved the birth weight of infants [61].

5. Conclusions

The sample of Chilean pregnant women showed a high consumption of saturated fat and low consumption of *n*-3 PUFA (ALA, EPA and DHA), which is reflected in the low DHA content of phospholipids from erythrocyte membranes, which are considered a good marker of the nutritional status of this fatty acid. The imbalance of *n*-6/*n*-3 PUFA and the low content of erythrocyte DHA, which results in a restrictive fetal supply of the fatty acid, could negatively affect fetal development with future possible effects on cognitive performance, such as the learning and memory skills of children. It is critical to evaluate new strategies aiming to improve the intake of *n*-3 PUFA throughout pregnancy and the breast feeding periods. It is necessary to develop dietary interventions aimed at improving the quality of consumed foods, with particular emphasis on specific fatty acids, such as *n*-3 PUFA.

Acknowledgments: The authors are grateful to the Nutrition and Dietetics School, Obstetrics and Gynecology Department, Clinical Hospital, and the Department of Nutrition, Faculty of Medicine, University of Chile. We are particularly grateful to Susana Mayer and Jedy Vivero for their valuable contribution in the process of dietary analyses. This work was supported by the Nutrition and Dietetics School, Department of Nutrition, Faculty of Medicine, University of Chile, and Benexia Company.

Author Contributions: Karla A. Bascuñán, Rodrigo Valenzuela and Rodrigo Chamorro designed the study and analyzed and interpreted the data. Karla A. Bascuñán, Rodrigo Valenzuela, Alejandra Valencia, Cynthia Barrera, Jorge Sandoval and Claudia Puigrredon performed clinical and nutritional evaluations. Karla A. Bascuñán, Rodrigo Chamorro and Alejandra Valencia conducted the dietary analysis. Karla A. Bascuñán, Rodrigo Chamorro, Rodrigo Valenzuela and Alfonso Valenzuela wrote the manuscript. All authors reviewed and approved the final version of the manuscript.

Conflicts of Interest: The authors declare no conflict of interest. The founding sponsors had no role in the design of the study; in the collection, analyses, or interpretation of data; in the writing of the manuscript, and in the decision to publish the results.

References

1. Michaelsen, K.F.; Jorgensen, M.H. Dietary fat content and energy density during infancy and childhood; the effect on energy intake and growth. *Eur. J. Clin. Nutr.* **1995**, *49*, 467–483.

2. Michaelsen, K.F.; Dewey, K.G.; Perez-Exposito, A.B.; Nurhasan, M.; Lauritzen, L.; Roos, N. Food sources and intake of *n*-6 and *n*-3 fatty acids in low-income countries with emphasis on infants, young children (6–24 months), and pregnant and lactating women. *Matern. Child. Nutr.* **2011**, *7*, 124–140.

3. Cunnane, S.C. Problems with essential fatty acids: Time for a new paradigm? *Prog. Lipid Res.* **2003**, *42*, 544–568.

4. Nakamura, M.T.; Nara, T.Y. Structure, function, and dietary regulation of delta6, delta5, and delta9 desaturases. *Annu. Rev. Nutr.* **2004**, *24*, 345–376.

5. Innis, S.M. Essential fatty acids in growth and development. *Prog. Lipid Res.* **1991**, *30*, 39–103.
6. Youdim, K.A.; Martin, A.; Joseph, J.A. Essential fatty acids and the brain: Possible health implications. *Int. J. Dev. Neurosci.* **2000**, *18*, 383–399.
7. O'Brien, J.S.; Fillerup, D.L.; Mead, J.F. Quantification and fatty acid and fatty aldehyde composition of ethanolamine, choline, and serine glycerophosphatides in human cerebral grey and white matter. *J. Lipid Res.* **1964**, *5*, 329–338.
8. Crawford, M.A.; Hassam, A.G.; Stevens, P.A. Essential fatty acid requirements in pregnancy and lactation with special reference to brain development. *Prog. Lipid Res.* **1981**, *20*, 31–40.
9. Clandinin, M.T.; Chappell, J.E.; Leong, S.; Heim, T.; Swyer, P.R.; Chance, G.W. Intrauterine fatty acid accretion rates in human brain: Implications for fatty acid requirements. *Early Hum. Dev.* **1980**, *4*, 121–129.
10. Martinez, M. Tissue levels of polyunsaturated fatty acids during early human development. *J. Pediatr.* **1992**, *120*, S129–S138.
11. Hibbeln, J.R.; Nieminen, L.R.; Blasbalg, T.L.; Riggs, J.A.; Lands, W.E. Healthy intakes of *n*-3 and *n*-6 fatty acids: Estimations considering worldwide diversity. *Am. J. Clin. Nutr.* **2006**, *83*, 1483S–1493S.
12. Carlson, S.E.; Colombo, J.; Gajewski, B.J.; Gustafson, K.M.; Mundy, D.; Yeast, J.; Georgieff, M.K.; Markley, L.A.; Kerling, E.H.; Shaddy, D.J. DHA supplementation and pregnancy outcomes. *Am. J. Clin. Nutr.* **2013**, *97*, 808–815.
13. Dunstan, J.A.; Simmer, K.; Dixon, G.; Prescott, S.L. Cognitive assessment of children at age 2.5 years after maternal fish oil supplementation in pregnancy: A randomised controlled trial. *Arch. Dis. Child. Fetal Neonatal Ed.* **2008**, *93*, F45–F50.
14. Birch, E.E.; Carlson, S.E.; Hoffman, D.R.; Fitzgerald-Gustafson, K.M.; Fu, V.L.; Drover, J.R.; Castaneda, Y.S.; Minns, L.; Wheaton, D.K.; Mundy, D.; *et al.* The diamond (DHA intake and measurement of neural development) study: A double-masked, randomized controlled clinical trial of the maturation of infant visual acuity as a function of the dietary level of docosahexaenoic acid. *Am. J. Clin. Nutr.* **2010**, *91*, 848–859.
15. Al, M.D.; van Houwelingen, A.C.; Kester, A.D.; Hasaart, T.H.; de Jong, A.E.; Hornstra, G. Maternal essential fatty acid patterns during normal pregnancy and their relationship to the neonatal essential fatty acid status. *Br. J. Nutr.* **1995**, *74*, 55–68.
16. Brenna, J.T.; Carlson, S.E. Docosahexaenoic acid and human brain development: Evidence that a dietary supply is needed for optimal development. *J. Hum. Evol.* **2014**.
17. Innis, S.M. Perinatal biochemistry and physiology of long-chain polyunsaturated fatty acids. *J. Pediatr.* **2003**, *143*, S1–S8.
18. Larque, E.; Gil-Sanchez, A.; Prieto-Sanchez, M.T.; Koletzko, B. Omega 3 fatty acids, gestation and pregnancy outcomes. *Br. J. Nutr.* **2012**, *107*, S77–S84.
19. Burdge, G.C.; Calder, P.C. Conversion of alpha-linolenic acid to longer-chain polyunsaturated fatty acids in human adults. *Reprod. Nutr. Dev.* **2005**, *45*, 581–597.
20. Makrides, M.; Gibson, R.A. Long-chain polyunsaturated fatty acid requirements during pregnancy and lactation. *Am. J. Clin. Nutr.* **2000**, *71*, 307S–311S.

21. Sauerwald, U.C.; Fink, M.M.; Demmelmair, H.; Schoenaich, P.V.; Rauh-Pfeiffer, A.A.; Koletzko, B. Effect of different levels of docosahexaenoic acid supply on fatty acid status and linoleic and alpha-linolenic acid conversion in preterm infants. *J. Pediatr. Gastroenterol. Nutr.* **2012**, *54*, 353–363.

22. Zhang, J.; Wang, C.; Gao, Y.; Li, L.; Man, Q.; Song, P.; Meng, L.; Du, Z.Y.; Miles, E.A.; Lie, O.; *et al.* Different intakes of n-3 fatty acids among pregnant women in 3 regions of China with contrasting dietary patterns are reflected in maternal but not in umbilical erythrocyte phosphatidylcholine fatty acid composition. *Nutr. Res.* **2013**, *33*, 613–621.

23. Denomme, J.; Stark, K.D.; Holub, B.J. Directly quantitated dietary (n>-3) fatty acid intakes of pregnant canadian women are lower than current dietary recommendations. *J. Nutr.* **2005**, *135*, 206–211.

24. Innis, S.M.; Elias, S.L. Intakes of essential n-6 and n-3 polyunsaturated fatty acids among pregnant canadian women. *Am. J. Clin. Nutr.* **2003**, *77*, 473–478.

25. Meyer, B.J.; Mann, N.J.; Lewis, J.L.; Milligan, G.C.; Sinclair, A.J.; Howe, P.R. Dietary intakes and food sources of omega-6 and omega-3 polyunsaturated fatty acids. *Lipids* **2003**, *38*, 391–398.

26. Otto, S.J.; Houwelingen, A.C.; Antal, M.; Manninen, A.; Godfrey, K.; Lopez-Jaramillo, P.; Hornstra, G. Maternal and neonatal essential fatty acid status in phospholipids: An international comparative study. *Eur. J. Clin. Nutr.* **1997**, *51*, 232–242.

27. Makrides, M. Is there a dietary requirement for DHA in pregnancy? *Prostaglandins Leukot. Essent. Fatty Acids* **2009**, *81*, 171–174.

28. European Society for Opinion and Marketing Research. *The ESOMAR Standard Demographic Classification*; ESOMAR: Amsterdam, The Netherlands, 1997.

29. Cerda, R.; Barrera, C.; Arena, M.; Bascuñán, K.A.; Jimenez, G. *Atlas Fotográfico de Alimentos y Preparaciones Típicas Chilenas. Encuesta Nacional de Consumo Alimentario 2010*, 1st ed.; Gobierno de Chile,Ministerio de Salud: Santiago, Chile, 2010.

30. Atalah, E.; Castillo, C.; Castro, R.; Aldea, A. Proposalof a new standard for the nutritional assessment of pregnant women. *Rev. Med. Chil.* **1997**, *125*, 1429–1436.

31. WHO/FAO/UNU. *Human Energy Requirements*, Report of a Joint FAO/WHO/UNU Expert Consultation: Rome, Italy, October 2014.

32. Food and Nutrition Board, Institute of Medicine. *Dietary Reference Intakes: Guiding Principles for Nutrition Labeling and Fortification*; Institute of Medicine of the National Academies: Washington, DC, USA, 2001; pp. 1–224.

33. Bligh, E.G.; Dyer, W.J. A rapid method of total lipid extraction and purification. *Can. J. Biochem. Physiol.* **1959**, *37*, 911–917.

34. Ruiz-Gutierrez, V.; Cert, A.; Rios, J.J. Determination of phospholipid fatty acid and triacylglycerol composition of rat caecal mucosa. *J. Chromatogr.* **1992**, *575*, 1–6.

35. Morrison, W.R.; Smith, L.M. Preparation of fatty acid methyl esters and dimethylacetals from lipids with boron fluoride—Methanol. *J. Lipid Res.* **1964**, *5*, 600–608.

36. De Vriese, S.R.; Matthys, C.; de Henauw, S.; de Backer, G.; Dhont, M.; Christophe, A.B. Maternal and umbilical fatty acid status in relation to maternal diet. *Prostaglandins Leukot. Essent. Fatty Acids* **2002**, *67*, 389–396.

37. Donahue, S.M.; Rifas-Shiman, S.L.; Olsen, S.F.; Gold, D.R.; Gillman, M.W.; Oken, E. Associations of maternal prenatal dietary intake of *n*-3 and *n*-6 fatty acids with maternal and umbilical cord blood levels. *Prostaglandins Leukot Essent. Fatty Acids* **2009**, *80*, 289–296.

38. Brenna, J.T.; Salem, N., Jr.; Sinclair, A.J.; Cunnane, S.C. Alpha-linolenic acid supplementation and conversion to n-3 long-chain polyunsaturated fatty acids in humans. *Prostaglandins Leukot Essent. Fatty Acids* **2009**, *80*, 85–91.

39. Janssen, C.I.; Kiliaan, A.J. Long-chain polyunsaturated fatty acids (LCPUFA) from genesis to senescence: The influence of LCPUFA on neural development, aging, and neurodegeneration. *Prog. Lipid Res.* **2014**, *53*, 1–17.

40. Coti Bertrand, P.; O'Kusky, J.R.; Innis, S.M. Maternal dietary (*n*-3) fatty acid deficiency alters neurogenesis in the embryonic rat brain. *J. Nutr.* **2006**, *136*, 1570–1575.

41. Green, P.; Glozman, S.; Kamensky, B.; Yavin, E. Developmental changes in rat brain membrane lipids and fatty acids. The preferential prenatal accumulation of docosahexaenoic acid. *J. Lipid Res.* **1999**, *40*, 960–966.

42. Salem, N., Jr.; Litman, B.; Kim, H.Y.; Gawrisch, K. Mechanisms of action of docosahexaenoic acid in the nervous system. *Lipids* **2001**, *36*, 945–959.

43. Helland, I.B.; Smith, L.; Saarem, K.; Saugstad, O.D.; Drevon, C.A. Maternal supplementation with very-long-chain *n*-3 fatty acids during pregnancy and lactation augments childrenÊ$\frac{1}{4}$s IQ at 4 years of age. *Pediatrics* **2003**, *111*, e39–e44.

44. Hibbeln, J.R.; Davis, J.M.; Steer, C.; Emmett, P.; Rogers, I.; Williams, C.; Golding, J. Maternal seafood consumption in pregnancy and neurodevelopmental outcomes in childhood (ALSPAC study): An observational cohort study. *Lancet* **2007**, *369*, 578–585.

45. Judge, M.P.; Harel, O.; Lammi-Keefe, C.J. A docosahexaenoic acid-functional food during pregnancy benefits infant visual acuity at four but not six months of age. *Lipids* **2007**, *42*, 117–122.

46. Parra-Cabrera, S.; Moreno-Macias, H.; Mendez-Ramirez, I.; Schnaas, L.; Romieu, I. Maternal dietary omega fatty acid intake and auditory brainstem-evoked potentials in mexican infants born at term: Cluster analysis. *Early Hum. Dev.* **2008**, *84*, 51–57.

47. Parra-Cabrera, S.; Stein, A.D.; Wang, M.; Martorell, R.; Rivera, J.; Ramakrishnan, U. Dietary intakes of polyunsaturated fatty acids among pregnant mexican women. *Matern. Child. Nutr.* **2011**, *7*, 140–147.

48. McCann, J.C.; Ames, B.N. Is docosahexaenoic acid, an *n*-3 long-chain polyunsaturated fatty acid, required for development of normal brain function? An overview of evidence from cognitive and behavioral tests in humans and animals. *Am. J. Clin. Nutr.* **2005**, *82*, 281–295.

49. Simopoulos, A.P. Importance of the omega-6/omega-3 balance in health and disease: Evolutionary aspects of diet. *World Rev. Nutr. Diet.* **2011**, *102*, 10–21.

50. Atalah, S.E.; Araya, B.M.; Rosselot, P.G.; Araya, L.H.; Vera, A.G.; Andreu, R.R.; Barba, G.C.; Rodriguez, L. Consumption of a DHA-enriched milk drink by pregnant and lactating women, on the fatty acid composition of red blood cells, breast milk, and in the newborn. *Arch. Latinoam. Nutr.* **2009**, *59*, 271–277.

51. Guesnet, P.; Alessandri, J.M. Docosahexaenoic acid (DHA) and the developing central nervous system (CNS)—Implications for dietary recommendations. *Biochimie* **2011**, *93*, 7–12.

52. Castillo, C.; Balboa, P.; Raimann, X.; Nutrición, R. Modificaciones a la leche del programa nacional de alimentación complementaria (PNAC) en chile. *Rev. Chil. Ped.* **2009**, *80*, 508–512.

53. Contreras, A.; Herrera, Y.; Rodríguez, L.; Pizarro, T.; Atalah, E. Acceptability and consumption of a dairy drink with omega-3 in pregnant and lactating women of the national supplementary food program. *Rev. Chil. Nutr.* **2011**, *38*, 313–320.

54. Hanson, M.; Gluckman, P.; Nutbeam, D.; Hearn, J. Priority actions for the non-communicable disease crisis. *Lancet* **2011**, *378*, 566–567.

55. Zeisel, S.H. Is maternal diet supplementation beneficial? Optimal development of infant depends on motherÊ¼s diet. *Am. J. Clin. Nutr.* **2009**, *89*, 685S–687S.

56. Yang, Z.; Huffman, S.L. Nutrition in pregnancy and early childhood and associations with obesity in developing countries. *Matern. Child. Nutr.* **2013**, *9*, 105–119.

57. Pasquare, F.A.; Bettinetti, R.; Fumagalli, S.; Vignati, D.A. Public health benefits and risks of fish consumption: Current scientific evidence v. mediacoverage. *Public Health Nutr.* **2013**, *16*, 1885–1892.

58. Kim, K.B.; Nam, Y.A.; Kim, H.S.; Hayes, A.W.; Lee, B.M. Alpha-linolenic acid: Nutraceutical, pharmacological and toxicological evaluation. *Food Chem. Toxicol.* **2014**, *70C*, 163–178.

59. Valenzuela, B.R.; Barrera, R.C.; Gonzalez-Astorga, M.; Sanhueza, C.J.; Valenzuela, B.A. Alpha-linolenic acid (ALA) from *Rosa canina*, sacha inchi and chia oils may increase ALA accretion and its conversion into *n*-3 LCPUFA in diverse tissues of the rat. *Food Funct.* **2014**, *5*, 1564–1572.

60. Plourde, M.; Cunnane, S.C. Extremely limited synthesis of long chain polyunsaturates in adults: Implications for their dietary essentiality and use as supplements. *Appl. Physiol. Nutr. Metab.* **2007**, *32*, 619–634.

61. Mardones, F.; Urrutia, M.T.; Villarroel, L.; Rioseco, A.; Castillo, O.; Rozowski, J.; Tapia, J.L.; Bastias, G.; Bacallao, J.; Rojas, I. Effects of a dairy product fortified with multiple micronutrients and omega-3 fatty acids on birth weight and gestation duration in pregnant chilean women. *Public Health Nutr.* **2008**, *11*, 30–40.

Fish Intake during Pregnancy and Foetal Neurodevelopment—A Systematic Review of the Evidence

Phoebe Starling, Karen Charlton, Anne T. McMahon and Catherine Lucas

Abstract: Fish is a source of several nutrients that are important for healthy foetal development. Guidelines from Australia, Europe and the USA encourage fish consumption during pregnancy. The potential for contamination by heavy metals, as well as risk of listeriosis requires careful consideration of the shaping of dietary messages related to fish intake during pregnancy. This review critically evaluates literature on fish intake in pregnant women, with a focus on the association between neurodevelopmental outcomes in the offspring and maternal fish intake during pregnancy. Peer-reviewed journal articles published between January 2000 and March 2014 were included. Eligible studies included those of healthy pregnant women who had experienced full term births and those that had measured fish or seafood intake and assessed neurodevelopmental outcomes in offspring. Medline, Scopus, Web of Science, ScienceDirect and the Cochrane Library were searched using the search terms: pregnant, neurodevelopment, cognition, fish and seafood. Of 279 papers sourced, eight were included in the final review. Due to heterogeneity in methodology and measured outcomes, a qualitative comparison of study findings was conducted. This review indicates that the benefits of diets providing moderate amounts of fish during pregnancy outweigh potential detrimental effects in regards to offspring neurodevelopment. It is important that the type of fish consumed is low in mercury.

Reprinted from *Nutrients*. Cite as: Starling, P.; Charlton, K.; McMahon, A.T.; Lucas, C. Fish Intake during Pregnancy and Foetal Neurodevelopment—A Systematic Review of the Evidence. *Nutrients* **2015**, *7*, 2001–2014.

1. Introduction

Fish is a source of several nutrients that are important during pregnancy for healthy foetal development including iodine, long chain omega-3 polyunsaturated fatty acids (LCn-3PUFAs), and vitamins A, D and B12 [1]. Guidelines from Australia [2], Europe [3] and the USA [4] encourage the consumption of fish during pregnancy. Recent studies indicate that pregnant women lack sufficient knowledge regarding the importance of iodine and LCn-3 PUFAs [5,6], nutrients that are present in fish and seafood. In addition, it appears Australian women are falling short of LCn-3PUFA intake recommendations during pregnancy [6,7]. On average, Australian women are consuming 33 g of fish per day and pregnant women an average of 28 g of fish per day, below Food Standards Australia New Zealand (FSANZ) recommended intakes [8]. As well as being a source of essential nutrients, fish are also a potential source of contaminants including mercury, polychlorinated biphenyls and dioxins [9]. Guidelines emphasising the health risks of methyl-mercury, with little mention of important nutrients found in fish, may be contributing to women consuming less than the recommended fish servings during pregnancy [10]. Thus the risks and benefits resulting from fish consumption need to be considered and scientific evidence should direct advice given to pregnant women to help them make the safest choice.

There are many documented health benefits from fish consumption with regard to foetal health, including improved neurodevelopment, increased birth weight and a reduced risk of spontaneous abortion [11,12]. This review focuses on neurodevelopmental outcomes for the foetus as much of the published research into fish consumption during pregnancy has focused on methyl-mercury, LCn-3PUFAs and iodine, all known to impact foetal neurodevelopment [13,14]. The aim of this review was to critically appraise literature investigating fish intake in pregnant women to assess the hypothesis that fish consumption during pregnancy positively influences foetal neurodevelopment. This review concludes with a discussion highlighting some of the methodological issues in researching associations between diet and infant neurodevelopment.

2. Experimental Section

2.1. Eligibility Criteria

Articles published in peer-reviewed journals between January 2000 and March 2014 were included in this review. Eligible studies were those with healthy pregnant women, full term births and offspring with no anomalies or diseases. Articles that investigated the relationship between the maternal consumption of fish or seafood and neurodevelopmental outcomes in offspring were included. Animal studies, studies not reported in English, and studies of populations exposed to contaminants were excluded. Articles directed at identifying suitable models to explain the relationship between components in fish or developing tools to analyse the risk-benefit of fish consumption without measuring neurodevelopmental outcomes were not deemed eligible for this review.

2.2. Search Strategy

Medline, Scopus, Web of Science, ScienceDirect and the Cochrane Library were searched using terms outlined in Table 1.

The Dietitians Association of Australia Process Manual for review of the Australian Dietary Guidelines [15] was the basis for reviewing the articles and guided the concluding evidence statement. The quality rating of the studies eligible for review was assessed based on the NHMRC guidelines for review of scientific literature [16].

Table 1. Database search strategy.

	Search terms	Keywords searched	BOOLEAN operator
Term 1	Pregnant or pregnancy	Pregnan*	AND
Term 2	Fish or seafood	Fish seafood	OR AND
Term 3	Neurodevelopment or neurodevelopmental or cognition or cognitive	Neurodevelopment* cogniti*	OR

3. Results

The initial search identified 279 articles after duplicates were removed, eight of which were suitable for inclusion. The PRISMA statement process was followed [17] as shown in Figure 1.

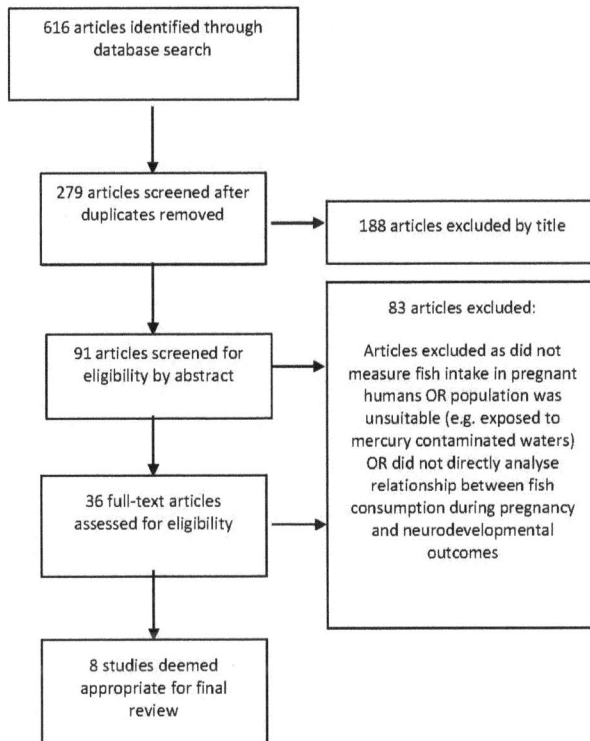

Figure 1. Flow diagram for inclusion of journal articles [17].

The search strategy did not yield any randomised controlled trials of fish intake in pregnant women and associated foetal neurodevelopmental outcomes. All eight studies included in the final review were observational in design. A summary of these articles and their quality rating is presented in Table 2.

Studies were heterogeneous in methodology in regard to the covariates, neurological assessment tools, length of follow up statistical analyses. In addition, the type and amounts of fish consumed differed across study locations. Due to this heterogeneity a qualitative rather than quantitative approach was deemed appropriate for comparison and presentation of findings.

A study by Oken *et al.* tested children at six months of age using Visual Recognition Memory (VRM) paradigm and found a significant improvement of 2.8 points for each additional serving of fish (85–140 g) consumed by the mother during pregnancy [19]. Mendez *et al.* found that the length of breastfeeding influenced whether a significant difference was found in offspring neurodevelopment when comparing high and low fish intakes during pregnancy [24]. Authors reported that fish consumption two to three times per week during pregnancy was beneficial for children who were breastfed for less than six months. However, no statistical improvement was indicated for those children who were breastfed for longer than six months [24]. Gale *et al.* demonstrated no adverse effects on offspring neurodevelopment with maternal fish consumption during pregnancy equal to or greater than once per week. This study reported an improved verbal Intelligence Quotient (IQ) in offspring aged nine years in children born to mothers who consumed up to two servings of fish per week compared with children born to mothers who had not consumed any fish during late pregnancy (32 weeks gestation). This association was not significant for fish consumption in early pregnancy (15 weeks gestation) suggesting that fish consumption may be of more benefit during the third trimester [21].

A report from the Avon Longitudinal Study of Parents and Children (ALSPAC) found that fish consumption during pregnancy of one to three servings per week was shown to provide a modest but significant improvement in developmental scores of the offspring for language and social activity at fifteen to eighteen months of age [18]. A longer follow up of the ALSPAC cohort demonstrated a reduction in the percentage of children with suboptimal IQ at eight years of age amongst mothers with a high seafood intake (greater than 340 g) during pregnancy [20].

Table 2. Summary and quality rating for reviewed articles.

Reference	Daniels et al, 2004 [18]	Oken et al, 2005 [19]	Hibbeln et al, 2007 [20]	Gale et al, 2008 [21]
Type of study	Observational cohort (Avon Longitudinal Study of Parents and Children-ALSPAC)	Prospective cohort (Project Viva)	Observational cohort (ALSPAC)	Observational cohort
NHMRC Level of evidence [20]	Level III-3	Level III-3	Level III-3	Level III-3
Population	Pregnant women living in Bristol & surrounds, United Kingdom (UK).	Pregnant women recruited in Massachusetts, United States of America (USA)	Pregnant women in Bristol & surrounds, UK.	Pregnant women recruited in Southampton, UK.
N—sample size	7421 mother-child pairs.	135 mother-child pairs	5449 children assessed.	217 mother-child pairs.
Method	Measured fish intake during at 32 weeks gestation by Food Frequency Questionnaire (FFQ) during. Breastfeeding, child fish consumption, maternal dental & lifestyle questionnaires. Neurodevelopmental testing of child completed by mother using ALSPAC adaption of the MacArthur Communicative Development Inventory (MCDI) at 15 months and Denver Developmental Screening Test (DDST) at 18 months of age.	Fish and seafood intake measured via a validated FFQ (calibrated for LCn-3PUFAs in blood) at 28 weeks gestation. Infant cognition measured using Visual Recognition Memory (VRM) paradigm at 6 months of age.	Seafood consumption assessed at 32 weeks gestation via FFQ. Postal questionnaires on diet, education, social, behavioural and developmental outcomes at child age: 6, 18, 30, 42, and 81 months. Wechsler Intelligence Scale for Children III used to assess Intelligence Quotient (IQ) at 8 years and Strengths and Difficulties Questionnaire (SDQ) conducted. Presented as percentage of children in the lowest quartile for WISC-III and ALSPAC development test subscales or in the suboptimum range of behavioural scores for the SDQ. Tested at 42 months, 7 and 8 years.	Two FFQs during pregnancy (at 15 weeks and 32 weeks) were used to estimate fish intake in early and late pregnancy. Cognitive & behavioural outcomes in offspring at 9 years using the Wechsler Abbreviated Scale of Intelligence. The SDQ was used to measure maladaptive behaviour.
Intervention/comparator	Fish intake: rarely/never, once a fortnight, 1–3 times per week, 4 or more times per week. Assumed each fish serve was 4.5 ounces (~0 g, 64 g, 255 g and 510 g per week).	Second trimester fish servings: more than 2 weekly fish servings compared to 2 or less. Did not convert servings to grams.	Comparing no seafood intake and 1–340 g per week with more than 340 g per week (3 servings is estimated as 340 g).	Fish servings per week in early and late pregnancy: never, less than 1, 1–2 times, 3 or more times. Oily fish servings in both early and late pregnancy: never, less than 1, 1 or more. Amount not specified in grams

Table 2. *Cont.*

Reference	Daniels et al., 2004 [18]	Oken et al., 2005 [19]	Hibbeln et al., 2007 [20]	Gale et al., 2008 [21]
Outcome	Fish consumption during pregnancy resulted in modest but significant improvement in developmental scores for language & social activity at 15–18 months age. Odds ratio (OR) and 95% confidence interval (CI) for high test score for MCDI: Vocabulary comprehension = 1.5 (1.1–2.0) for one or more serves compared to no serves. Social activity = 1.6 (1.2–2.2) for 1/fortnight, 1.7 (1.3–2.2) for 1–3/week and 1.8 (1.4–2.4) for 4+ serves/week compared to no serves.	Non-significant increase in VRM of 2.8 points for each additional weekly fish serving (95% CI = 0.2 to 5.4). When mercury confounder was adjusted for, this association became significant: 4.0 (1.3 to 6.7). Mothers consuming greater than 2 fish serves per week had infants with the greatest VRM scores.	Seafood intake during pregnancy was associated with a significant reduction in percentage of children with suboptimal IQ and behaviour test scores in 9 of 23 outcomes. Non-seafood consumers during pregnancy had children who scored lower on tests of verbal IQ at 8 years: OR (CI) for no seafood = 1.48 (1.16–1.90); some seafood 1.09 (0.92–1.20) compared with >340 g per week [overall trend: $p = 0.004$].	Oily fish consumption more than once per week versus no oily fish reduced the risk of hyperactivity. No association with fish consumption in early pregnancy and full scale IQ, however, total fish intake in late pregnancy of 1 to 2 serves per week was associated with having a child with higher IQ at age 9 years. Higher intakes (3 or more serves per week) did not show a statistically significant improvement. Regression coefficients (95% CI) for fish consumption and full scale IQ: less than once per week *vs.* no fish = 7.76 (0.38 to 15.1), once or twice per week vs. no fish = 6.91 (0.19 to 13.6). Verbal IQ & fish consumption: Increase of 7.32 (0.26 to 14.4) with fish consumption once or twice per week. 8.07 (0.28 to 15.9) with three or more serves per week.
Quality	Neutral	Positive	Neutral	Positive
Type of study	Prospective population-based cohort	Prospective cohort (Project Viva)	Prospective birth cohort	Birth cohort study
NHMRC Level of evidence [20]	Level III-3	Level III-3	Level III-3	Level III-3
Population	Pregnant women recruited throughout Denmark.	Pregnant women recruited in Massachusetts, USA.	Pregnant women living in Menorca, Spain.	Pregnant women recruited in Japan.
N—sample size	25,446 mothers-child pairs.	341 mother-child pairs.	392 mother-child pairs	498 mother-infant pairs

54

Table 2. Cont.

Reference	Daniels et al., 2004 [18]	Oken et al., 2005 [19]	Hibbeln et al., 2007 [20]	Gale et al., 2008 [21]
Method	Validated FFQ conducted at 25 weeks gestation to estimate fish intake. Standardised interview with mother used to assess child neurodevelopment at 6 and 18 months. Measured the odds of improved development scores due to fish intake. No individual comparison for each category—pooled estimate only.	Fish intake during pregnancy estimated via semi-quantitative FFQ. Peabody Picture Vocabulary Test (PPVT) and Wide Range Assessment of Visual Motor Abilities (WRAVMA) tested at ~38 months age of child and analysed for association with fish intake.	FFQ of typical diet during pregnancy completed 3 months after delivery and fish and shellfish/squid intake estimated. Neurodevelopment (as well as diet and physical activity) assessed when child was 4 years of age using the McCarthy Scales of Children's Abilities (MCSA) tests—global cognitive scale & 5 subscales (perceptive-performance, memory, verbal, quantitative and motor).	Fish intake measured via FFQ 4 days after birth of child. Trained examiners conducted Neurodevelopmental testing of child was completed via a Neonatal Behavioural Assessment 3 days post birth (28 behavioural & 18 reflex items).
Comparator and Comparison	Fish intake in quintiles Weekly servings Categories: no fish (0 g), 1–2 servings (1–340 g per week), or 3 or more servings per week (over 340 g).	Fish consumption: No fish serves, less than or equal to 2 servings per week, greater than 2 servings per week.	Maternal fish intake of more than 2–3 times per week compared to up to once per week. No mention of intake in grams.	Maternal seafood intake in grams (average intake = 300–360 g per week).
Outcome	Highest 3 quintiles of fish intake resulted in improved motor, social/cognitive and total development scores at 18 months: OR (95%CI) = 1.28 (1.20, 1.38) for highest versus lowest quintile. This association was less obvious at 6 months (only the highest quintile showed significant improvement).	Offspring of women who ate fish more than twice a week scored significantly higher on WRAVMA drawing and total scores compared with no serves. OR (95%CI) for WRAVMA drawing = 6.0 (1.8, 10.2) for more than two serves per week compared with no serves. WRAVMA total score = 5.3 (0.9, 9.6) for more than two serves per week compared to no serves.	Pregnant women fish consumption greater than 2–3 times per week had children with significantly higher cognition and motor development scores compared to women consuming fish less than once a week. This association was only significant in children breastfed for up to 6 months. Greater than 3 serves per week was not associated with improved outcomes.	Seafood intake weakly ($p = 0.1$) correlated with motor development. Other measures of neurodevelopment not significant in either direction.
Quality	Neutral	Positive	Positive	Neutral

55

A smaller ($n = 498$) Japanese study did not demonstrate a positive or negative association between maternal fish intake during pregnancy and neurodevelopment as measured by the Neonatal Behavioural Assessment tool in infants at three days of age [25]. Conversely, results from a US cohort study demonstrated a significant improvement in IQ with consumption of more than two maternal servings of fish intake per week as assessed via 'milestone' achievement in children aged six months and eighteen months [23]. Results from a large Danish national birth cohort ($n = 25,446$) indicated a significant improvement in motor, cognitive and total developmental scores for eighteen month old children who were born to women within the highest three quintiles of fish intake during pregnancy. At six months, this improvement was only significant for children of women in the highest quintile of fish consumption, suggesting that age of testing may be relevant [22].

The overall quality rating score for the reviewed studies are presented in Table 2. The eight eligible studies were graded as negative, neutral or positive overall based on NHMRC guidelines for scientific literature reviews [16]. All studies were found to be either positive or neutral in regards to quality rating. Seven of the eight reviewed articles showed a beneficial impact on certain measures of offspring neurodevelopment with fish intake ranging from less than one to three or more servings of fish per week. Thus, the evidence in these cohort studies supports the current recommendations for fish consumption during pregnancy [2–4]. The level of this evidence is Grade C as per the ratings outlined in Table 3, adapted from Williams *et al.* [15] indicating that the body of evidence is supportive of fish intake during pregnancy.

Table 3. Evidence Rating Table [13].

Component	Rating	Comments
Evidence Base	Satisfactory	NHMRC Level III (cohort studies) with moderate risk of bias [20].
Consistency	Good	Seven out of eight studies demonstrated a positive association between fish intake and foetal neurodevelopment.
Clinical impact	Satisfactory	Trend towards improved neurodevelopment with significant results in several domains.
Generalisability	Good	All studies in pregnant women.
Applicability	Poor	A variety of populations studied from different countries where type of fish and the level of contaminants would likely vary.

4. Discussion

This systematic review of observational cohort studies demonstrates an association between consumption of one or more servings of fish per week during pregnancy and better offspring neurodevelopment outcomes. Suzuki *et al.* [21] was the only study to report a neutral effect of seafood intake on all neurodevelopmental outcomes. However, in that study neurodevelopment was assessed when the infant was only three days old. The seven studies, which demonstrated a benefit in neurodevelopment, had a follow up time ranging from six months to nine years. Thus it is possible that longer follow up may be needed to determine significant associations. This concept is supported by Oken *et al.* which found an improvement in neurodevelopmental scores at six months in only the highest quintile of fish intake while this improvement was evident in the highest three quintiles at eighteen months [22].

Mendez *et al.* [24] found that seafood consumption that excluded fish intake had a detrimental effect on neurodevelopment, while fish intake alone led to improved outcomes. Thus it is possible that the study of Suzuki *et al.* [25] may have detected a benefit had fish been considered separately from total seafood. Gale *et al.* [21] reported differences in outcomes associated with oily fish intake and total fish intake in early compared to late pregnancy. This suggests that the type of fish and timing of consumption during pregnancy may impact on neurodevelopmental outcomes of offspring. However, this information is limited to a single study, which was conducted in a relatively small sample (n = 217). More research in this area is required to draw sound conclusions.

It is important to note the number methodological limitations in research on diet and infant neurodevelopment that are present in these studies. This prevents the conclusion of a definitive relationship without further research, preferably clinical randomised controlled trials, and a proper meta-analysis.

Measuring dietary intake in cohort studies is problematic due to the difficulty in obtaining detailed information without causing significant subject burden. All identified observational cohort studies in the current review used food frequency questionnaires (FFQs) to assess fish intake. No studies reported adjusting results from the FFQ for energy intake, a recommendation made by Freedman *et al.* 2011 [26] to prevent attenuation. Three studies [19,21,24] reported on the frequency of consumption without specifying the weight of fish servings while the remaining studies made assumptions based on standard serving sizes, as to the quantity of fish consumed at each occasion. This limits the accuracy of a quantifiable conclusion as due to individual variability in the perception of a 'serving size'.

Assessing cognitive development differences in infancy and childhood is fraught with difficulties due to the nature of childhood development and the accurate measurement of such. Firstly, children develop in 'spurts' rather than in a continuous fashion, which means they may slip in and out of the 'normal' reference ranges, particularly in the earlier years [27,28]. To combat this, it has been suggested that testing occurs at more than one time point [27] and that testing should extend beyond the first two years, preferable to school aged children in order to detect more subtle differences [28]. Only 4 studies tested at multiple time points [18,21,22,24], four beyond two years [20,21,23,24], and only two looked at children of school age [20,21].

Secondly, there are multiple interrelated factors which impact on neurodevelopment, and not all confounders were accounted for in all analyses. Maternal intelligence, alcohol consumption, smoking and breastfeeding practices were included as covariates in all studies. However, factors including ethnicity, paternal intelligence, the home environment, drug use, dietary patterns, supplement use and maternal responsiveness were not always measured. The ALSPAC study reports by Daniels *et al.* [18] and Hibbeln *et al.* [20] included the home environment as a confounder, but not paternal IQ. Conversely, the two studies by Oken *et al.* adjusted for paternal IQ but not the home environment [22,23]. The remaining four studies did not correct for either paternal IQ or home environment. No studies adjusted for maternal responsiveness which has been shown to be related to developmental outcomes independent of sociodemographic factors [28]. An intake of fish may reflect a health conscious diet and thus the positive effects may not be directly attributed to the fish but rather to the diet as a whole. Oken *et al.* considered maternal diet by classifying women as following a "prudent" or "western" dietary pattern [23]. Hibbeln *et al.* [20] also adjusted for maternal diet, while Mendez *et al.* [24] adjusted for both maternal and child diets. Other studies did not effectively account for dietary intake and are thus at risk of bias. Oken *et al.* [22], Mendez *et al.* [24] and Hibbeln *et al.* [20] measured supplement usage during pregnancy. Hibbeln *et al.* [20] reported that only 1.7% of women consumed fish oil supplements not affecting outcomes, however, this study did not consider supplements other than fish oil. Only Mendez *et al.* [24] included supplement usage as a confounder.

There is no universal standard for which neurodevelopmental tests are most appropriate for use in children of varying ages and at what age meaningful differences in neurocognitive development can be detected [29]. Performance in assessments can be significantly altered if the participant is hungry, tired or fearful of being in a strange place or being tested [27]. The accuracy of the tests for the population depends on when the test was standardised and within what population. In particular the Denver test, utilised in the ALSPAC study [18] has been criticised for its low specificity and potentially outdated 'norm' as it was standardised in 1980 [30]. Research on the reliability of parental reports on child development is conflicting [31], Daniels *et al.* [18], Hibbeln *et al.* [20] and Oken *et al.* [22] used developmental testing carried out by the mother and thus results may not be as reliable as those reported by other studies, which used trained professionals.

Due to the risks associated with consuming fish and seafood during pregnancy related to food safety and heavy metal contamination, pregnant women may question the necessity of including these foods in their diets, when nutrition supplements are readily accessible in Western countries [32]. A systematic review of randomised control trials examining LCn-3PUFA supplementation during pregnancy found no clear association between supplement use and infant cognitive outcomes [33]. This may be attributable to the synergistic effects of food [34] and associated with fish being a source of other nutrients which are important for infant development such as iodine and vitamin D. Presently, there have been no randomised control trials examining neurocognitive outcomes associated with prenatal multivitamin use and infant neurodevelopment, and these are unlikely to occur given ethical implications of such [35]. Recent research has suggested that effects of methyl-mercury on infant brain development may be mediated by LCn-3PUFA [36]. Because it is possible to consume fish and seafood safely during pregnancy, through following recommendations to limit high mercury species, it is prudent to recommend that pregnant women consume these foods, rather than rely on supplementation, in order to maximise infant neurodevelopment outcomes.

5. Conclusions

This review assessed the hypothesis that fish intake during pregnancy improves offspring neurodevelopmental outcomes. A review of the available evidence indicates that intake of fish during pregnancy is associated with positive foetal neurodevelopmental outcomes, as supported by seven of eight articles reviewed, which showed a beneficial impact on foetal neurodevelopment with one or more servings of fish per week compared with no fish intake. Based on the results from these observational studies the current recommendation of two to three servings per week appears appropriate. Randomised clinical trials have been conducted using fish oil supplementation in pregnancy, but not with fish considered as a whole food. Existing evidence is currently insufficient to inform advice regarding fish intake during pregnancy. Further well designed studies are required to strengthen the evidence base regarding the type and quantity of maternal fish consumption during pregnancy and associated neurodevelopmental outcomes in the offspring, while considering the contribution of mercury from fish-containing diets.

Author Contributions: Phoebe Starling conducted the literature review, summarized the findings and drafted the initial manuscript. Karen Charlton, Anne McMahon and Catherine Lucas provided guidance on search terms, the review process, quality rating, and provided editorial assistance with the final manuscript.

Conflicts of Interest: The authors declare no conflict of interest.

References

1. Simpson, J.L.; Bailey, L.B.; Pietrzik, K.; Shane, B.; Holzgreve, W. Micronutrients and women of reproductive potential: required dietary intake and consequences of dietary deficienty or excess. Part II—Vitamin D, Vitamin A, Iron, Zinc, Iodine, Essential Fatty Acids. *J. Maternal-Fetal Neonatal Med.* **2011**, *24*, 1–24.

2. National Health and Medical Research Council. *Australian Dietary Guidelines*; National Health and Medical Research Council: Canberra, Australia, 2013.

3. European Food Safety Authority. Scientific Opinion on health benefits of seafood (fish and shellfish) consumption in relation to health risks associated with exposure to methylmercury. *EFSA J.* **2014**, *12*, 1–80.

4. U.S. Department of Agriculture and U.S Department of Health and Human Services. *Dietary Guidelines for Americans*, 7th ed.U.S Government Printing Office: Washington, DC, USA, 2010.

5. Charlton, K.E.; Yeatman, H.; Brock, E.; Lucas, C.; Gemming, L.; Goodfellow, A.; Ma, G. Improvement in iodine status of pregnant Australian women 3 years after introduction of a mandatory iodine fortification programme. *Prev. Med.* **2013**, *57*, 26–30.

6. Emmett, R.; Akkersdyk, S.; Yeatman, H.; Meyer, B.J. Expanding awareness of docosahexaenoic acid during pregnancy. *Nutrients* **2013**, *5*, 1098–1109.

7. Sinikovic, D.; Yeatman, H.; Cameron, D.; Meyer, B. Women's awareness of the importance of long chain omega-3 polyunsaturated fatty acid consumption during pregnancy: Knowledge of risks, benefits and information accessibility. *Public Health Nutr.* **2009**, *12*, 562–569.

8. Taylor, A.L.; Collins, C.E.; Patterson, A.J. The relationship between contaminant exposure from fish and nutrient intakes in Australian women by pregnancy status. *Nutr. Diet.* **2014**, *71*, 229–235.

9. Costa, L.G. Contaminants in fish: Risk-benefit considerations. *Arh. Hig. Rada. Toksikol.* **2007**, *58*, 367–374.

10. Oken, E. Decline in fish consumption among pregnant women after a national mercury advisory. *Obstet. Gynecol.* **2003**, *102*, 346–351.

11. Zimmermann, M.B. The role of iodine in human growth and development. *Semin. Cell. Dev. Biol.* **2011**, *22*, 645–652.

12. Jensen, C.L. Effects of *n*-3 fatty acids during pregnancy and lactation. *Am. J. Clin. Nutr.* **2006**, *83*, 1452S–1457S.

13. Bose-O'Reilly, S.; McCarty, K.M.; Steckling, N.; Lettmeier, B. Mercury exposure and children's health. *Curr. Probl. Pediatr. Adolesc. Health Care* **2010**, *40*, 186–215.

14. Dennehy, C. Omega-3 Fatty Acids and Ginger in Maternal Health: Pharmacology, Efficacy, and Safety. *J. Midwifery Womens Health* **2011**, *56*, 584–590.

15. Williams, P.; Allman-Farinelli, M.; Collins, C.; Gifford, J.; Byron, A. A review of the evidence to address targeted questions to inform the revision of the Australian dietary guidelines 2009. In *Process Manual*; National Health and Medical Research Council: Canberra, Australia, 2011.

16. NHMRC. *How to Review the Evidence: Systematic Identification and Review of the Scientific Literature*; NHMRC, Ed.; Biotext: Canberra, Australia, 2000.

17. Moher, D.; Liberati, A.; Tetziaff, J.; Altman, D.G.; The PRISMA group. Preferred Reporting Items for Systematic Reviews and Meta-Analyses: The PRISMA Statement. *Ann. Int. Med.* **2009**, *151*, 264–269.

18. Daniels, J.L.; Longnecker, M.P.; Rowland, A.S.; Golding, J. Fish intake during pregnancy and early cognitive development of offspring. *Epidemiology* **2004**, *15*, 394–402.

19. Oken, E.; Wright, R.O.; Kleinman, K.P.; Bellinger, D.; Amarasiriwardena, C.J.; Hu, H.; Rich-Edwards, J.W.; Gillman, M.W. Maternal fish consumption, hair mercury, and infant cognition in a U.S. cohort. *Environ. Health Perspect.* **2005**, *113*, 1376–1380.

20. Hibbeln, J.R.; Davis, J.M.; Steer, C.; Emmett, P.; Rogers, I.; Williams, C.; Golding, J. Maternal seafood consumption in pregnancy and neurodevelopmental outcomes in childhood (ALSPAC study): An observational cohort study. *Lancet* **2007**, *369*, 578–585.

21. Gale, C.R.; Robinson, S.M.; Godfrey, K.M.; Law, C.M.; Schlotz, W.; O'Callaghan, F.J. Oily fish intake during pregnancy—Association with lower hyperactivity but not with higher full-scale IQ in offspring. *J. Child. Psychol. Psychiatry Allied Discipl.* **2008**, *49*, 1061–1068.

22. Oken, E.; Osterdal, M.L.; Gillman, M.W.; Knudsen, V.K.; Halldorsson, T.I.; Strom, M.; Bellinger, D.C.; Hadders-Algra, M.; Michaelsen, K.F.; Olsen, S.F. Associations of maternal fish intake during pregnancy and breastfeeding duration with attainment of developmental milestones in early childhood: A study from the Danish National Birth Cohort. *Am. J. Clin. Nutr.* **2008**, *88*, 789–796.

23. Oken, E.; Radesky, J.S.; Wright, R.O.; Bellinger, D.C.; Amarasiriwardena, C.J.; Kleinman, K.P.; Hu, H.; Gillman, M.W. Maternal fish intake during pregnancy, blood mercury levels, and child cognition at age 3 years in a US cohort. *Am. J. Epidemiol.* **2008**, *167*, 1171–1181.

24. Mendez, M.A.; Torrent, M.; Julvez, J.; Ribas-Fit, N.; Kogevinas, M.; Sunyer, J. Maternal fish and other seafood intakes during pregnancy and child neurodevelopment at age 4 years. *Public Health Nutrition* **2009**, *12*, 1702–1710.

25. Suzuki, K.; Nakai, K.; Sugawara, T.; Nakamura, T.; Ohba, T.; Shimada, M.; Hosokawa, T.; Okamura, K.; Sakai, T.; Kurokawa, N.; Murata, K.; Satoh, C.; Satoh, H. Neurobehavioral effects of prenatal exposure to methylmercury and PCBs, and seafood intake: Neonatal behavioral assessment scale results of Tohoku study of child development. *Environ. Res.* **2010**, *110*, 699–704.

26. Freedman, L.S.; Schatzkin, A.; Midthune, D.; Kipnis, V. Dealing with dietary measurement error in nutritional cohort studies. *J. Natl. Cancer Inst.* **2011**, *103*, 1086–1092.

27. Marks, K.; Glascoe, F.P.; Aylward, G.P.; Shevell, M.I.; Lipkin, P.H.; Squires, J.K. The Thorny Nature of Predictive Validity Studies on Screening Tests for Developmental-Behavioral Problems. *Pediatrics* **2008**, *122*, 866–868.

28. Singer, L.T. Randomized clinical trials in infancy: Methodologic issues. *Semin. Neonatol.* **2001**, *6*, 393–401.

29. Dietrich, K.N.; Eskenazi, B.; Schantz, S.; Yolton, K.; Rauh, V.A.; Johnson, C.B.; Alkon, A.; Canfield, R.L.; Pessah, I.N.; Berman, R.F. Principles and practices of neurodevelopmental assessment in children: Lessons learned for the centers for children's environmental health and disease prevention research. *Environ. Health Perspect.* **2005**, *113*, 1437–1446.

30. Glascoe, F.P.; Byrne, K.E.; Ashford, L.G.; Johnson, K.L.; Chang, B.; Strickland, B. Accuracy of the Denver-II in Developmental Screening. *Pediatrics* **1992**, *89*, 1221–1225.

31. Emond, A.; Bell, J.C.; Heron, J.; The, A.S.T. Letter to the editor—Using parental questionnaires to identify developmental delay. *Dev. Med. Child. Neurol.* **2005**, *47*, 646–648.

32. Bloomingdale, A.; Guthrie, L.B.; Price, S.; Wright, R.O.; Platek, D.; Haines, J.; Oken, E. A qualitative study of fish consumption during pregnancy. *Am. J. Clin. Nutr.* **2010**, *92*, 1234–1240.

33. Dziechciarz, P.; Horvath, A.; Szajewska, H. Effects of *n*-3 Long-Chain Polyunsaturated Fatty Acid Supplementation during Pregnancy and/or Lactation on Neurodevelopment and Visual Function in Children: A Systematic Review of Randomized Controlled Trials. *J. Am. Coll. Nutr.* **2010**, *29*, 443–454.

34. Jacobs, D.R.; Tapsell, L.C. Food, not nutrients, is the fundamental unit in nutrition. *Nutr. Rev.* **2007**, *65*, 439–450.

35. Zhou, S.J.; Anderson, A.J.; Gibson, R.A.; Makrides, M. Effect of iodine supplementation in pregnancy on child development and other clinical outcomes: A systematic review of randomized controlled trials. *Am. J. Clin. Nutr.* **2013**, *98*, 1241–1254.

36. Strain, J.; Yeates, A.J.; van Wijngaarden, E.; Thurston, S.W.; Mulhern, M.S.; McSorley, E.M.; Watson, G.E.; Love, T.M.; Smith, T.H.; Yost, K.; *et al.* Prenatal exposure to methyl mercury from fish consumption and polyunsaturated fatty acids: associations with child development at 20 mo of age in an observational study in the Republic of Seychelles. *Am. J. Clin. Nutr.* **2015**, *101*, 530–537.

Micronutrients in Pregnancy in Low- and Middle-Income Countries

Ian Darnton-Hill and Uzonna C. Mkparu

Abstract: Pregnancy is one of the more important periods in life when increased micronutrients, and macronutrients are most needed by the body; both for the health and well-being of the mother and for the growing foetus and newborn child. This brief review aims to identify the micronutrients (vitamins and minerals) likely to be deficient in women of reproductive age in Low- and Middle-Income Countries (LMIC), especially during pregnancy, and the impact of such deficiencies. A global prevalence of some two billion people at risk of micronutrient deficiencies, and multiple micronutrient deficiencies of many pregnant women in LMIC underline the urgency to establishing the optimal recommendations, including for delivery. It has long been recognized that adequate iron is important for best reproductive outcomes, including gestational cognitive development. Similarly, iodine and calcium have been recognized for their roles in development of the foetus/neonate. Less clear effects of deficiencies of zinc, copper, magnesium and selenium have been reported. Folate sufficiency periconceptionally is recognized both by the practice of providing folic acid in antenatal iron/folic acid supplementation and by increasing numbers of countries fortifying flours with folic acid. Other vitamins likely to be important include vitamins B12, D and A with the water-soluble vitamins generally less likely to be a problem. Epigenetic influences and the likely influence of micronutrient deficiencies on foetal origins of adult chronic diseases are currently being clarified. Micronutrients may have other more subtle, unrecognized effects. The necessity for improved diets and health and sanitation are consistently recommended, although these are not always available to many of the world's pregnant women. Consequently, supplementation programmes, fortification of staples and condiments, and nutrition and health support need to be scaled-up, supported by social and cultural measures. Because of the life-long influences on reproductive outcomes, including inter-generational ones, both clinical and public health measures need to ensure adequate micronutrient intakes during pregnancy, but also during adolescence, the first few years of life, and during lactation. Many antenatal programmes are not currently achieving this. We aim to address the need for micronutrients during pregnancy, the importance of micronutrient deficiencies during gestation and before, and propose the scaling-up of clinical and public health approaches that achieve healthier pregnancies and improved pregnancy outcomes.

Reprinted from *Nutrients*. Cite as: Darnton-Hill, I.; Mkparu, U.C. Micronutrients in Pregnancy in Low- and Middle-Income Countries. *Nutrients* **2015**, *7*, 1744–1768.

1. Introduction

Optimal outcomes of pregnancy and their importance to the mother, the future child, families and societies, is contingent on appropriate care, adequate antenatal preparation and sufficient nutrition. The consequences of antenatal nutritional deficiencies can be devastating to the mother, child and effect future generations. As such, it is critical that expectant mothers enter pregnancy with the best possible macronutrient and micronutrient status and then receive adequate antenatal nutrition for their health, and for the well-being of their offspring. This short review examines micronutrient deficiencies in women in Low and Middle Income Countries, and programmatic responses.

Maternal nutrition has profound effects on foetal growth, development, and subsequent infant birthweight, and the health and well-being of the woman herself [1]. Maternal undernutrition, maternal mortality rates, infant mortality and morbidity rates have declined since the 1990s as a result of increasing attention to improving the quality of the antenatal period and improving obstetric care and social change. However, there is still a great need for further improvements. The nutritional status and size of the pregnant woman is the result of past health and nutrition, including her own birth size and subsequent health and societal influences.

Poor dietary patterns, and options, in the periconceptional period are known to lead to pre-term delivery, shorter birth-length and earlier gestation [1] and poor potential neurodevelopmental outcomes for the foetus [2]. Given the impact of poor maternal diet, both public health and clinical measures need to be in place, especially in low socio-economic environments. These need to address all stages of the women's life-cycle, and especially during the pregnancy. There is increased risk if that pregnancy occurs during adolescence, is spaced too closely to a preceding pregnancy, or is one of multiple pregnancies. Nutritional, dietary and health interventions need to be complemented by improved obstetric care and support, and exposure to "nutrition-sensitive" interventions such as access to education, improvement in women's status and improved agricultural and environmental determinants [3].

While the global burden of diseases caused by deficiencies of micronutrients during pregnancy is relatively modest globally, the cumulative individual impact can be considerable. This is especially so for adolescent pregnancies and women of lower economic or minority status in low and middle-income economic settings [4]. The aim of this short review is to describe micronutrient deficiencies and programmes in LMIC where the vast majority of micronutrient deficiencies occur, and appropriate public health and maternal antenatal care in such settings to address such deficiencies. Where relevant, research literature from more affluent countries is also used.

2. Micronutrient Deficiencies in Women of Reproductive Age

Globally, approximately two billion people, the majority women and young children, are affected, by micronutrient deficiencies, with even higher rates during pregnancy [5]. Concurrent deficiencies of more than one or two micronutrients are well documented among young pregnant women, (and young children), especially in LMIC [6–9]. Deficiencies in maternal micronutrient status are a result of: poor quality diets; high fertility rates; repeated pregnancies; short inter-pregnancy intervals; and, increased physiological needs. These factors are aggravated by often inadequate health systems with poor capacity, by poverty and inequities, and by socio-cultural factors such as early marriage and adolescent pregnancies, and some traditional dietary practices [3,4,10–12]. A systematic review identifying all studies that had been published between 1988 and 2008 reporting on micronutrient intakes in women living in such environments, showed that for women, the reported mean/median intakes in over 50% of the studies were below the Estimated Average Requirements (EAR) for micronutrient intakes, except for vitamin A, vitamin C, and niacin, where the reported intakes were around a third of the EAR, 29%, 34% and 34% respectively [11].

Pregnancy during adolescence is a relatively common event in much of the world [13] and the young women are usually incomplete in their own growth and often deficient in micronutrients [14,15]. Pregnancies at this time will make reproductive outcomes more likely to be negative as well as impacting on the health, nutrition and well-being of the adolescent. Studies of micronutrient status in adolescents, including when pregnant, have found poor micronutrient intakes and status [14], including in the UK [16], and increased risk of small-for-gestational-age (SGA) and low birthweight [LBW] infants at birth [10]. Adolescent pregnancy, besides negatively affecting the young mother's own growth and nutritional status [17], is associated with a 50% increased risk of stillbirths and neonatal deaths, and increased risk of preterm birth, low birthweight, and asphyxia [18]. A review assessing the association between inter-pregnancy intervals with maternal, newborn, and child health outcomes found that short inter-pregnancy intervals (<6 months) were also associated with a higher probability of maternal anaemia (32%) and stillbirths (40%) whereas longer intervals (>60 months) were associated with an increased risk of pre-eclampsia [19].

3. Micronutrients during Pregnancy

Information concerning vitamin and mineral metabolism and requirements during pregnancy are surprisingly imprecise, largely because of the complexity of maternal metabolism during pregnancy [4,20] and interactions between micronutrients. Overall nutrient requirements are increased during pregnancy due to the greater needs of the mother's own increase in body tissue reserves and metabolic demands, and the development of placenta and the foetus [21,22]. Requirements for many, but not all, micronutrients also increase during pregnancy [21]. However the increased requirements will depend on existing nutritional status, rate of weight gain and availability of adequate nutrition and co-existing disease. For micronutrients especially, adequacy can be difficult to assess due to plasma volume increases and often-poor biomarkers [23,24]. Nutrient-binding proteins that transport micronutrients also demonstrate decreased concentrations [21].

Iron and iron deficiency anaemia: iron deficiency anaemia (IDA) leading to a decrease in oxygen carrying capacity is one of the most common pregnancy-related complications [23,25]. The majority of the 1.62 billion people currently affected by anaemia are women or young children [25]. The global prevalence in pregnant women has fallen only slightly since 1995 from 43% to 38% [25]. The global prevalence of severe anaemia on the other hand, which poses the greatest risk for maternal mortality, has shown a greater relative reduction but still only from 2.0% to 0.9%, and overall the risk is far higher in women of LMIC [25]. About half of all anaemia is estimated to be attributable to iron deficiency, depending on the geographic and disease environment. Much of the other (approximately) half is caused by diseases such as malaria, HIV and parasites, and by deficiencies of other micronutrients such as vitamin A, folate and zinc [22], again according to the local environments.

The apparent increased risk of anaemia during pregnancy is confounded by the plasma volume expansion at about six weeks into pregnancy [23], although red blood cell mass does not increase proportionately to the expanding plasma volume. Plasma volume increases by about 48% while red cell mass only increases by about 18% [23]. Iron deficiency itself, even before manifest as anaemia, affects both mother and child [23] and in the mother includes cognitive impairment, decreased physical activity and reduced immunity, and possibly more subtle impairments. Where there is real iron deficiency, this decreases the mother's ability to synthesize hemoglobin and transport oxygen [26]. The foetus developing *in-utero* has no direct contact with the atmosphere and depends on the mother for oxygen, although foetal hemoglobin does also have a higher affinity for oxygen which helps to ensure that the developing foetus' oxygen requirements can be met [27].

Young children who are the offspring of anaemic mothers, or are anaemic themselves, usually have poor development. A recent overview reported on a relatively recent meta-analysis that established the strong causal link between maternal iron deficiency and adverse outcomes [28]. Amongst other things, iron deficiency is thought to affect the optimal development of the foetal brain [20] and in mice at least, gestational iron deficiency of the mother differentially alters the structure and function of white and grey matter brain regions of the offspring [29]. A recent study found that psychosocial stimulation benefitted development in non-anaemic children but not in anaemic, iron-deficient children [30]. This would suggest in addition to iron treatment, children with IDA may require more intense or longer interventions than for young children neither anaemic nor iron deficient. There have been studies now with many years of follow-up that have demonstrated direct positive association between maternal Hb levels during pregnancy and educational achievements of off-spring later in life. One, from Finland, has demonstrated improvements 31 years later [31]. The study authors suggest that that iron prophylaxis even at fairly late stages of pregnancy may be beneficial for the offspring [31]. However, while iron deficiency is to be avoided in pregnancy, iron supplements and increased iron stores in the third trimester have been linked to maternal complications such as gestational diabetes and increased oxidative stress and risk of preeclampsia [32]. The author notes that anaemia and iron deficiency anaemia are not synonymous, including among low income and minority women in their reproductive years [32].

Iodine: Unlike most essential dietary nutrients, iodine status is not linked so much to socio-economic development but more to geography [33]. Its critical significance during pregnancy is, rather than on maternal health directly, due to the devastating impact on the foetus of deficiency, including cretinism and impaired growth. Nevertheless, reproductive outcomes are affected with increased risk of stillbirths, abortions, and congenital abnormalities. Maternal urinary iodine has also been positively associated with birth weight, length and head circumference in male offspring in a recent study of a Bangladeshi population of pregnant women [2], as well as the well-recognized impact on offspring cognitive impairment as described below.

Calcium: Calcium supplementation is associated with a reduction in pre-eclampsia as well as LBW and pre-term birth [18]. Gestational hypertensive disorders are the second main causes of maternal morbidity and mortality, as well as being associated with an increased risk of pre-term birth and foetal growth restriction [34]. As calcium supplementation during pregnancy reduces the incidence of gestational hypertension by 35%, pre-eclampsia by 52%–55% and pre-term births by 24% [35], the World Health Organization (WHO) now recommends 1.5 g to 2.0 g of elemental calcium per day for pregnant women with low dietary calcium intakes.

Other minerals: Other trace element deficiencies that have been described as possibly associated with complications in pregnancy, childbirth or foetal development include copper, magnesium, selenium and zinc [22]. While a Cochrane review found that zinc supplementation in pregnancy may result in a 14% reduction in preterm birth [36], this decrease was not accompanied by a similar reduction in stillbirths, neonatal death, SGA, or low birthweight. The Lancet Series on Maternal and Young Child Undernutrition concluded there is insufficient evidence at this point for policy to be made on zinc supplementation during pregnancy [18].

Folate: folate deficiency leading to megaloblastic anemia is the second most common cause of anaemia during pregnancy [23]. Folate, a B-vitamin, has an important role in the synthesis and maintenance of DNA and therefore has an increased requirement throughout pregnancy supporting optimal growth and development of the foetus, as well as due to blood volume expansion and tissue growth of the mother [37]. Folate deficiency during pregnancy, especially around the time of conception, is strongly correlated with increased risk of neural tube defects such as spina bifida [38]. A recent study showed significant reductions in rates of both pre-eclampsia in mothers and SGA (small for gestational age) newborns with maternal folic acid supplementation (but no other associations between pregnancy and birth outcomes) [39].

Vitamin D: Vitamin D deficiency is estimated to affect one billion people globally and is increasingly recognized as being common amongst pregnant women [20]. Despite its important role in bone homeostasis, brain development and modulation of the immune system, the impact of antenatal vitamin D is still poorly understood [40], not least because of uncertainties with appropriate biomarkers and cut-off points. A systematic review suggested that women with circulating 25-hydroxyvitamin D (25(OH)D) concentrations <50 nmol/L in pregnancy have an increased risk of preeclampsia, gestational diabetes mellitus, preterm birth and SGA newborns [41]. A Cochrane review found a significant relationship between an increase in serum vitamin D concentrations at term and borderline reduction in low birthweight [42] but there is yet not enough evidence for policy as the number of high-quality trials is thought to be currently too small to draw conclusions on its usefulness and safety [18].

Other vitamins: Deficiencies of yet other vitamins such as vitamin B12 and perhaps vitamin A may be important but evidence is sparse or conflicting [22,43]. There was an earlier recommendation by the FAO (Food and Agricultural Organization)/WHO of a 40% increase in the vitamin B-12 dietary allowance to meet foetal demands and increased metabolic needs [21]. As pregnancy does not require additional vitamin E and it is common in most diets, additional vitamin E is unlikely to be required [21]. Observational or experimental data linking water-soluble vitamins to any risk of maternal mortality are apparently unavailable [21]; these vitamins, such as vitamin C, thiamin, niacin and riboflavin and others, do however appear to decline in serum or plasma levels, likely due to extra uptake by the foetus or haemodilution, or in the case of niacin also increased urinary excretion [21]. Most return to normal within a week of delivery [21]. Possible side-effects of overdosage of vitamin E and vitamin C in pregnancy are discussed below (Section 7.2).

4. Interactions among Micronutrients

Interactions between micronutrient-dependent physiological and biological actions can be both positive, e.g., zinc and vitamin A, and negative, as e.g., with zinc or copper and iron [43]. Addition of zinc to iron and folic acid supplements have been shown to attenuate or even negate the positive association with outcomes due to iron, probably related to the inhibitory role of zinc in iron absorption [44]. Maintaining a balance between antioxidants such as selenium, and pro-oxidants (such as iron can be) has also been described as desirable, beyond the need to meet recommended intakes [20].

Because pregnant women in resource-poor areas are at risk of multiple micronutrient deficiencies [43], both the effects of single micronutrient deficiencies, and multiple ones, as well as interactions among them, all need to be considered. As described above, micronutrient deficiencies during pregnancy are associated with adverse pregnancy outcomes, especially in women of lower socioeconomic status who tend to have more than one deficiency, and those of young age who are at risk of being undernourished and underweight [11,18]. When important clinically, such micronutrient/micronutrient interactions complicate public health recommendations and interventions, as some will be synergistic and some will be antagonistic [20,22]. Framing specific recommendations can be further complicated by human variability in uptake and utilization of micronutrients, and genomics and epigenetic changes due to early deficiencies during gestation. One recent meta-analysis e.g., strongly suggested the *MTHFD1* G1958A polymorphism appears to be associated with increased maternal risk for NTDs (neural tube defects) in Caucasian populations [45]. Neural tube defects present as a wide range of phenotypes and the aetiology is multifactorial "with a large number of unclear genetic components, environmental conditions, and their interactions playing critical roles" [45]. This seems likely possible also for other micronutrients important in pregnancy outcomes. Multi-micronutrient supplementation is discussed below.

5. Offspring of Micronutrient-Deficient Mothers

Although pregnancy is the focus of this review, the effects of micronutrient deficiencies on their offspring also need to be addressed as part of the mother-child dyad. Perhaps the most noteworthy natural experiment demonstrating this necessity came about as a result of the Dutch famine of 1944 which provided a unique opportunity to study the long term consequences of maternal nutritional status and health outcomes in offspring [46,47]. Before the famine ended in 1945, rations were as low as 500 Kcal per person [47]. Expectant mothers who were subjected to the famine became severely macro- and micronutrient deficient. The famine was directly observed to affect fertility, infant birth weight, maternal weight gain, and the development of the neonate's central nervous system [47].

Assessing the impact of antenatal micronutrient status of pregnant women (especially when improved by supplementation) on the outcomes for their offspring is a challenge due to the need to follow the women through pregnancy and then the offspring, often in less than ideal settings for such research. In an important study from Nepal, intellectual functioning, including working memory, inhibitory control, and fine motor functioning among offspring at 7 to 9 years of age were positively associated with prenatal iron/folic acid supplementation in an area of high iron deficiency [8]. Related and similar findings of positive impact on the child of maternal antenatal supplementation have been found in Bangladesh [48], China [49] and in HIV-infected mothers in Tanzania [50]. A study from rural Viet Nam found that low maternal 25-hydroxyvitamin D levels in late pregnancy were associated with reduced language developmental outcomes at six months of age [40]. Maternal antenatal zinc supplementation may have beneficial long-term consequences for neural development associated with autonomic regulation of cardiovascular function in children at 54 months whose zinc-deficient pregnant mothers had received supplementation [51]. Even in areas of mild-to-moderate iodine deficiency, subtle reductions in the intelligent quotient of children in those areas may be reduced on average by 8–13.5 IQ points but can be corrected in populations by salt iodization [33]. On the other hand, there is increasing evidence of a positive impact of multiple micronutrient supplementation to deficient mothers on the growth and development of their offspring, although mechanisms are still unclear and findings inconsistent. This is probably because of different formulations and dosages of the supplements, rather than lack of effect.

6. Gestational Micronutrient Deficiencies and Later Risk of Chronic Disease

It has been noted that whereas micronutrient deficiencies are known to be associated with various shorter-term adverse outcomes of pregnancy, their effects on long-term health and later chronic disease of the children of such pregnancies are largely unknown. It is now generally accepted that early life nutritional exposures, combined with changes in lifestyle in adult life, can result in an increased risk of chronic diseases [52,53]. The excellent review by Christian and Stewart [52] that considered various strands of evidence, including animal studies, concludes that there are also strong suggestive links between intrauterine micronutrient status and the potential risk of chronic diseases but the underlying mechanisms are largely unclear. However, it is known that micronutrient status in foetal and early life can alter metabolism, vasculature, and organ growth and function, and so is likely to have consequences for increased risk of cardiometabolic disorders, adiposity, altered kidney function, and ultimately type 2 diabetes and cardiovascular diseases [52]. Epigenetic influences, as mentioned previously, heritable long-term changes in gene expression which are not caused by changes in gene sequence [54], may also play a significant role in long-term pregnancy outcomes. Christian and Stewart [52] have suggested a conceptual framework for how maternal diet and micronutrient status may effect the development of chronic disease; the most likely, given present knowledge, seem to be vitamin A, folate, iron and zinc and perhaps calcium and magnesium as shown in their conceptual framework (Figure 1).

Maternal micronutrient deficiency

Hormonal adaptations
Fe, Zn, Ca
- Increased stress hormones
- Decreased somatotrophic hormones (IGF, insulin)

Epigenetic gene regulation
Folate, vitamin B-12

Restricted fetal growth and development

Renal function
Fe, Zn, vitamin A, folate
- Impaired nephrogenesis / Reduced nephron endowment
- Reduced GFR
- Increased sodium sensitivity

Cardiovascular function
Fe, Zn, vitamin A, folate
- Impaired vascularization
- Malformations
- Cardiac hypertrophy

Pancreas / β-cell function
Fe, Zn, folate, vitamin B-12
- Reduction in number and area of β-cells

Body composition
Mg, Zn, Fe, Ca, folate, vitamin B-12
- Reduced lean body mass
- Altered fat deposition or metabolism
- Sedentary behavior
- Altered appetite regulation

Pulmonary function
Vitamin A, vitamin D
- Reduced bronchial branching & alveoli
- Reduced elastin
- Reduced VEGF
- Chronic respiratory infections
- Reduced lung capacity

Hypertension

Insulin resistance and β-cell dysfunction

Cardiometabolic risk

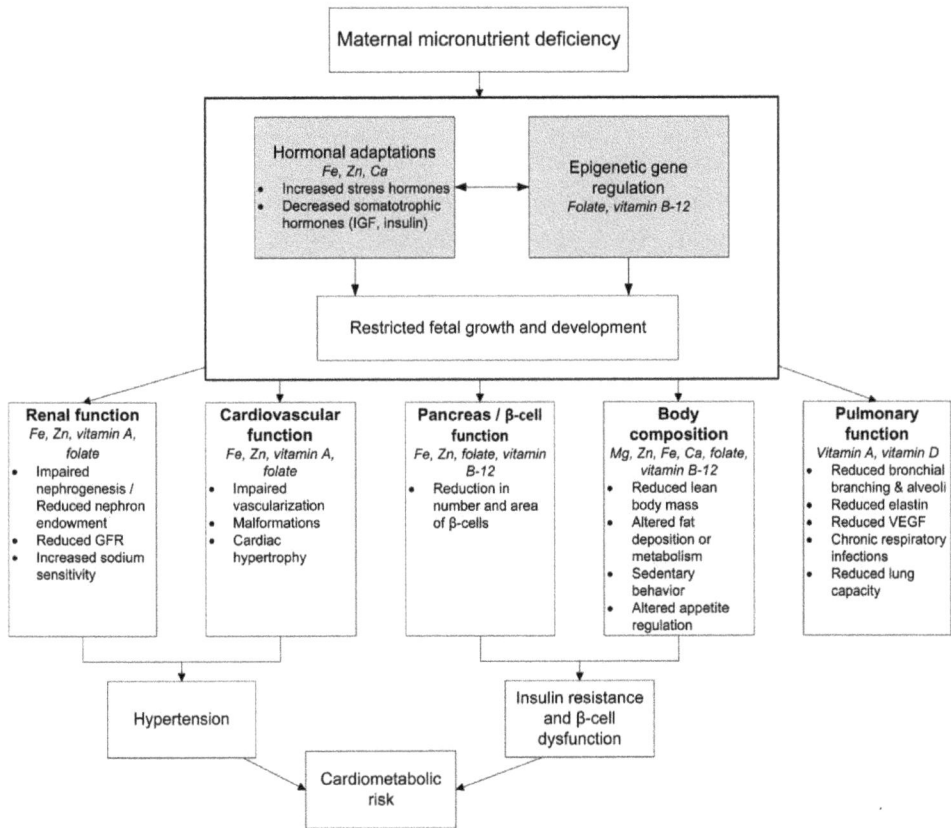

Figure 1. Conceptual framework by Christian and Stewart [52] for how maternal diet and micronutrient status may affect the development of chronic disease in the offspring. Gray boxes represent hypothesized pathways through which various micronutrient deficiencies may influence the growth, development, or function of the indicated systems.

Numerous studies have found significantly higher morbidity and mortality rates amongst individuals who were exposed to the nutritional shortages during gestational developmental periods, compared to unexposed individuals as e.g., in the above-mentioned Dutch famine [46,55,56]. Exposure during early gestation was associated with increased glucose intolerance, increased prevalence of coronary heart disease, elevated atherogenic lipid profile, increased risk of obesity, increased risk of schizophrenia, and disturbances in blood coagulation [47,55,56]. Some of these morbidities were found to transcend generations, with higher rates of obesity and associated co-morbidities observed in second-generation offspring of males who were exposed to the famine prenatally [57,58]. It is known that nutritional deficiencies during pregnancy may result in epigenetic modifications to the human genome, resulting in changes to gene expression, without alterations to gene sequence. In the review by Christian and Stewart [52], of how deficient maternal micronutrient status might influence the development of chronic disease in the children, they suggest that micronutrient status might influence regulatory pathways, such as hormonal adaptations and epigenetic gene regulation that can influence restricted growth and development in the developing foetus (Figure 1). In population-based prospective cohort studies, maternal hyper-homocysteinaemia (a biomarker of folate deficiency) was, for example, also linked to a higher risk of adiposity and type 2 diabetes in mothers and their offspring, both of which have future negative outcomes, and in the shorter term, lead to negative birth outcomes [39].

An emerging trend, in terms of noncommunicable diseases, is that of increasing numbers of overweight and obese mothers such as is now happening in LMIC, often at the same time, as their underweight children—the so-called "double burden of malnutrition". This is important because of increasing evidence e.g., from the Danish National Birth Cohort studies, that obese women have a higher risk of micronutrient deficiencies [59], and so micronutrient deficiencies associated with pregnancy in overweight/obese women are becoming increasingly an issue in both affluent and lower- and middle-income countries. High-dose supplementation with vitamin C and vitamin E has been found to not prevent preeclampsia but to increase the rate of babies born with low birthweight [59]. A later systematic review confirmed the lack of effect on preeclampsia and also found an increased risk of developing gestational hypertension and premature rupture of membranes, with a decreased risk of *abruptio placentae* [60,61]. There does not appear to be evidence to recommend supplementation with vitamins C and E.

7. Addressing the Problem

Short-term clinical interventions for micronutrient deficiencies may be critical for the immediate pregnancy and should obviously be addressed on presentation. Particularly in countries with under-resourced Health Systems, concurrent antenatal preventive measures also need to be in place and must be strengthened and scaled-up for optimizing maternal, neonatal and young child outcomes. The extended roles of other opportunities throughout the life course such as the adolescent young woman [28] are being increasingly recognized as further opportunities. The distinction will be made here between clinical interventions, those occurring during the pregnancy and delivery such as antenatal supplementation e.g., with iron and folic acid and obstetric care, and those occurring before the pregnancy and periconceptionally, such as preventive weekly iron and folic acid supplementation [62] which are seen as more public health and nutrition interventions.

7.1. Clinical

There have been significant strides in addressing perinatal nutritional issues, especially at the public health level. Consequently, the risk of nutritional insufficiency in pregnant women in most middle and high-income populations has been drastically reduced but remains a real risk in many LMIC women. Clinical care is used here in the sense of care before pregnancy, during the actual pregnancy, and during delivery and the neonatal phase. For convenience, "antenatal" refers to the pregnant women's care, whereas "perinatal" is larger including the periconceptional time and even before, as well as including immediately after birth. In terms of micronutrients, these clinical interventions include oral tablet supplementation, improved diets and nutrition education, food supplementation, monitoring of anaemia levels where facilities permit, management of weight gain, and encouragement to plan for breastfeeding, and related activities such as delayed cord clamping to improve neonatal iron stores.

7.1.1. Supplementation with Micronutrient Tablets

The Recommended Dietary Allowance RDA of iron increases by about 50% during pregnancy (from 18 mg to 27 mg). Due to the fact that the median dietary intake of iron in pregnant women is considerably lower than the Estimated Dietary Requirement (EAR) for iron, even in an affluent country like the USA, and often lower still in LMIC, it is recommended that pregnant women take iron supplements [63,64]. Antenatal iron and folic acid supplementation is a well-established intervention but the coverage and impact has been poor despite clear WHO recommendations for both anaemic and non-anaemic pregnant women and by national bodies [63–65]. Some other countries, especially more affluent ones, often have their own policies [64,65] including not recommending iron and folic acid at all in non-anaemic pregnant women. However, many women in such countries are anyway receiving a multiple micronutrient supplement [65], and there is a good body of research suggesting this should be recommended for pregnant women in LMICs [10,18,66] and there is growing support for the potential replacement of iron-folic acid supplements in pregnancy with multiple micronutrient supplements in populations at risk [18]. All bodies, multilateral or national, recommend supplementation to be complemented by healthy antenatal diets.

The reasons for the generally poor coverage of the existing recommended iron/folic acid tablets have been extensively reviewed [3]. They include: poor antenatal attendance especially in the first two trimesters; the effects of lower status of women; the taste and side effects of iron-containing tablets (especially lower quality ones); logistical issues; lack of conviction of positive impact by health workers; fear of larger babies where there is inadequate obstetric care; and so on [3]. Nevertheless, where coverage is good, the results are impressive and can be expected to have an impact on the mother's health, reducing anaemia and improving birth outcomes, and a likely impact on infant and young child outcomes, as noted above. A study in rural western China found that antenatal supplementation with iron-folic acid was associated with longer gestation and a reduction in early neonatal mortality compared with only folic acid, whereas multiple micronutrient supplements were associated with a modest increased birth weight compared with folic acid [67]. Despite the weight gain, there was no significant reduction in early neonatal mortality [67]. In 2012, the World Health Assembly endorsed nutrition targets for 2025 that included a 50% reduction in the number of women of reproductive age affected by anaemia compared with 2011 [25].

There is accumulating evidence that folic acid by supplementation has an additional protective effect against adverse pregnancy outcomes, as well as the now well-established reduction in neural tube defects (NTD) [18]. Studies have suggested improved neurodevelopmental outcomes in children of mothers with higher blood folate concentrations or mothers receiving antenatal folic acid supplements [37]. The RDA increases by 50% during pregnancy, from 400 µg/day to 600 µg/day [20]. This is hard to accomplish without consumption of folic acid-fortified foods or folic acid supplements. For this reason, periconceptional supplementation of 400 µg/day of folic acid is recommended internationally for women of childbearing age in order to minimize neural tube defects [20]. Except in some settings, coverage has not usually been impressive, especially to those of poor socio-economic status and adolescents who are amongst those most at risk of unplanned pregnancies. For example, the CDC reports that about 50% of U.S. pregnancies are unintended and most women are not aware that they are pregnant until they are about two months into the pregnancy. However, the neural tube closes between 23–27 days after conception [20], and so this is already too late. An alternative approach that has been considered is to recommend folic acid supplements for all women who are of child-bearing age. However, long term folic acid supplementation on the off chance that an unplanned conception occurs has significant implementation and cost implications. Where pregnancies are generally carefully planned, as was the case in one experience in China, folic acid supplementation has been successful. However, the public health food-based population approach of fortification is now the accepted intervention in most countries, and where instituted, has shown a dramatic reduction in the incidence of NTDs [38].

There are also several other clinical considerations to be made when supplementing with folic acid. For example, folate may mask symptoms of megaloblastic anemia, which could be an indicator of vitamin B-12 deficiency [68]. Indicators of low vitamin B-12 are associated with adverse pregnancy outcomes, anaemia, low birthweight, and intrauterine retardation [9]. By the possible masking of vitamin B-12 deficiency, folic acid could make it difficult to detect and remedy B-12 deficiency, but the evidence for this happening with fortification of cereal staples is mixed. Oral supplementation of urban Indian women with vitamin B-12 throughout pregnancy and early lactation significantly increased vitamin B-12 status of both mothers and infants [9] and so worth considering where vitamin B12 intakes are marginal. There are also concerns from observational data of possible increases in rates of some cancers with higher levels of folic acid in the diet due to the relatively high levels used in fortification [20].

As noted, WHO now recommends calcium supplementation to reduce the risk of hypertensive diseases in pregnancy. However calcium requires large and frequent tablets, as well as the 60 mg of iron and 400 µg of folic acid and where the iron and calcium may negatively react intra-intestinally [34]. Recently a novel micronutrient powder containing micro-encapsulated pH-sensitive calcium in addition to iron and folic acid has been designed to facilitate early intestinal release of the iron and delayed calcium release [34].

In affluent countries, where supplementation with antenatal multimicronutrient supplements is relatively common and often recommended [65], use of targeted antenatal micronutrients probably has the potential to decrease infant morbidity and mortality in anaemic and deficient women, especially low-income urban women [69]. In a Canadian study, self-reported vitamin supplementation was associated with decreased odds of miscarriage although other associated positive health-related behaviours also likely contributed [70]. On the other hand, an earlier systematic review found that taking vitamin supplements prior to pregnancy or in early pregnancy, did not prevent miscarriage or stillbirth but the mothers appeared to be less likely to develop pre-eclampsia (but were more likely to have a multiple pregnancy) [71]. The evidence is not yet entirely clear, as iron and folic acid supplements in Indonesian women significantly reduced the risk of early neonatal death [72]. Similarly a double-blind cluster-randomized trial, also in Indonesia, found that maternal multiple micronutrient supplementation, as compared with iron/folic acid, reduced early infant mortality, especially in undernourished and anaemic women [73]. The size of the pregnant women appears to modify the effect and well-nourished women may be less appropriate for supplementation where there is inadequate clinical support.

Supplementation with multiple micronutrient formulations has a certain logic to it given the multiple micronutrient deficiencies that frequently occur together and the interactions between micronutrient-dependent physiological and biological actions [43]. Current evidence has been described as suggesting that vitamins and minerals have added bio-functionality which may be particularly important in pregnancy with synergisms e.g., between folic acid and vitamin B12, possibly enhancing their biological potential—in this case to further reduce the occurrence of NTDs [20].

An independent systematic review and meta-analysis of 12 randomized, controlled trials comparing multiple micronutrient supplementation with iron-folic acid supplementation found that both supplements were equally effective in reducing anaemia (even though iron content was often lower in the multimicronutrient supplement) and resulted in a small, significant increase in mean birthweight; larger micronutrient doses appeared to have a greater impact [10]. The findings of other intervention trials, especially effectiveness trials, have been variable, although efficacy is largely accepted. Many factors affect the impact, such as baseline iron and/or anaemia levels, diet, the disease environment and importantly it seems the size of the pregnant woman. A recent study in Chinese women e.g., showed that compared with controls taking folic acid, prenatal iron/folic acid or multiple micronutrient supplements improved iron status later in pregnancy but did not affect perinatal anaemia in women with no or mild anaemia [74].

Nevertheless, "despite encouraging high compliance to community-based supplementation, a proportion of mothers remain anaemic, suggesting a need to also address parasitic and other infections and malaria" [10,13]. It is also worth noting that meaningful improvements with antenatal multiple micronutrients in height and cognitive development in children by two years of age have been observed, although these findings have been less consistent. Nevertheless, following these findings, it was concluded that replacing iron-folic acid supplements with multiple micronutrients in the package of health care, including improved obstetric care of health and nutrition interventions, would improve the impact of supplementation on birthweight, small-for-gestational age neonates, and perhaps child growth and development [10]. Despite some initial concern in some settings of (non-significant) risk of increased neonatal mortality [75] (not found in other reviews e.g., Haider *et al.* [66]), the conclusion immediately above was later endorsed by the Lancet Series (2013) following further evidence supporting the approach [18]. Trials are underway in a number of countries at present. Supplementation with multivitamins (vitamin B complex, vitamin C and vitamin E) also significantly decreases the risk of adverse pregnancy outcomes among HIV-infected women [76].

A consensus appears to be emerging on the usefulness of antenatal supplementation with multimicronutrients, especially for improvements in birthweights [10,18], at least in LMIC. Replacement of iron-folic acid with multiple micronutrient supplements in pregnancy, as a public health recommendation in at-risk populations, seems warranted, although further evidence from effectiveness assessments might be needed to guide a universal policy change [18]. However, delivery platforms for micronutrient antenatal care are a constraint in many settings e.g., a recent study in PNG showed how socio-cultural, health care staff attitudes and economic factors all affect antenatal care attendance and that only a third of women receive any antenatal care during pregnancy [77]. Clearly, however effective micronutrient interventions are for pregnant women, other factors, including logistics need to be addressed in many settings.

7.1.2. Food Supplementation

Food supplementation, especially in emergency and resource-poor settings is increasingly evidence-based. Emergency rations and supplies in particular have invested considerable resources in ensuring that the micronutrient content of such supplements are adequate while recognizing that in undernourished pregnant mothers it is the low energy (caloric) content of the available diets that is the main risk. The MINIMat randomized trial in Bangladesh tested the hypothesis that antenatal multiple micronutrient supplementation and an early invitation to food supplementation would improve birth outcomes [78]. They found that among these pregnant women from poor communities, supplementation with multiple micronutrients, as well as just iron and folic acid, combined with food supplementation, resulted in decreased childhood mortality. A recent review concluded that a dietary pattern containing several protein-rich food sources, fruit, and some whole grains is associated with a reduced risk of preterm delivery [1]. A platform used with limited experience (in pregnant women) has been the use of multimicronutrient powders (added to food) during the antenatal period, or more recently lipid-based supplements that supply both dietary energy, protein and micronutrients [79]. Studies show that use of micronutrient fortified supplementary foods, especially those containing milk and/or essential fatty acids during pregnancy, increase mean birthweight by around 60–73 g [80]. Fortified food supplements containing milk and essential fatty acids, along with micronutrients, offer benefits for improving maternal status and pregnancy outcome [80]. Fortified beverages containing only multiple micronutrients have been shown to reduce micronutrient deficiencies such as anaemia and iron deficiency. Food supplementation, while clearly effective in undernourished mothers will not be discussed further here, as it is mainly an intervention to increase dietary energy and the micronutrients needed to accompany it are largely known. Other antenatal *clinical* advice and monitoring, while clearly essential to the mother's health and reproductive outcomes, are also not discussed here but recognized as part of the larger care of the mother, of which adequate micronutrient status is but one part.

7.2. Public Health Measures

Public health and nutrition measures aim to improve pregnancy outcomes in general, especially for those women with limited access to good antenatal clinical care, and to reduce the risk of periconceptional micronutrient deficiencies, among other ancillary benefits. The most commonly used approaches, in terms of micronutrients includes: blanket supplementation, and sometimes targeted supplementation, policies and programmes; fortification; and, general measures to improve diets and micronutrient intakes and general health.

7.2.1. Supplementation

Public health supplementation includes blanket approaches e.g., all women of reproductive age, especially adolescents, receiving weekly iron and folic acid supplements [62]. The use of weekly iron and folic acid supplements through schools or factories has proven efficacy and is recommended by the WHO [62]. As a preventive measure it has not been taken up by governments and requires more implementation experience in national programmes, despite already promising experiences in some countries such as the Philippines and Vietnam. Targeted, preconceptional supplementation such as folic acid supplements for young women intending to get pregnant has had limited use and success, not least because the majority of pregnancies are not planned, as discussed above. Targeted iron/folic acid supplementation to pregnant women has a long history and continues to be recommended nationally and by the WHO but has been relatively unsuccessful due to poor covergae, especially in LMIC, as also discussed above.

Oral iodized oil has also been used for this purpose but as a public health measure has been supplanted by iodized salt programmes. Where coverage by iodized salt is sub-optimal, WHO recommends that pregnant (and lactating) women should be given an oral supplement of iodized oil [81]. Although 38 million newborns are born iodine-deficient in LMIC, affluent countries are also increasingly at risk unless supplementary measures e.g., iodine fortification of bread or supplementation of pregnant women are undertaken. Even in affluent countries such as the UK and Australia, poor iodine intake in pregnancy predicts lower child IQ [82] and in a small recent study in South Eastern Australia, less than half (46%) of pregnant women were following national recommendations and only 18.5% believed they needed a supplement and only a third (34.5%) had been given adequate advice by their medical practitioner [83]. In the USA, iodine supplements are used by only 22% of pregnant women [82]. Such findings explain the continued global emphasis on salt fortification with iodine [84], despite the challenges of other recommendations for populations to reduce their salt intake to reduce the prevalence of hypertension.

7.2.2. Nutrition Education, Dietary Improvement and Improved Public Health Measures

Other interventions that impact on the micronutrient status during pregnancy include dietary measures and other public health and social interventions such as deworming, education and horticultural activities. While the risk of being born low birthweight is significantly greater with moderate preconception anaemia [85], it has also been noted that in many unsafe settings, mothers purposefully "eat-down" aiming to have a smaller neonate. A failure of nutrition education has also been implicated in poor diets as well as some dietary taboos [21] and soil-transmitted helminthes [86]. Nevertheless, where access and availability to foods is possible, improving diets by including such items as eggs and animal-source foods are likely to provide protein, energy and micronutrients. However, such foods are not often available to the very poor, or there are cultural constraints, which is why food supplements to such pregnant women is now a recommendation [3,18].

International guidelines recommend routine safe and protective prevention and treatments, during pregnancy, to reduce hookworm, malaria and other infections such as schistosomiasis [87]. Despite the effectiveness of such programmes, and because women with high levels of hookworm or malaria infections are at high risk of anaemia [86], there continues to be a need for more general scaling-up of coverage in affected populations. A recent randomized trial (that included pregnant women with anaemia and iron deficiency at baseline) in a malaria endemic area found major gains in birthweight, without apparent effect on *Plasmodium* infection and urged that universal coverage of iron supplementation (60 mg per day) should be scaled-up, preferably with cover by IPT (intermittent preventive treatment of malaria) [88]. A systematic review and meta-analysis recently concluded that more evidence is needed to the long-standing, and often contentious, role of giving iron in malaria-endemic populations and so concluded that currently it is prudent to provide iron in combination with malaria prevention during pregnancy [89]. There is increasing consensus in this view, along with the need for concomitant improved obstetric care and diet.

Attention to adolescent girls as an important preventive strategy is increasingly recognized, despite some strong cultural and social constraints. It has been observed that, even in affluent settings, adolescents are more likely than adults to consume energy-dense, micronutrient-poor diets and to have adverse pregnancy outcome such as increased risk of SGA [16]. The risk is likely to be even greater in food-insecure populations such as in Central Africa [90]. Other non-direct micronutrient interventions that could be expected to have a positive impact on nutrition and health of pregnant women (at least where most births are within a marital relationship), include interventions to increase the age at marriage and first pregnancy are important, and can reduce repeat adolescent pregnancies by 37% [18]. The African Union has recently launched a new campaign to end child marriage in Africa [91] which, if successful would be expected to have positive reproductive outcomes.

Table 1, derived from Bhutta *et al.* [18], shows micronutrient interventions that have an adequate evidence base to be recommended for women of reproductive age and during pregnancy (as well as maternal supplementation with balanced energy and protein including through supplementation).

7.2.3. Fortification

Fortification can be considered a dietary intervention and one that has recently been recommended by the Lancet Maternal and Young Child Undernutrition series and has been in practice for over sixty years in many affluent countries [18]. Bhutta *et al.* [18] concluded that "fortification has the greatest potential to improve the nutritional status of a population when implemented within a comprehensive nutrition strategy, including for pregnant women and has the advantage of reaching women before pregnancy". Iodized salt programs are now implemented in many countries worldwide, and the past two decades have shown considerable progress, so that globally, 76% of households are now adequately consuming iodized salt. On the other hand, nearly 30% of school-aged children are estimated to have insufficient iodine intakes and global progress appears to be slowing [84]. The need for continual global scaling-up and consolidation of existing programmes has already been commented upon. There have also been efficacy, and limited effectiveness studies of doubly fortified salt with iodine and encapsulated iron.

The provision of balanced energy protein supplementary foods to underweight pregnant women was also considered to have enough evidence of reduction in SGA and stillbirths and improved birthweights for widespread implementation, whereas maternal vitamin D and zinc supplementation, while promising, were considered to have insufficient evidence [18].

Fortification of cereal flours with iron and often other micronutrients such as some B group vitamins, and more recently zinc and even selenium, has been in existence e.g., in the USA, for over 60 years, and now 80 countries globally have legislation to mandate fortification of at least one industrially milled cereal grain (79 countries have legislation to fortify wheat flour; 12 countries to fortify maize products; and five countries to fortify rice) [38]. Costa Rica is the only country that mandates fortification of all three grains, and Papua New Guinea is the only country that requires only rice fortification. Currently the 79 countries that mandate required fortification of wheat flour produced in industrial mills require at least iron and folic acid, except Australia, which does not include iron, and Congo, the Philippines, Venezuela, and the United Kingdom, which do not include folic acid. Additionally, seven countries fortify at least half their industrially milled wheat flour through voluntary efforts and it has been estimated that about a third (31%) of the world's industrially milled wheat flour is now fortified with at least iron or folic acid through these mandatory and voluntary efforts [38]. Other success stories include the fortification of sugar with vitamin A in Central America. A continuing challenge is that populations most at risk of deficiency either cannot afford fortified foods or, especially in lower-income countries, they are not available to them. Nevertheless, fortification is likely to be an increasingly major part of the reduction of micronutrient deficiencies, including during pregnancy.

Table 1. Nutrition/micronutrient interventions for women of reproductive age and during pregnancy (based on Bhutta *et al.* in the Lancet series of 2013 which has estimates of size of the significant effects and the evidence from which they come [18]).

Intervention	Setting	Comments (Only Significant Findings and Original Systematic Review References)
Folic acid supplementation		
WRA *	LMIC ** and affluent countries	[92]
Pregnant women	Mostly more developled countries	[93]
Iron and iron-folic acid supplementation		
WRA	Both LMIC and affluent countries. Interventions mainly given in school settings to adolescents and evidence mostly from effectiveness studies	Intermittent iron supplementation (once or twice a week)—reduces anaemia rates [94]
Pregnant women	Both LMIC and affluent countries. Intervention	Reduction in LBW ***, reduction in anaemia rates at term and improved Hb [95]
Multiple micronutrients (MMN) supplementation		
Pregnant women	LMIC and affluent countries. Studies compared MMN with two or fewer micronutrients	Reduction in LBW and currently insignificant data for neurodevelopmental outcomes in offspring [96]
Calcium supplementation		
Pregnant women	LMIC and affluent countries. Mostly effectiveness trials	Reduction in pre-eclampsia as well as LBW and pre-term birth [97]
Iodine through salt iodization programmes		
Pregnant women	Mostly LMIC. Mostly effectiveness trials.	Cretinism at 4y reduced, improved birthweight, developmental scores higher in young children [98]

* WRA = women of reproductive age; ** LMIC = Low- and Middle-Income Countries; *** LBW = Low birth weight.

8. Conclusions

The deficiencies in micronutrients that affect many women of reproductive age are now known to be associated with adverse maternal and perinatal outcomes. These adverse outcomes can have longer-term impacts into adulthood [18,99,100]. Personal, social and economic costs are high [3]. Maternal undernutrition has been described as one of the most neglected aspects of nutrition in public health globally [99,100]. Consequently, low-cost public health interventions that might help to ameliorate the impact of poor nutrition and diets, high disease burdens and the socio-cultural factors contributing to the high levels of these micronutrient deficiency problems during pregnancy, and before, continue to need scaling-up in scope and coverage [101].

Important factors besides inadequate diet and diseases that are indirectly related to maternal, foetal, and neonatal nutritional status and pregnancy outcomes include young age at first pregnancy and repeated pregnancies. Young girls who are not physically mature enter pregnancy with depleted nutrition reserves and often anaemia [102] and other micronutrient deficiencies [3,43]. While micronutrient deficiencies can undoubtedly have profound influences on the health of the mother and her child, there remain considerable areas of uncertainty and controversy that has made the development of robust public health recommendations a challenge [20]. Along with the noted challenges to get compliance, especially periconceptionally and in settings with limited health care capacity, and questions of how optimal micronutrient formulations and dosages are established, Berti *et al.* [20] have called for "adequately powered, randomized controlled trials with long periods of follow-up" to "establish causality and the best formulation, dose, duration and period of supplementation during pregnancy". However, the methodological issues in doing this would be considerable, especially in establishing causality. Consequently, factors that are known to be important, such as entering a pregnancy adequately nourished, being aged beyond adolescence, and good health and obstetric care, and nutrition education and support, should be scaled-up actively in the meantime.

If proven to be effective and safe in national health care systems, supplementation with multimicronutrients, at least in pregnancy, could complement preventive supplementation with weekly iron and folic acid in vulnerable populations. This could help break the intergenerational reality of low birthweight infants growing up disadvantaged and stunted and so at high-risk of repeating the same cycle. Whereas there has been a lot, if insufficient, attention paid to iron deficiency anaemia in pregnant women, most of the other involved micronutrients, are less well characterized [20,43]. Micronutrients likely to be important for maternal, infant and child outcomes include iron, iodine, folate, vitamin B12, vitamin D, calcium, and selenium, probably zinc and maybe others, along with appropriate dietary energy intakes. In addition to programmes to reduce micronutrient deficiencies such as micronutrient supplementation and food fortification, needed complementary interventions should optimally improve overall maternal nutrition, address household food insecurity, reduce the burden of maternal infections such as HIV and malaria, improve sanitation, and actively address gender and social disadvantage.

Author Contributions: Ian Darnton-Hill developed the concept and then both authors, Ian Darnton-Hill and Uzonna Mkparu wrote the text, including reworking the manuscript according to reviewer feedback and both doing final review and editing.

Conflicts of Interest: The authors declare no conflict of interest.

References

1. Grieger, J.A.; Grzeskowiak, L.E.; Clifton, V.L. Preconception dietary patterns in human pregnancies are associated with preterm delivery. *J. Nutr.* **2014**, *144*, 75–80.
2. Rydbeck, F.; Rahman, A.; Grander, M.; Ekström, E.C.; Vahter, M.; Kippler, M. Maternal urinary iodine concentration up to 1.0 mg/L is positively associated with birth weight, length, and head circumference of male offspring. *J. Nutr.* **2014**, *144*, 1438–1444.
3. Darnton-Hill, I.; Webb, P.; Harvey, P.W.J.; Hunt, J.M.; Dalmiya, N.; Chopra, M.; Ball, M.J.; Bloem, M.W.; de Benoist, B. Micronutrient deficiencies and gender: Social and economic costs. *Am. J. Clin. Nutr.* **2005**, *819*, 1198S–1205S.
4. Darnton-Hill, I. Global burden and significance of multiple micronutrient deficiencies in pregnancy. In *Meeting Micronutrient Requirements for Health and Development*; Nestlé Nutrition Institute Workshop Series; Bhutta, Z.A., Hurrell, R.F., Rosenberg, I.H., Eds.; Karger: Basel, Switzerland, 2012; Volume 70, pp. 49–60.
5. IFPRI. Actions and accountability to accelerate the World's progress on Nutrition. In *Global Nutrition Report 2014*; International Food Policy Research Institute: Washington, DC, USA, 2014.
6. Black, R. Micronutrient deficiency—An underlying cause of morbidity and mortality. *Bull. World Health Org.* **2003**, *81*, 79.
7. Allen, L.H.; Peerson, J.M.; The Maternal Micronutrient Supplementation Study Group. Impact of multiple micronutrient *versus* iron-folic acid supplements on maternal anemia and micronutrient status in pregnancy. *Food Nutr. Bull.* **2009**, *30*, S527–S532.
8. Christian, P.; Murray-Kolb, L.E.; Khatry, S.; Katz, J.; Schaefer, B.A.; Cole, P.M.; LeClerq, S.C.; Tielsch, J.M. Prenatal micronutrient supplementation and intellectual and motor function in early school-aged children in Nepal. *J. Am. Med. Assoc.* **2010**, *304*, 2716–2723.
9. Duggan, C.; Srinivasan, K.; Thomas, T.; Samuel, T.; Rajendran, R.; Muthayya, S.; Finkelstein, J.L.; Lukose, A.; Fawzi, W.; Allen, L.H.; *et al.* Vitamin B-12 supplementation during pregnancy and early lactation increases maternal, breast milk, and infant measures of vitamin B-12 status. *J. Nutr.* **2014**, *144*, 758–764.
10. Shrimpton, R.; Huffman, S.L.; Zehner, E.R.; Darnton-Hill, I.; Dalmiya, N. Multiple micronutrient supplementation during pregnancy in developing country settings: Policy and program implications of the results of a meta-analysis. *Food Nutr. Bull.* **2009**, *30*, S556–S573.
11. Torheim, L.E.; Ferguson, E.L.; Penrose, K.; Arimond, M. Women in resource-poor settings are at risk of inadequate intakes of multiple micronutrients. *J. Nutr.* **2010**, *140*, 2051S–2058S.
12. Matthews, Z.; Channon, A.; Neal, S.; Osrin, D.; Madise, N.; Stones, W. Examining the "urban advantage" in maternal health care in developing countries. *PLoS Med.* **2010**, *7*, e1000327.
13. Shrimpton, R. Global policy and programme guidance on maternal nutrition: What exists, the mechanisms for providing it, and how to improve them? *Paediatr. Perinat. Epidemiol.* **2012**, *26*, 315S–325S.

14. Ahmed, F.; Khan, M.R.; Akhtaruzzaman, M.; Karim, R.; Williams, G.; Banu, C.P.; Nahar, B.; Darnton-Hill, I. Effect of long-term intermittent supplementation with multiple micronutrients compared with iron-and-folic acid supplementation on Hb and micronutrient status of non-anaemic adolescent schoolgirls in rural Bangladesh. *Br. J. Nutr.* **2012**, *108*, 1484–1493.

15. Thurnham, D.I. Nutrition of adolescent girls in low- and middle-income countries. *Sight Life* **2013**, *27*, 26–37.

16. Baker, P.N.; Wheeler, S.J.; Sanders, T.A.; Thomas, J.E.; Hutchinson, C.J.; Clarke, K.; Berry, J.L.; Jones, R.L.; Seed, P.T.; Poston, L. A prospective study of micronutrient status in adolescent pregnancy. *Am. J. Clin. Nutr.* **2009**, *89*, 1114–1124.

17. Rah, J.H.; Christian, P.; Shamim, A.A.; Arju, U.T.; Labrique, A.B.; Rashid, M. Pregnancy and lactation hinder growth and nutritional status of adolescent girls in rural Bangladesh. *J. Nutr.* **2008**, *138*, 1505–1511.

18. Bhutta, Z.A.; Das, J.K.; Rizvi, A.; Gaffey, M.F.; Walker, N.; Horton, S.; Webb, P.; Black, R.E.; for the Lancet Nutrition Interventions Review Group; the Maternal and Child Nutrition Study Group. Evidence-based interventions for improvement of maternal and child nutrition: What can be done and at what cost? *Lancet* **2013**, *382*, 452–477.

19. Conde-Agudelo, A.; Rosas-Bermudez, A.; Castaño, F.; Norton, M.H. Effects of birth spacing on maternal, perinatal, infant, and child health: A systematic review of causal mechanisms. *Stud. Fam. Plan.* **2012**, *43*, 93–114.

20. Berti, C.; Biesalski, H.K.; Gärtner, R.; Lapillone, A.; Pietrzik, K.; Poston, L.; Redman, C.; Koletzko, B.; Cetin, I. Micronutrients in pregnancy: Current knowledge and unresolved questions. *Clin. Nutr.* **2011**, *30*, 689–701.

21. Ladipo, O.A. Nutrition in pregnancy: Mineral and vitamin supplements. *Am. J. Clin. Nutr.* **2000**, *72*, 280S–290S.

22. Black, R.E. Micronutrients in pregnancy. *Br. J. Nutr.* **2001**, *85*, S193–S197.

23. Sifakis, S.; Pharmakides, G. Anemia in pregnancy. *Ann. N. Y. Acad. Sci.* **2000**, *900*, 125–136.

24. Raiten, D.J.; Namasté, S.; Brabin, B.; Combs, G.; L'Abbé, M.R.; Wasantwisut, E.; Darnton-Hill, I. Executive summary: Biomarkers of nutrition for development (BOND): Building a consensus. *Am. J. Clin. Nutr.* **2011**, *94*, 633S–650S.

25. Stevens, G.A.; Finucane, M.M.; de-Regil, L.M.; Paciorek, C.J.; Flaxman, S.R.; Branca, F.; Peña-Rosas, J.P.; Bhutta, Z.A.; Ezzati, M.; Nutrition Impact Model Study Group (Anaemia). Global, regional, and national trends in haemoglobin concentration and prevalence of total and severe anaemia in children and pregnant and non-pregnant women for 1995–2011: A systematic analysis of population-representative data. *Lancet Glob. Health* **2013**, *1*, e16–e25.

26. Riggs, A.F. Hemoglobins. *Curr. Opin. Struct. Biol.* **1991**, *1*, 915–921.

27. Allen, D.W.; Wyman, J.; Smith, C.A. The oxygen equilibrium of fetal and adult human hemoglobin. *J. Biol. Chem.* **1953**, *203*, 81–87.

28. Black, R.E.; Victora, C.G.; Walker, S.P.; Bhutta, Z.A.; Christian, P.; de Onis, M.; Ezzati, M.; Grantham-McGregor, S.; Katz, J.; Martorell, R.; *et al.* Maternal and child undernutrition and overweight in low-income and middle-income countries. *Lancet* **2013**, *382*, 427–451.

29. Greminger, A.R.; Lee, D.L.; Shrager, P.; Mayer-Pröschel, M. Gestational iron deficiency differentially alters the structure and function of white and gray matter brain regions of developing rats. *J. Nutr.* **2014**, *144*, 1058–1066.

30. Tofail, F.; Hamadani, J.D.; Mehrin, F.; Ridout, D.A.; Huda, S.N.; Grantham-McGregor, S.M. Psychosocial stimulation benefits development in nonanemic children but not in anemic, iron-deficient children. *J. Nutr.* **2013**, *143*, 885–893.

31. Fararouei, M.; Robertson, C.; Whittaker, J.; Sovio, U.; Ruokonen, A.; Pouta, A.; Hartkainen, A.L.; Jarvelin, M.R.; Hyppönen, E. Maternal Hb during pregnancy and offspring's educational achievement: A prospective cohort study over 30 years. *Br. J. Nutr.* **2010**, *104*, 1363–1368.

32. Scholl, T.O. Iron status during pregnancy: Setting the stage for mother and infant. *Am. J. Clin. Nut* **2005**, *81*, 1218S–1222S.

33. Rohner, F.; Zimmermann, M.; Jooste, P.; Pandav, C.; Caldwell, K.; Raghavan, R.; Raiten, D.J. Biomarkers Of Nutrition for Development—Iodine review. Supplement: Biomarkers of Nutrition for Development (BOND) Expert Panel reviews, Part 1. *J. Nutr.* **2014**, *144*, 1322S–1342S.

34. Phillips, A.M.; Zlotkin, S.H.; Baxter, J.A.; Martinuzzi, F.; Kadria, T.; Roth, D.E. Design and development of a combined calcium-iron-folic acid prenatal supplement to support implementation of the new World Health Organization recommendations for calcium supplementation during pregnancy. *Food Nutr. Bull.* **2014**, *35*, 221–229.

35. Imdad, A.; Bhutta, Z.A. Intervention strategies to address multiple micronutrient deficiencies in pregnancy. In *Meeting Micronutrient Requirements for Health and Development*; Nestlé Nutrition Institute Workshop Series; Bhutta, Z.A., Hurrell, R.F., Rosenberg, I.H., Eds.; Karger: Basel, Switzerland, 2012; Volume 70, pp. 61–73.

36. Mori, R.; Ota, E.; Middleton, P.; Tobe-Gai, R.; Mahomed, K.; Bhutta, Z.A. Zinc supplementation for improving pregnancy and infant outcome. *Cochrane Database Syst. Rev.* **2012**, *7*.

37. Stamm, R.A.; Houghton, L.A. Nutrient intake values for folate during pregnancy and lactation vary widely around the world. *Nutrients* **2013**, *5*, 3920–3947.

38. Food Fortification Initiative. Why fortify? Improved health. Available online: http://www.ffinetwork.org/why_fortify/health.html (accessed on 27 July 2014).

39. Kim, M.W.; Ahn, K.H.; Ryu, K.J.; Hong, S.C.; Lee, J.S.; Nava-Ocampo, A.A.; Oh, M.J.; Kim, H.J. Preventive effects of folic acid supplementation on adverse maternal and fetal outcomes. *PLoS One* **2014**, *9*, e97273.

40. Hanieh, S.; Ha, T.T.; Simpson, J.A.; Thuy, T.T.; Khuong, N.C.; Thoang, D.D.; Tran, T.D.; Tuan, T.; Fisher, J.; Biggs, B.A.; *et al.* Maternal vitamin D status and infant outcomes in rural Vietnam: A prospective cohort study. *PLoS One* **2014**, *9*, e99005.

41. Wei, S.Q.; Qi, H.P.; Luo, Z.C.; Fraser, W.D. Maternal vitamin D status and adverse pregnancy outcomes: A systematic review and meta-analysis. *J. Matern Fetal Neonatal Med.* **2013**, *26*, 889–899.

42. De-Regil, L.M.; Palacios, C.; Ansary, A.; Kulier, R.; Peña-Rosas, J.P. Vitamin D supplementation for women during pregnancy. *Cochrane Database Syst. Rev.* **2012**.

43. Allen, L.H. Multiple micronutrients in pregnancy and lactation: An overview. *Am. J. Clin. Nutr.* **2005**, *81*, S1206–S1212.

44. Olivares, M.; Pizarro, F.; Ruz, M. New insights about iron bioavailability inhibition by zinc. *Nutrition* **2007**, *23*, 292–295.

45. Jiang, J.; Zhang, Y.; Wei, L.; Sun, Z.; Liu, Z. Association between *MTHFD1* G1958A and neural tube defects susceptibility: A meta-analysis. *PLoS One* **2014**, *996*, e101169.

46. Roseboom, T.; de Rooij, S.; Painter, R. The Dutch famine and its long-term consequences for adult health. *Early Hum. Dev.* **2006**, *82*, 485–491.

47. Lumey, L.H.; Stein, A.D.; Kahn, H.S.; van der Pal-de Bruin, K.M.; Blauw, G.J.; Zybert, P.A.; Susser, E.S. Cohort Profile: The Dutch Hunger Winter Families Studies. *Int. J. Epidemiol.* **2007**, *36*, 1196–1204.

48. Tofail, F.; Persson, L.A.; el Arifeen, S.; Hamadani, J.D.; Mehrin, F.; Ridout, D.; Ekström, E.-C.; Huda, S.N.; Grantham-McGregor, S.M. Effects of prenatal food and micronutrient supplementation on infant development: A randomized trial from the Maternal and Infant Nutrition Interventions, Matlab (MINIMat) study. *Am. J. Clin. Nutr.* **2008**, *87*, 704–711.

49. Li, Q.; Yan, H.; Zeng, L. Effects of maternal multimicronutrient supplementation on the mental development of infants in rural western China: Follow-up evaluation of a double-blind, randomized, controlled trial. *Pediatrics* **2009**, *123*, e685–e692.

50. McGrath, N.; Bellinger, D.; Robins, J.; Msamanga, G.I.; Tronick, E.; Fawzi, W.W. Effect of maternal multivitamin supplementation on the mental and psychomotor development of children who are born to HIV-1-infected mothers in Tanzania. *Pediatrics* **2006**, *117*, e216–e225.

51. Caulfield, L.E.; Zavaleta, N.; Chen, P.; Lazarte, F.; Albornoz, C.; Putnick, D.L.; Bornstein, M.H.; DiPetro, J.A. Maternal zinc supplementation during pregnancy affects autonomic function of Peruvian children assessed at 54 months of age. *J. Nutr.* **2010**, *141*, 327–332.

52. Christian, P.; Stewart, C.P. Maternal micronutrient deficiency, fetal development, and risk of chronic disease. *J. Nutr.* **2010**, *140*, 437–445.

53. Barker, D.J.P. Developmental origins of chronic disease. *Publ. Health* **2012**, *126*, 185–189.

54. Heijmans, B.T.; Tobi, E.W.; Lumey, L.H.; Slagboom, E. The Epigenome. *Epigenetics* **2009**, *4*, 526–531.

55. Lumey, L.H.; Stein, A.D.; Kahn, H.S.; Romijn, J.A. Lipid profiles in middle-aged men and women after famine exposure during gestation: The Dutch Hunger Winter Families Study. *Am. J. Clin. Nutr.* **2009**, *89*, 1737–1743.

56. Lindeboom, M.; Portrait, F.; van den Berg, G.J. Long-run effects on longevity of a nutritional shock early in life: The Dutch Potato famine of 1846–1847. *J. Health Econ.* **2010**, *29*, 617–629.

57. Heijmans, B.T.; Tobi, E.W.; Stein, A.D.; Putter, H.; Blauw, G.J.; Susser, E.S.; Slagboom, E.; Lumey, L.H. Persistent epigenetic differences associated with prenatal exposure to famine in humans. *Proc. Natl. Acad. Sci. USA* **2008**, *105*, 17046–17049.

58. Veenendaal, M.V.; Painter, R.C.; de Rooij, S.R.; Bossuyt, P.M.; van der Post, J.A.; Gluckman, P.D.; Hanson, M.A.; Roseboom, T.J. Transgenerational effects of prenatal exposure to 1944–1945 Dutch famine. *BJOG* **2013**, *120*, 548–554.

59. Bodnar, L.M.; Parrott, M.S. Intervention strategies to improve outcome in obese pregnancies: Micronutrients and dietary supplements. In *Maternal Obesity*; Gillman, M.W., Poston, L., Eds.; Cambridge University Press: Cambridge, UK, 2012; Chapter 16; pp. 199–207.

60. Poston, L.; Briley, A.L.; Seed, P.T.; Kelly, F.J.; Shennan, A.H. Vitamin C and vitamin E in pregnant women at risk for pre-eclampsia (VIP trial): Randomised placebo-controlled trial. *Lancet* **2006**, *367*, 1145–1154.

61. Conde-Agudelo, A.; Romero, R.; Kusanovic, J.P.; Hassan, S. Supplementation with vitamins C and E during pregnancy for the prevention of preeclampsia and other adverse maternal and perinatal outcomes: A systematic review and metaanalysis. *Am. J. Obstet. Gynaecol.* **2011**, *204*, 503.e1–503.e12.

62. WHO. Intermittent Iron and Folic Acid Supplementation in Menstruating Women: Guideline 2011. Available online: http://www.who.int/nutrition/publications/micronutrients/guidelines/guideline_iron_folicacid_suppl_women/en/ (accessed on 25 July 2014).

63. WHO. Daily Iron and Folic Acid Supplementation in Pregnant Women: Guideline 2012. Available online: http://www.who.int/nutrition/publications/micronutrients/guidelines/daily_ifa_supp_pregnant_women/en/ (accessed on 25 July 2014).

64. Institute of Medicine, Food and Nutrition Board. *Dietary Reference Intakes for Vitamin A, Vitamin K, Arsenic, Boron, Chromium, Copper, Iodine, Iron, Manganese, Molybdenum, Nickel, Silicon, Vanadium, and Zinc: A Report of the Panel on Micronutrients*; National Academy Press: Washington, DC, USA, 2001.

65. The American College of Obstetricians and Gynecologists. Nutrition during Pregnancy 2013. Available online: http://www.acog.org/Patients/FAQs/Nutrition-During-Pregnancy (accessed on 25 July 2014).

66. Haider, B.A.; Yakoob, M.Y.; Bhutta, Z.A. Effect of multiple micronutrient supplementation during pregnancy on maternal and birth outcomes. *BMC Public Health* **2011**, *11*, S19.

67. Zeng, L.; Cheng, Y.; Kong, L. Impact of micronutrient supplementation during pregnancy on birth weight, duration of gestation, and perinatal mortality in rural western China: A double blind cluster randomized controlled trial. *BMJ* **2008**, *337*.

68. Johnson, M.A. If high folic acid aggravates B-12 deficiency what should be done about it? *Nutr. Rev.* **2008**, *65*, 451–458.

69. Scholl, T.O.; Hediger, M.L.; Bendich, A.; Schall, J.I.; Smith, W.K.; Krueger, P.M. Use of multivitamin/mineral prenatal supplements: Influence on the outcome of pregnancy. *Am. J. Epidemiol.* **1997**, *146*, 134–141.

70. Hasan, R.; Olshan, A.F.; Herring, A.H.; Savitz, D.A.; Siega-Riz, A.M.; Hartmann, K.E. Self-reported vitamin supplementation in early pregnancy and risk of miscarriage. *Am. J. Epidemiol.* **2009**, *169*, 1312–1318.

71. Rumbold, A.; Middleton, P.; Crowther, C.A. Vitamin supplementation for preventing miscarriage. *Cochrane Database Syst. Rev.* **2005**.

72. Titaley, C.R.; Dibley, M.J.; Roberts, C.L.; Hall, J.; Agho, K. Iron and folic acid supplements and reduced early neonatal deaths in Indonesia. *Bull. World Health Organ.* **2010**, *88*, 500–508.

73. Shankar, A.H.; Jahari, A.B.; Sebayang, S.K.; Aditiawarman; Aprianti, M.; Harefa, B.; Muadz, H.; Soesbandoro, S.D.; Tjiong, R.; Fachry, A.; *et al.* Effect of maternal multiple micronutrient supplementation on fetal loss and infant death in Indonesia: A double-blind cluster-randomised trial. *Lancet* **2008**, *371*, 215–227.

74. Mei, Z.; Serdula, M.K.; Liu, J.M.; Flores-Ayala, R.C.; Wang, L.; Ye, R.; Grummer-Strawn, L.M. Iron-containing micronutrient supplementation of Chinese women with no or mild anemia during pregnancy improved iron status but did not affect perinatal anemia. *J. Nutr.* **2014**, *144*, 943–948.

75. Christian, P.; Osrin, D.; Manandhar, D.S.; Khatry, S.K.; de L Costello, A.M.; West, K.P., Jr. Antenatal micronutrient supplements in Nepal. *Lancet* **2005**, *366*, 711–712.

76. Kawai, K.; Kupka, R.; Mugusi, F.; Aboud, S.; Okuma, J.; Villamor, E.; Spiegelman, D.; Fawzi, W.W. A randomized trial to determine the optimal dosage of multivitamin supplements to reduce adverse pregnancy outcomes among HIV-infected women in Tanzania. *Am. J. Clin. Nutr.* **2010**, *91*, 391–397.

77. Andrew, E.V.W.; Pell, C.; Angwin, A.; Auwun, A.; Daniels, J.; Mueller, I.; Phuanukoonnon, S.; Pool, R. Factors affecting attendance at and timing of formal antenatal care: Results from a qualitative study in Madang, Papua New Guinea. *PLoS ONE* **2014**, *9*, e93025.

78. Persson, L.A.; Arifeen, S.; Ekström, E.C.; Rasmussen, K.M.; Frongillo, E.A.; Yunus, M.; for the MINIMat Study Team. Effects of prenatal micronutrient and early food supplementation on maternal hemoglobin, birth weight, and infant mortality among children in Bangladesh. The MINIMat Randomized trial. *JAMA* **2012**, *307*, 2050–2059.

79. Moran, V.H.; Dewey, K. (Eds.) Consequences of malnutrition in early life and strategies to improve maternal and child diets through targeted fortified products. *Matern. Child Nutr.* **2011**, *7*, 19–43.

80. Yang, Z.; Huffman, S.L. Review of fortified food and beverage products for pregnant and lactating women and their impact on nutritional status. *Matern. Child Nutr.* **2011**, *7*, 1–142.

81. Andersson, M.; de Benoist, B.; Delange, F.; Zupan, J.; (WHO Secretariat on behalf of participants to the Expert Consultation). Prevention and control of iodine deficiency in pregnant and lactating women and in children less than 2-years-old: Conclusions and recommendations of the Technical Consultation. *Publ. Health Nutr.* **2007**, *10*, 1606–1611.

82. ICCIDD. IDD Newsletter 2013. Available online: http://www.ign.org/newsletter/idd_may13_australia.pdf (accessed on 25 July 2014).

83. Martin, J.C.; Savige, G.S.; Mitchell, E.K. Health knowledge and iodine intake in pregnancy. *Aust N. Z. J. Obstet. Gynaecol.* **2014**.

84. Mannar, M.G.V. Making salt iodization truly universal by 2020. *IDD Newsl.* **2014**, *42*, 12–15.

85. Ronnenberg, A.G.; Wood, R.J.; Wang, X.; Xing, H.; Chen, C.; Chen, D.; Guang, W.; Huang, A.; Wang, L.; Xu, X. Preconception hemoglobin and ferritin concentrations are associated with pregnancy outcome in a prospective cohort of Chinese women. *J. Nutr.* **2004**, *134*, 2586–2591.

86. Gyorkos, T.W.; Gilbert, N.L. Blood drain: Soil-transmitted helminthes and anemia in pregnant women. *PLoS Negl. Trop. Dis.* **2014**, *8*, e2912.

87. McClure, E.M.; Meshnik, S.R.; Mungai, P.; Malhotra, I.; King, C.L.; Goldenberg, R.L.; Hudgens, M.G.; Siega-Riz, A.M.; Dent, A.E. The association of parasitic infections in pregnancy and maternal and fetal anemia: A cohort study in coastal Kenya. *PLoS Negl. Trop. Dis.* **2014**, *8*, e2724.

88. Mwanga, M.N.; Roth, J.M.; Smit, M.; Trijsburg, L.; Mwangi, A.M.; Demir, A.Y.; Mens, P.; Prentice, A.M.; Andang'o, P.E.A.; Verhoef, H.; *et al.* Safety and efficacy of antenatal iron supplementation in a malaria-endemic area in Kenya: A randomised trial. In Proceedings of the Micronutrient Forum, Addis Ababa, Ethiopia, 2–6 June 2014.

89. Sangaré, L.; van Eijk, A.M.; ter Kuile, F.O.; Walson, J.; Stergachis, A. The association between malaria and iron status or supplementation in pregnancy: A systematic review and meta-analysis. *PLoS One* **2014**, *9*, e87743.

90. Kurth, F.; Bélard, S.; Mombo-Ngoma, G.; Schuster, K.; Adegnika, A.A.; Bouyou-Akotet, M.K.; Kremsner, P.G.; Ramharter, M. Adolescence as risk factor for adverse pregnancy outcome in Central Africa—A cross-sectional study. *PLoS One* **2010**, *5*, e14367.

91. Onabanjo, J.; Kalasa, B.; Abdel-Ahad, M. *Op-Ed by UNFPA "Why Ending Child Marriage in Africa Can No Longer Wait"*; Inter Press Service: Johannesburg, South Africa, 2014.

92. De-Regil, L.M.; Fernandez-Gaxiola, A.C.; Dowswell, T.; Pena-Rosas, J.P. Effects and safety of periconceptional folate supplementation for preventing birth defects. *Cochrane Database Syst. Rev.* **2010**, *10*.

93. Lassi, Z.S.; Salam, R.A.; Haider, B.A.; Bhutta, Z.A. Folic acid supplementation during pregnancy for maternal health and pregnancy outcomes. *Cochrane Database Syst. Rev.* **2013**, *3*.

94. Fernandez-Gaxiola, A.C.; de-Regil, L.M. Intermittent iron supplementation for reducing anaemia and its associated impairments in menstruating women. *Cochrane Database Syst. Rev.* **2011**, *12*.

95. Pena-Rosas, J.P.; de-Regil, L.M.; Dowswell, T.; Viteri, F.E. Daily oral iron supplementation during pregnancy. *Cochrane Database Syst. Rev.* **2012**, *12*.

96. Haider, B.A.; Bhutta, Z.A. Multiple-micronutrient supplementation for women during pregnancy. *Cochrane Database Syst. Rev.* **2012**, *11*.

97. Imdad, A.; Bhutta, Z.A. Effects of calcium supplementation during pregnancy on maternal, fetal and birth outcomes. *Paediatr. Perinat. Epidemiol.* **2012**, *26*, 138–152.

98. Zimmermann, M.B. The effects of iodine deficiency in pregnancy and infancy. *Paediatr. Perinat. Epidemiol.* **2012**, *26*, 108–117.

99. Ramakrishnan, U.; Manjrekar, R.; Rivera, J.; Gonzáles-Cossio, T.; Martorell, R. Micronutrients and pregnancy outcome: A review of the literature. *Nutr. Res.* **1999**, *19*, 103–159.

100. Bhutta, Z.A.; Haider, B.A. Prenatal micronutrient supplementation: Are we there yet? *CMAJ* **2009**, *180*, 1188–1189.

101. Bryce, J.; Coitinho, D.; Darnton-Hill, I.; Pelletier, D.; Pinstrup-Andersen, P.; for the Maternal and Child Undernutrition Study Group. Maternal and child undernutrition: Effective action at national level. *Lancet* **2008**, *371*, 510–526.

102. Mehra, S.; Agrawal, D. Adolescent health determinants for pregnancy and child health outcomes among the urban poor. *Indian Pediatr.* **2004**, *41*, 137–145.

Dietary and Health Profiles of Spanish Women in Preconception, Pregnancy and Lactation

Marta Cuervo, Carmen Sayon-Orea, Susana Santiago and Jose Alfredo Martínez

Abstract: The nutritional status and lifestyle of women in preconception, pregnancy and lactation determine maternal, fetal and child health. The aim of this cross-sectional study was to evaluate dietary patterns and lifestyles according the perinatal physiological status in a large sample of Spanish women. Community pharmacists that were previously trained to collect the data recruited 13,845 women. General information, anthropometric measurements, physical activity, unhealthy habits and dietary data were assessed using a validated questionnaire. Mean values and percentages were used as descriptive statistics. The *t*-test, ANOVA or chi-squared test were used to compare groups. A score that included dietary and behavioral characteristics was generated to compare lifestyles in the three physiological situations. The analysis revealed that diet quality should be improved in the three stages, but in a different manner. While women seeking a pregnancy only met dairy recommendations, those who were pregnant only fulfilled fresh fruits servings and lactating women only covered protein group requirements. In all cases, the consumption allowances of sausages, buns and pastries were exceeded. Food patterns and unhealthy behaviors of Spanish women in preconception, pregnancy and lactation should be improved, particularly in preconception. This information might be useful in order to implement educational programs for each population group.

Reprinted from *Nutrients*. Cite as: Cuervo, M.; Sayon-Orea, C.; Santiago, S.; Martínez, J.A. Dietary and Health Profiles of Spanish Women in Preconception, Pregnancy and Lactation. *Nutrients* **2014**, *6*, 4434–4451.

1. Introduction

Nutrition in the periconceptional period, pregnancy and lactation is very important for the mother and child health status [1], and there is consistent evidence about the association between nutrition and lifestyles during pregnancy and health outcomes [2].

In preconception nutrition care, besides folic acid supplementation [3], it is important to have an adequate intake of iron, iodine, calcium, vitamins A and D, essential fatty-acids and dietary supplements, when necessary [4,5]. Besides, a greater adherence to the Mediterranean-type dietary pattern may enhance fertility [6]. On the other hand, high consumption of caffeine and alcohol, smoking, use of illegal drugs and mothers being overweight or underweight have been associated with higher difficulty conceiving [7,8].

Early nutrition factors might be involved in the long-term development of obesity [9], cardiovascular disease, diabetes and other non-communicable diseases [10], according to the developmental origin of health and disease (DoHad) theory [11]. Besides, maternal weight status during pregnancy has been linked to adverse birth outcomes, such as fetal growth, birth defects or preterm delivery [12,13]. Traditionally, nutritional epidemiology in pregnancy has centered on food consumption patterns [14–17] and specific macronutrients [18] or micronutrients inadequacy [19]. In general, pregnant women in developed countries are at risk of suboptimal intakes of folate, iron and vitamin D [20].

The diet quality and lifestyles of lactating mothers have an important role, not only in recovering nutritional status after pregnancy [21], but also in other health outcomes for mother and child [22]. A healthy and varied diet during lactation ensures a balanced maternal nutrition and the optimal concentration of some nutrients of human milk [23]. Specifically, concentrations of many vitamins, iodine and fatty acids [24] in human milk depend on or are influenced by maternal diet [23].

In Spain, a previous longitudinal study conducted in 80 women who were planning immediate pregnancy in preconception, were pregnant or were at six months postpartum concluded that dietary patterns did not change significantly from preconception to postpartum [25]. However, nutritional epidemiology studies in Spanish women at these physiological situations are scarce [7,26–29] and mostly are centered in iron [30] and iodine intake [31]. Besides, other studies have reported smoking habits [32–34], socioeconomic factors or self-care [27,35–37], mainly in Spanish pregnant women.

The period before, during and after pregnancy provides a great opportunity to assess nutritional status and to offer women practical advice to improve diet quality, become more physically active and to help them manage body weight effectively [38]. All women should be offered support to breastfeed their babies to increase the duration and exclusivity of breastfeeding [39]. In this context, it is necessary to assess nutritional status in order to provide an adequate dietary advice in preconception, pregnancy and lactation. To our knowledge, there are no previous studies that have examined at the same time these periods in Spain. Therefore, the two aims of the present work were to assess dietary patterns and unhealthy behaviors in a large sample of Spanish women in preconception, pregnancy and lactation and to propose a short healthy lifestyle score for these three life periods.

2. Experimental Section

2.1. Subject Recruitment

This cross-sectional, population-based study included 13,845 Spanish women in preconceptional pregnancy or lactation periods, who participated in a national plan of nutritional education, between November 2009 and March 2010. This program was conducted in order to provide information to these population groups about the importance of how women's health behaviors could influence the development and health of their offspring. The study took place in 2794 pharmacies all over Spain, from both urban and rural areas. The information was collected through a validated questionnaire for this population [28]. Volunteers were recruited by community pharmacists (one pharmacist per pharmacy) and had a face-to-face interview with them. Subsequently, each potential volunteer was specifically asked if she would be willing to take part anonymously in the study. After ensuring that participants understood the information, only those who voluntarily accepted were enrolled. Voluntary completion of the questionnaire was considered to imply verbal informed consent. This study was conducted with the approval of the Spanish Council of Pharmacist (ref 14100127) on 29 June 2009, and the Board of the Institute of Food Sciences and Nutrition of the University of Navarra (ref 90), according to the guidelines laid down in the Declaration of Helsinki for anonymous surveys [40]. Additionally, this nutritional program has the recognition of Health Interest Activity by the Spanish Ministry of Health and Social Policy [41].

Prior to data collection, community pharmacists were recruited through the Spanish Pharmacists Council. To assure harmonization among interviewers, all of them received a training session by videoconference and an extensive document with explanations and a decision tree to interpret each question and other information needed about the survey [42]. This information was also available for all pharmacists involved in the study on a website [41]. Furthermore, this approach has been successfully applied in a previous study concerning an elderly population [43,44].

2.2. The Survey

The first question of the survey was the self-reported physiological status of woman: preconception, pregnancy or lactation. Pregnancy intention was assessed by response to the following question: "Time looking for pregnancy: less than 6 months, between 6 and 11 months or more or equal to 12 months". Pregnant woman were asked if pregnancy status was medically confirmed. Type of pregnancy (unique, twins, triplets or more) and week of gestation were also recorded. We considered the lactation period as 6 months postpartum, and women were asked about the type of feeding in that period: breastfeeding, formula feeding or mixed.

To assess the nutritional status and food habits of women, information about anthropometric measurements, self-perception of nutrition and health educational level, physical activity, unhealthy lifestyle habits and diet data were inquired. The anthropometric measurements were taken by community pharmacists at pharmacies (actual weight and height). Body mass index (BMI) was calculated by dividing weight in kilograms by the square of height in meters. Self-reported pre-gestational weight was also registered in pregnant and lactating women. Anthropometric and physical activity data collection has been validated [28]. Anthropometric measurements validation was assessed by testing the accuracy of measurements collected by community pharmacists and comparing them to measurements collected by trained research staff. Physical activity information included the number of hours spent in lying, sitting and moving activities, paying special attention so that the sum of the hours of a day were 24 in total. We validated this physical activity information using as another gold standard physical activity questionnaire, previously validated for Spanish adults [28]. Subsequently, the individual activity factor was calculated for each subject applying activity factors set by the Food Agriculture Organization, World Health Organization [45].

Information about age, physical activity, educational level (no studies, primary, high school, university graduate), self-perception of health (very good, good, regular, bad, very bad, I do not know), self-perception of actual nutrition (very balanced, balanced, medium balanced, non-balanced, I do not know) and unhealthy lifestyles was obtained from self-reported information. Unhealthy lifestyle comprised smoking status (never, former/passive, actual), alcohol consumption (yes, no) and use of illicit drugs (never, former, actual). Participants were also asked if they followed a special diet (low calorie, low fat, low carbohydrates, low sodium diets or any type of vegetarian diets). Qualitative information on self-reported nutrient supplementation was also assessed with the baseline questionnaire, specifically: enriched milk in calcium or vitamins, folic acid/vitamin B_{12} supplements or enriched foods, iodine supplements/iodine salt, iron supplements or enriched foods, multivitamins and others (supplements or foods enriched in fiber, prebiotics or probiotics).

Concerning the diet, semi-quantitative information was assessed by a validated food frequency questionnaire (FFQ) in which basic foods were classified into twelve food groups, where 4 responses were possible: daily, weekly, monthly or never. After that, the daily frequency of food consumption was calculated. To assess the validity of food patterns information, we used as gold standard, the FFQ of the SUN project (Seguimiento Universidad de Navarra project), which has been validated for Spanish adult population [28]. The correlation coefficients obtained ranged between $r = 0.4$ and $r = 0.6$. The "questionnaire application guide" included information on the typical serving size for each basic food [44]. In order to estimate if the three groups fulfilled the dietary recommendations for Spanish women [46], nuts, legumes, fish, eggs and meat were grouped as protein group, and bread and rice, pasta and potatoes were grouped as the cereal group.

2.3. Data Collection

Community pharmacists, previously trained, collected the information by a face-to-face interview with the volunteers and introduced the answers in a specific platform located on the website created for this study (under a password). Data were refined, processed and analyzed in an anonymous and confidential way. From 14,972 participants that were initially included in the study, 1127 were excluded because of implausible or missing values on important variables. Therefore, the final sample for the analyses was 13,845.

2.4. Statistical Analyses and Additional Calculations

Mean values and standard deviations (SD) for continuous variables and percentages for categorical variables were used as descriptive statistics. Analysis of variance (ANOVA) or the chi-squared test (χ^2 tests) were used to compare the baseline characteristics of the participants according to the physiological status.

Mean and SD were calculated for each food group in the three categories of physiological status. ANOVA tests were used to compare the means of consumption in the three categories, while t-tests were conducted to compare the mean of consumption of every food group with the dietary guidelines of the Spanish Society of Community Nutrition (Sociedad Española de Nutricion Comunitaria (SENC)) in each of the three periods [46].

We also generated a healthy lifestyle score to obtain an estimation of selected healthy behavior characteristics [47,48], based on the recommendations proposed by the SENC (Spanish Society of Community Nutrition) [46] and Mediterranean diet adherence [49]. The Mediterranean diet is a plant-based dietary pattern, where each food group is eaten in moderation, and the cultural lifestyle that accompanies this food pattern embodies a sense of community, physical activity and adequate rest. This diet includes vegetables, fruits, olive oil, legumes and nuts, in abundance; intake of fish, dairy products and wine with moderation; and small portions of meat and poultry and sweets [50]. Points were allocated as follows: participants earn a point if (1) olive oil was used as the principal fat; (2) the protein group was consumed ≥ 1/day; (3) cereals were consumed 3–6/day; (4) salads and vegetables were consumed at least 2 servings/day; (5) fresh fruits were consumed ≥ 2 servings/day; (6) sausages were consumed <1/day; (7) buns and pastries were consumed <2/week; (8) they were never smokers (actual smokers deduct one point); (9) they were never drug users (actual drug users deduct one point); (10) activity factor above the median; and (11) they were normal weight (BMI between 18.5 and 24.9 kg/m^2) (weight was based on pre-pregnancy data). Therefore, the range of the scores that could be earned was from −2 to 11 points. ANOVA was used to compare the means of the healthy lifestyle score in the three categories.

Simple linear regression and then stepwise multiple linear regression analysis were used to evaluate the predictive strength of the lifestyle variables, using as the dependent variable the total healthy lifestyle score. All p-values presented are two-tailed; $p < 0.05$ was considered statistically significant. Analyses were performed using STATA/SE version 12.0 (StataCorp, College Station, TX, USA).

3. Results

The main characteristics of participants according to their physiological status are presented in Table 1. The mean age of the women included in the study was 31.8 (SD: 4.7) years. Women in the lactation period reported a higher activity factor, and a higher percentage of this group of women perceived their health status as very good. Furthermore, a higher percentage of this group were never smokers and never drug users. Only 48.9% of childbearing women were consuming folic acid (supplements or enriched food) and 14.1% multivitamins. As expected, women with the status of pregnancy consumed more supplements, such as iodine, folic acid and vitamin B_{12}, iron, multivitamins and minerals or others.

Table 2 shows the means of the consumption of every food group, and we compared these means between the three periods and found differences between them almost in all of the food groups ($p < 0.05$), except in eggs, cereal group, bread and salad and vegetables Additionally, we compared the means of consumption of each of the groups with the recommendations from the SENC for each specific physiological status.

Women in a preconceptional status did not reach the recommendation for consumption in the following food groups: proteins, cereals, salad vegetables and fresh fruits. On the other hand, women who were pregnant did not reach the recommendation for proteins, cereals, dairy and salad and vegetables. Finally, lactating women did not reach the recommendation for cereal, dairy, salad vegetables and fresh fruits. All of the women exceeded the recommendation for sausage and bun and pastry consumption.

The definition of the healthy lifestyle score is presented in Table 3. The mean healthy lifestyle score was 7.29 (SD: 1.65) points. When we compared the mean of the score in each group of women, we observed a statistically significant difference between groups, finding a higher score in those women who were in the lactation period 7.51 (95% CI: 7.47–7.56). In Figure 1, the means and the 95% CI of the healthy lifestyle score in each group of women are shown.

Table 1. Baseline characteristics according to physiological status (n = 13,845).

Characteristics	All	Pre-Conception	Pregnancy	Lactation	p [a]
N	13,845	4471	5087	4287	
Age (years)	31.8 (4.7)	31.4 (4.8)	31.9 (4.6)	32.2 (4.6)	<0.001
Height (cm)	164.0 (6.1)	164.0 (6.1)	164.1 (6.2)	164.1 (6.1)	0.621
Weight (kg)	61.3 (8.9)	61.4 (9.6)	61.2 (8.4)	61.3 (8.6)	0.432
BMI (kg/m^2)	22.8 (3.3)	22.9 (3.9)	22.7 (3.0)	22.8 (3.0)	0.926
Activity factor	1.43 (0.05)	1.43 (0.05)	1.41 (0.05)	1.45 (0.06)	<0.001
Education level (%)					
No studies	1.8	1.7	2.10	1.6	
Primary	16.0	13.2	16.8	18.1	<0.001
High school	35.1	34.1	34.9	36.4	
University graduate	47.1	51.1	46.2	43.9	
Self-perception of health (%)					
Very good	21.4	19.4	22.3	22.4	
Good	65.5	66.3	63.7	66.7	
Regular	11.3	12.1	12.1	9.6	<0.001
Bad	0.8	0.7	1.0	0.7	
Very bad	0.3	0.3	0.3	0.2	
Don't know	0.7	1.1	0.7	0.7	
*Self-perception of actual nutrition * (%)*					
Very Balanced	45.9	44.8	47.3	45.5	
Balanced	38.7	36.6	39.6	39.7	
Medium balanced	13.0	15.9	11.0	12.4	<0.001
Non balanced	0.6	0.7	0.4	0.9	
Don't know	1.8	2.1	1.7	1.5	
Tobacco					
Never	63.7	56.3	67.1	67.4	
Former/passive	22.9	23.2	23.9	21.3	<0.001
Actual	13.4	20.4	9.0	11.4	
Alcohol					
No	67.3	51.0	75.4	74.6	<0.001
Yes	32.7	49	24.6	25.4	
Illicit Drugs					
Never	97.8	96.9	98.2	98.4	
Former	1.3	1.6	1.3	1.1	<0.001
Actual	0.9	1.5	0.5	0.5	
*Special Diets ** *					
No	85.0	83.8	85.7	85.4	0.021
Yes	15.0	16.2	14.3	14.6	

Table 1. *Cont.*

Characteristics	All	Pre-Conception	Pregnancy	Lactation	p [a]
Diet supplementation (yes %)					
Enriched milk with calcium/vitamins	24.1	21.1	24.9	26.2	
Folic acid/vitamin B_{12}	49.5	48.9	74.7	20.4	
Iodine/Iodine salt	30.5	26.1	41.3	22.3	
Iron	32.5	16.0	46.1	33.7	<0.001
Multivitamin and minerals	21.3	14.1	26.7	22.4	
Other supplements	39.7	35.9	48.9	32.7	
No supplementation	18.3	26.1	5.8	25.2	
Main fat consumed					
Olive oil	92.2	91.2	92.9	92.4	0.008
Others	7.8	8.8	7.1	7.6	

* Women were asked how they considered their actual nutrition in comparison with other women in their same physiological status. ** Including low-calorie, low-sugar, low-fat, low-salt, vegan, lacto-ovo vegetarian and others. Values are expressed as the mean (SD), unless otherwise stated. [a] Continuous variables were compared using analyses of variance. Categorical variables were compared using the chi-squared test.

Table 2. Mean (SD) of daily serving consumption in women according to physiological status.

Servings/Day	Physiological Status						p
	Preconception		Pregnancy		Lactation		
	Mean (SD)	SENC [†]	Mean (SD)	SENC [†]	Mean (SD)	SENC [†]	
N	4471	2	5087	2	4287	2	
Protein group	1.96 [‡] (1.64)	2	1.96 [‡] (1.18)		1.98 (1.13)		<0.001
Meat	0.58 (0.58)		0.59 (0.51)		0.61 (0.50)		<0.001
Fish	0.42 (0.50)		0.44 (0.47)		0.43 (0.40)		<0.001
Eggs	0.36 (0.31)		0.34 (0.23)		0.35 (0.27)		0.10
Legumes	0.32 (0.50)		0.33 (0.39)		0.32 (0.39)		0.001
Nuts	0.27 (0.56)		0.27 (0.48)		0.26 (0.52)		0.04
Cereal group	2.39 [‡] (1.56)	3	2.38 [‡] (1.51)	4	2.42 [‡] (1.53)	4	0.34
Bread	1.72 (1.23)		1.71 (1.23)		1.73 (1.22)		0.78
Rice, pasta and potatoes	0.66 (0.71)		0.67 (0.68)		0.70 (0.73)		0.01
Dairy	2.00 (1.19)	2	2.26 [‡] (1.26)	3	2.30 [‡] (1.33)	4	<0.001
Salad and vegetables	1.22 [‡] (1.00)	2	1.26 [‡] (1.01)	2	1.24 [‡] (0.98)	2	0.10
Fresh fruits	1.82 [‡] (1.33)	2	2.06 (1.36)	2	1.93 [‡] (1.34)	2	<0.001
Sausages	0.46 * (0.58)	Occasionally	0.36 * (0.50)	Occasionally	0.43 * (0.54)	Occasionally	<0.001
Buns and pastries	0.43 * (0.88)	Occasionally	0.35 * (0.59)	Occasionally	0.40 * (0.67)	Occasionally	<0.001

[†] Recommendations from the SENC (Sociedad Española de Nutricion Comunitaria (Spanish Society of Community Nutrition)), using as a reference the minimum serving of recommended range for each group. * Exceeded the recommendation from SENC. [‡] Did not reach the recommendation from SENC.

In the stepwise multiple linear regression analysis, the factors that were more associated with the healthy lifestyle score were tobacco, fresh fruits, salad and vegetables, buns and pastries and activity factor. The coefficient of determination of these variables in the simple regression model was $R^2 = 0.299$ (tobacco), $R^2 = 0.267$ (fresh fruits), $R^2 = 0.209$ (salad and vegetables), $R^2 = 0.156$ (buns and pastries) and $R^2 = 0.112$ (activity factor) (Table 4).

Table 3. Definition of the healthy lifestyle score.

Characteristics	Condition to Score	Points
Olive oil as principal fat	Yes	1
Protein group [1,4]	$\geq$1 serving/day	1
Cereal group [2,5]	3–6 servings/day	1
Salad and vegetables [6]	$\geq$2 servings/day	1
Fresh fruits [7]	$\geq$2 servings/day	1
Sausages [8]	$\leq$1 serving/day	1
Buns and pastries [3,9]	<2 servings/week	1
Tobacco	Never	1
	Former	0
	Actual	−1
Illicit drugs	Never	1
	Former	0
	Actual	−1
Activity factor	Above the median	1
Pre-gestational BMI	18.5–24.9 kg/m^2	1
Total		−2 to 11

[1] The protein group included: meat, eggs, fish, legumes and nuts. [2] The cereal group included: bread, rice, pasta and potatoes. [3] The buns and pastries group included all commercial pastries, sweets, doughnuts, *etc.* [4] A serving size for the protein group was defined as: one egg, 100–125 g of meat, 125–150 g of fish, 30 g of nuts, 60–80 g of legumes. [5] A serving size for the cereal group was defined as: 40–60 g of bread, 60–80 g of rice or pasta and 150–200 g of potatoes. [6] A serving size of salad or vegetables was defined as: 150–200 g of salad or 200 g of cooked vegetables. [7] A serving size of fruit was defined as: 120–200 g of fruit or 200 mL of natural juice. [8] A serving size of sausages was defined as 50 g. [9] A serving size of buns and pastries was defined as 50 g.

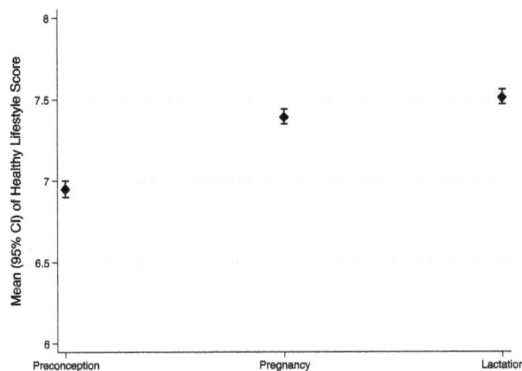

Figure 1. Mean and 95% confidence interval of healthy lifestyle score in each physiological status.

Table 4. Proportion of total variability in the healthy lifestyle score (R^2) explained by individual items.

Predictors *	Simple Linear Regression			Stepwise Regression (Cumulative R^2)
	Preconception	Pregnancy	Lactation	Total
N	4471	5087	4287	13,845
Healthy Score	R^2	R^2	R^2	R^2
Tobacco	0.340	0.254	0.268	0.299
Fresh fruits	0.256	0.274	0.265	0.512
Salads and vegetables	0.175	0.238	0.226	0.614
Buns and pastries	0.157	0.167	0.148	0.694
Activity factor	0.125	0.121	0.098	0.793
Pre-gestational BMI	0.102	0.060	0.076	0.855
Olive oil	0.077	0.071	0.070	0.879
Cereal group	0.054	0.076	0.076	0.947
Illicit drugs	0.068	0.054	0.044	0.964
Sausages	0.036	0.024	0.021	0.977
Protein group	0.026	0.026	0.022	1.00

* All of the predictors of the model were statistical significant in the stepwise regression.

4. Discussion

This cross-sectional study examined the healthy behaviors and dietary patterns of 13,845 Spanish women in preconception, pregnancy or lactation situations. Results revealed that a high proportion of women in these periods had a very good or good self-perception of their health and diet, but their dietary patterns and health behaviors are not optimal.

The recommendation of folic acid supplementation was not completely fulfilled in preconception: only 48.9% and 14.1% of childbearing women declared that they were consuming folic acid supplements and multivitamins, respectively. Previous investigation on the Infancia y Medio Ambiente (INMA) cohort showed that women initiate folic acid supplementation after the recommended period [51]. In Spain, according to a study published in 2007 by the Spanish Collaborative Study of Congenital Malformations [52], trends in folic acid supplementation before pregnancy have increased form from 9% to 17.4%, and the results of the Spanish Autonomic Regions were quite similar. Furthermore, the last national survey of the dietary intake of Spain ENIDE, 2010–2011 [53], reported that folic acid intake in women from 18–25 years was 234.2 µg/day and from 25–44 years was 265.04 µg and concluded that these results seem to be of concern, especially in women of childbearing age, due to the risk of neural tube defects. The preconceptional use of folate supplements varies with education and awareness of the importance of folic acid intake among women of reproductive age, the healthcare system, access to and/or distribution of pre-pregnancy folic acid supplements and/or fortification of staple foods with folic acid [54]. In 2004, a review found evidence for suboptimal use of periconceptional folic acid supplements globally [55]. Comparing to other European countries, recent studies reported different rates in France, where only 14.8% women had started folic supplementation before conception [56], 8%–25% in Poland [57] and 64% in Ireland [58]. In our sample, preconceptional women did not reach the recommended consumption of cereals, fruits and vegetables. Consumption of protein group was also slightly lower than dietary guidelines. Recent results of the Australian Longitudinal Study on Women's Health [17] found no evidence that women trying to conceive consume greater intakes of nutrient-rich foods prior to conception, and those who met key nutrient recommendations generally consume more fruit and dairy. Thus, these authors suggest that dietary guidelines should be revised for reproductive-aged women. In Spain, nutritional epidemiology on dietary patterns in childbearing women is scarce, but Cuco *et al.* (2006) [25] observed that diet in preconception does not vary significantly in pregnancy and postpartum.

Therefore, food intake information should be recorded in women who are planning a pregnancy in order to give early and effective nutritional education for a healthy pregnancy. Furthermore, previous investigations concluded that a healthy diet (such us the Mediterranean-type diet) seems to be an efficient alternative means of enhancing fertility [7] and may protect against being overweight and obesity during pregnancy [59]. Besides, it has been reported that women with a high adherence to a Mediterranean diet in early pregnancy had a significantly lower risk of delivering a fetal growth-restricted infant with respect to weight [29].

Concerning lifestyles, a higher percentage of women in preconception declared unhealthy habits, such as smoking and consumption of alcohol and illicit drugs (even occasionally), compared to pregnancy and lactation. Although the smoking rate has decreased in relation to previous studies in Spain [7,32,34], it is still high, even when pregnancy is confirmed [27,32,33,60]. Smoking women are more likely to be infertile and have an increased risk of miscarriage [8]. Notwithstanding this evidence and the global recommendation of folic acid supplementation in preconception, as well as the well-known negative influence of smoking, excess weight and other health risk behaviors on fertility and birth outcomes, there is necessarily more individual education and intervention in preconception care [2,4,61], especially among women with lower education level [62].

Previous investigations in Spain revealed that pregnant women have evidenced inadequate consumption of cereals and vegetables [27,35,60], which coincides with our results. Nevertheless, when comparing birth cohort studies in all of Europe, pregnant women in Spain consumed more vegetables, fruits and seafood [16]. Besides, the essential nutrient content of fruit, vegetables and grains (whole grains) increases fiber intake, which may help to alleviate constipation, a common complaint during pregnancy [2]. Furthermore, in our sample, the consumption of foods of the protein group and dairy were lower than Spanish dietary guidelines [46]. On the other hand, the percentage of pregnant women consuming iodine supplements was lower than previously reported [27]. Routine supplementation of iodine during pregnancy is widely recommended [63]. Studies conducted in Spain confirm that most women are iodine deficient during pregnancy and lactation and recommend iodine supplements in these stages, even also in preconception [64].

In our sample, lactating women did not meet the recommendations of cereals, vegetables, fruits and dairy. To our knowledge, there are no available specific studies on food patterns in lactating women in Spain, although Sanchez et al. [65] found that only 36% of lactating women meet energy, calcium and vitamin D recommendations. In this sense, it has been reported that energy intake increased immediately after birth, but six months after delivery, energy and nutritional intake decrease compared to preconception [66]. Thus, postpartum women should be advised to replenish nutritional stores, return to a healthy weight and prevent problems in subsequent pregnancies, as well as be encouraged to increase the consumption of whole grains, fruits and vegetables [2].

Additionally, in all cases, the recommended servings for sausages, buns and pastries were exceeded. These foods are usually high in saturated fatty acids or sugars, which should be limited in the diet, even more in pregnancy and lactating women, according to Spanish dietary guidelines [46].

Moreover, we devised an 11-item score to summarize several factors that are well known to be associated with healthier lifestyles, following the Mediterranean diet model [49]. Our results showed that women with the status of lactation and pregnancy had healthier lifestyles than women in with status of preconception. This outcome could be explained, because pregnancy is a period when the majority of women are in close contact with physicians, and they are more receptive to health messages [67]. However, we considered that better health advice should be given to all women in order to improve their dietary habits and lifestyles. Furthermore, it has been found that early antenatal health promotion workshops on lifestyle behaviors had a great impact on maternal and infant health outcomes [47]. We have to take into consideration that women with the status of preconception that were included in our study were all seeking to become pregnant. Recently, a new evidence-informed framework for maternal and new-born care [68] has been proposed, which highlights the components of a health system needed by childbearing women, including information, education and health promotion, for example on maternal nutrition, family planning and breastfeeding promotion.

In this context, a recent review by Anderson et al. [6] concluded that time to pregnancy might be impacted by factors that are modifiable, some of which have an effect that is conclusive on reproductive health, such as body weight, intake of folate and smoking. With regard to other factors, such as alcohol and caffeine, the literature is inconsistent. Therefore, health advice should be given to this population focusing on those modifiable factors.

Our study has certain limitations. Firstly, the cross-sectional design of our study did not allow us to measure behavior changes in participants over time. Besides, the origin of the recruitment (pharmacies) and the voluntary participation of the women may have resulted in selection bias, the sample not being totally representative, as women using pharmacies are expected to be aware of the importance of self-care and may have a higher education level and economic status. In Spain, all population groups have access to the national health system and to free (partial or total) drugs issued in the pharmacy. In particular, some prenatal supplements are partially financed, but multivitamins are not. Thus, although the results are not totally generalizable, they give valuable information about food patterns and lifestyles in a large sample of Spanish women ($n = 13,845$).

Another potential limitation is that the large number of examiners might cause an inter-observer variation; however, an effort was made to minimize this. Thus, all of the pharmacists were trained on the protocol interview, including an application guide to the questionnaire with detailed information about each item and a decision tree to interpret answers in each case [42]. Furthermore, a joint videoconference explaining the study was simultaneously broadcast to every provincial pharmacy college, and a website [41] was available for all pharmacists involved in the study to support consistency among interviewers. This kind of training session for health professionals usually has a positive impact on reflecting nutritional issues [69,70].

In addition, we were not able to present macronutrient and micronutrient intakes, because the FFQ includes only 12 items, so we assessed major food and supplementation habits in women, but not nutrient intake adequacy. Despite these limitations, this study adds interesting information about anthropometric measures, food patterns, physical activity (using a validated questionnaire) [28], as well as health behaviors in a large sample of Spanish women.

5. Conclusions

The present study suggests that food patterns and unhealthy behaviors in Spanish women in preconception, pregnancy and lactation should be improved, particularly in preconception.

Regarding dietary habits in the three subgroups, most of the food groups analyzed were not consumed within the recommendations of the Spanish dietary guidelines. On the other hand, women seeking pregnancy had, in general, worse health related habits. This information might be useful in order to implement educational programs for each population group. However, specific studies on micronutrient intake are needed to complement these data.

Acknowledgments: This work was supported by the Spanish Pharmacists Council. The authors thank all the women who agreed to participate voluntarily in this study and the pharmacists who collected the data. Furthermore, the support of CIBERobn is gratefully acknowledged.

Author Contributions: The authors contributions are as follows: Jose Alfredo Martínez, Marta Cuervo and Susana Santiago contributed to design the study; Marta Cuervo and Carmen Sayon-Orea analyzed the data; Marta Cuervo, Carmen Sayon-Orea and Susana Santiago drafted the manuscript; Jose Alfredo Martínez, Marta Cuervo, Carmen Sayon-Orea and Susana Santiago edited and critically reviewed the manuscript; Jose Alfredo Martínez was responsible for funding and economic management. All of the authors approved the final version of the manuscript.

Conflicts of Interest: The authors declare no conflict of interest.

References

1. Harnisch, J.M.; Harnisch, P.H.; Harnisch, D.R., Sr. Family medicine obstetrics: Pregnancy and nutrition. *Prim. Care* **2012**, *39*, 39–54.

2. Kaiser, L.; Allen, L.H.; American Dietetic Association. Position of the American dietetic association: Nutrition and lifestyle for a healthy pregnancy outcome. *J. Am. Diet. Assoc.* **2008**, *108*, 553–561.

3. Lumley, J.; Watson, L.; Watson, M.; Bower, C. Periconceptional supplementation with folate and/or multivitamins for preventing neural tube defects. *Cochrane Database Syst. Rev.* **2001**, *3*, CD001056.

4. Gardiner, P.M.; Nelson, L.; Shellhaas, C.S.; Dunlop, A.L.; Long, R.; Andrist, S.; Jack, B.W. The clinical content of preconception care: Nutrition and dietary supplements. *Am. J. Obstet. Gynecol.* **2008**, *199*, S345–S356.

5. Temel, S.; van Voorst, S.F.; Jack, B.W.; Denktas, S.; Steegers, E.A. Evidence-based preconceptional lifestyle interventions. *Epidemiol. Rev.* **2014**, *36*, 19–30.

6. Anderson, K.; Nisenblat, V.; Norman, R. Lifestyle factors in people seeking infertility treatment—A review. *Aust. N. Z. J. Obstet. Gynaecol.* **2010**, *50*, 8–20.

7. Toledo, E.; Lopez-del Burgo, C.; Ruiz-Zambrana, A.; Donazar, M.; Navarro-Blasco, I.; Martinez-Gonzalez, M.A.; de Irala, J. Dietary patterns and difficulty conceiving: A nested case-control study. *Fertil. Steril.* **2011**, *96*, 1149–1153.

8. Practice Committee of American Society for Reproductive Medicine in collaboration with Society for Reproductive Endocrinology and Infertility. Optimizing natural fertility: A committee opinion. *Fertil. Steril.* **2013**, *100*, 631–637.

9. Symonds, M.E.; Mendez, M.A.; Meltzer, H.M.; Koletzko, B.; Godfrey, K.; Forsyth, S.; van der Beek, E.M. Early life nutritional programming of obesity: Mother-child cohort studies. *Ann. Nutr. Metab.* **2013**, *62*, 137–145.

10. Hanson, M.; Gluckman, P. Developmental origins of noncommunicable disease: Population and public health implications. *Am. J. Clin. Nutr.* **2011**, *94*, 1754S–1758S.

11. Wadhwa, P.D.; Buss, C.; Entringer, S.; Swanson, J.M. Developmental origins of health and disease: Brief history of the approach and current focus on epigenetic mechanisms. *Semin. Reprod. Med.* **2009**, *27*, 358–368.

12. Bautista-Castano, I.; Henriquez-Sanchez, P.; Aleman-Perez, N.; Garcia-Salvador, J.J.; Gonzalez-Quesada, A.; Garcia-Hernandez, J.A.; Serra-Majem, L. Maternal obesity in early pregnancy and risk of adverse outcomes. *PLoS One* **2013**, *8*, e80410.

13. Li, N.; Liu, E.; Guo, J.; Pan, L.; Li, B.; Wang, P.; Liu, J.; Wang, Y.; Liu, G.; Baccarelli, A.A.; *et al.* Maternal prepregnancy body mass index and gestational weight gain on pregnancy outcomes. *PLoS One* **2013**, *8*, e82310.

14. Tobias, D.K.; Zhang, C.; Chavarro, J.; Bowers, K.; Rich-Edwards, J.; Rosner, B.; Mozaffarian, D.; Hu, F.B. Prepregnancy adherence to dietary patterns and lower risk of gestational diabetes mellitus. *Am. J. Clin. Nutr.* **2012**, *96*, 289–295.

15. Sotres-Alvarez, D.; Siega-Riz, A.M.; Herring, A.H.; Carmichael, S.L.; Feldkamp, M.L.; Hobbs, C.A.; Olshan, A.F.; National Birth Defects Prevention Study. Maternal dietary patterns are associated with risk of neural tube and congenital heart defects. *Am. J. Epidemiol.* **2013**, *177*, 1279–1288.

16. Mendez, M.A.; Kogevinas, M. A comparative analysis of dietary intakes during pregnancy in Europe: A planned pooled analysis of birth cohort studies. *Am. J. Clin. Nutr.* **2011**, *94*, 1993S–1999S.

17. Blumfield, M.L.; Hure, A.J.; Macdonald-Wicks, L.K.; Patterson, A.J.; Smith, R.; Collins, C.E. Disparities exist between national food group recommendations and the dietary intakes of women. *BMC Womens Health* **2011**, *11*, 37.

18. Blumfield, M.L.; Hure, A.J.; Macdonald-Wicks, L.; Smith, R.; Collins, C.E. Systematic review and meta-analysis of energy and macronutrient intakes during pregnancy in developed countries. *Nutr. Rev.* **2012**, *70*, 322–336.

19. Haider, B.A.; Bhutta, Z.A. Multiple-micronutrient supplementation for women during pregnancy. *Cochrane Database Syst. Rev.* **2012**, *11*, CD004905.

20. Blumfield, M.L.; Hure, A.J.; Macdonald-Wicks, L.; Smith, R.; Collins, C.E. A systematic review and meta-analysis of micronutrient intakes during pregnancy in developed countries. *Nutr. Rev.* **2013**, *71*, 118–132.

21. Amorim Adegboye, A.R.; Linne, Y.M. Diet or exercise, or both, for weight reduction in women after childbirth. *Cochrane Database Syst. Rev.* **2013**, *7*, CD005627.

22. James, D.C.; Lessen, R.; American Dietetic Association. Position of the American dietetic association: Promoting and supporting breastfeeding. *J. Am. Diet. Assoc.* **2009**, *109*, 1926–1942.

23. Valentine, C.J.; Wagner, C.L. Nutritional management of the breastfeeding dyad. *Pediatr. Clin. N. Am.* **2013**, *60*, 261–274.

24. Innis, S.M. Impact of maternal diet on human milk composition and neurological development of infants. *Am. J. Clin. Nutr.* **2014**, *99*, 734S–741S.

25. Cuco, G.; Fernandez-Ballart, J.; Sala, J.; Viladrich, C.; Iranzo, R.; Vila, J.; Arija, V. Dietary patterns and associated lifestyles in preconception, pregnancy and postpartum. *Eur. J. Clin. Nutr.* **2006**, *60*, 364–371.

26. Cárcel, C.; Quiles, J.; Rico, B.; Sanchis, T.; Quiles, J.; Rico, B.; Sanchis, T. Adecuación de la ingesta nutricional de embarazadas de segundo y tercer trimestre. *Rev. Esp. Nutr. Comunitaria* **2005**, *11*, 136–144.

27. Larranaga, I.; Santa-Marina, L.; Begiristain, H.; Machon, M.; Vrijheid, M.; Casas, M.; Tardon, A.; Fernandez-Somoano, A.; Llop, S.; Rodriguez-Bernal, C.L.; *et al.* Socio-economic inequalities in health, habits and self-care during pregnancy in Spain. *Matern. Child Health J.* **2013**, *17*, 1315–1324.

28. Goni, L.; Martínez, J.A.; Santiago, S.; Cuervo, M. Validación de una encuesta para evaluar el estado nutricional y los estilos de vida en las etapas preconcepcional, embarazo y lactancia. *Rev. Esp. Nutr. Comunitaria* **2013**, *19*, 105–113.

29. Chatzi, L.; Mendez, M.; Garcia, R.; Roumeliotaki, T.; Ibarluzea, J.; Tardon, A.; Amiano, P.; Lertxundi, A.; Iniguez, C.; Vioque, J.; *et al.* Mediterranean diet adherence during pregnancy and fetal growth: INMA (Spain) and RHEA (Greece) mother-child cohort studies. *Br. J. Nutr.* **2012**, *107*, 135–145.

30. Aranda, N.; Ribot, B.; Garcia, E.; Viteri, F.E.; Arija, V. Pre-pregnancy iron reserves, iron supplementation during pregnancy, and birth weight. *Early Hum. Dev.* **2011**, *87*, 791–797.

31. Vila, L.; Serra-Prat, M.; de Castro, A.; Palomera, E.; Casamitjana, R.; Legaz, G.; Barrionuevo, C.; Munoz, J.A.; Garcia, A.J.; Lal-Trehan, S.; *et al.* Iodine nutritional status in pregnant women of two historically different iodine-deficient areas of Catalonia, Spain. *Nutrition* **2011**, *27*, 1029–1033.

32. Palma, S.; Perez-Iglesias, R.; Pardo-Crespo, R.; Llorca, J.; Mariscal, M.; Delgado-Rodriguez, M. Smoking among pregnant women in Cantabria (Spain): Trend and determinants of smoking cessation. *BMC Public Health* **2007**, *7*, 65.

33. Delgado Pena, Y.P.; Rodriguez Martinez, G.; Samper Villagrasa, M.P.; Caballero Perez, V.; Cuadron Andres, L.; Alvarez Sauras, M.L.; Moreno Aznar, L.A.; Olivares Lopez, J.L.; Grupo Colaborativo CALINA. Socio-cultural, obstetric and anthropometric characteristics of newborn children of mothers who smoke in Spain. *An. Pediatr. (Barc.)* **2012**, *76*, 4–9.

34. Jimenez-Muro, A.; Samper, M.P.; Marqueta, A.; Rodriguez, G.; Nerin, I. Prevalence of smoking and second-hand smoke exposure: Differences between Spanish and immigrant pregnant women. *Gac. Sanit.* **2012**, *26*, 138–144.

35. Ferrer, C.; Garcia-Esteban, R.; Mendez, M.; Romieu, I.; Torrent, M.; Sunyer, J. Social determinants of dietary patterns during pregnancy. *Gac. Sanit.* **2009**, *23*, 38–43.

36. Rius, J.M.; Ortuno, J.; Rivas, C.; Maravall, M.; Calzado, M.A.; Lopez, A.; Aguar, M.; Vento, M. Factors associated with early weaning in a Spanish region. *An. Pediatr. (Barc.)* **2014**, *80*, 6–15.

37. Aurrekoetxea, J.J.; Murcia, M.; Rebagliato, M.; Lopez, M.J.; Castilla, A.M.; Santa-Marina, L.; Guxens, M.; Fernandez-Somoano, A.; Espada, M.; Lertxundi, A.; *et al.* Determinants of self-reported smoking and misclassification during pregnancy, and analysis of optimal cut-off points for urinary cotinine: A cross-sectional study. *BMJ Open* **2013**, *3*, e002034.

38. National Institute for Health and Care Excellence, NICE. *Weight Management before, during and after Pregnancy*; NICE: London, UK, 2010; p. 61.

39. Renfrew, M.J.; McCormick, F.M.; Wade, A.; Quinn, B.; Dowswell, T. Support for healthy breastfeeding mothers with healthy term babies. *Cochrane Database Syst. Rev.* **2012**, *5*, CD001141.

40. Claudot, F.; Fresson, J.; Coudane, H.; Guillemin, F.; Demore, B.; Alla, F. Research in clinical epidemiology: Which rules should be applied? *Rev. Epidemiol. Sante Publique* **2008**, *56*, 63–70.

41. Portalfarma. Available online www.portalfarma.com (accessed on 5 June 2014).

42. Plenufar IV: Educación Nutricional en la Etapa Preconcepcional, Embarazo y Lactancia. Guía para Completar la Encuesta Nutricional. Available online: http://www. portalfarma.com/Profesionales/campanaspf/categorias/Documents/PLFIV_AB_ GUIA%20APLICACION%20DE%20LA%20ENCUESTA.pdf (accessed on 5 June 2014).

43. Cuervo, M.; Garcia, A.; Ansorena, D.; Sanchez-Villegas, A.; Martinez-Gonzalez, M.; Astiasaran, I.; Martinez, J. Nutritional assessment interpretation on 22,007 Spanish community-dwelling elders through the mini nutritional assessment test. *Public Health Nutr.* **2009**, *12*, 82–90.

44. Consejo General de Colegios Oficiales de Farmacéuticos. *Plan de Educación Nutricional por el Farmacéutico (PLENUFAR 3): Alimentación y Salud en las Personas Mayores*; Eurograf Navarra S.L.: Pamplona. Spain, 2005; p. 112.

45. Food and Agriculture Organization of the United Nations/World Health Organization. *Human Vitamins and Mineral Requirements*; Report of a Joint FAO/WHO Expert Consultation; FAO: Rome, Italy; WHO: Geneva, Switzerland, 2002.

46. Sociedad Española de Nutrición Comunitaria (SENC). *Consejos para una Alimentación Saludable*; SENC: Madrid, Spain, 2007; p. 42.

47. Wilkinson, S.A.; McIntyre, H.D. Evaluation of the "healthy start to pregnancy" early antenatal health promotion workshop: A randomized controlled trial. *BMC Pregnancy Childbirth* **2012**, *12*, 131.

48. Rautiainen, S.; Wang, L.; Gaziano, J.M.; Sesso, H.D. Who uses multivitamins? A cross-sectional study in the physicians' health study. *Eur. J. Nutr.* **2014**, *53*, 1065–1072.

49. Hu, E.A.; Toledo, E.; Diez-Espino, J.; Estruch, R.; Corella, D.; Salas-Salvado, J.; Vinyoles, E.; Gomez-Gracia, E.; Aros, F.; Fiol, M.; *et al.* Lifestyles and risk factors associated with adherence to the Mediterranean diet: A baseline assessment of the PREDIMED trial. *PLoS One* **2013**, *8*, e60166.

50. Bach-Faig, A.; Berry, E.M.; Lairon, D.; Reguant, J.; Trichopoulou, A.; Dernini, S.; Medina, F.X.; Battino, M.; Belahsen, R.; Miranda, G.; *et al.* Mediterranean diet pyramid today. Science and cultural updates. *Public Health Nutr.* **2011**, *14*, 2274–2284.

51. Navarrete-Munoz, E.M.; Gimenez Monzo, D.; Garcia de La Hera, M.; Climent, M.D.; Rebagliato, M.; Murcia, M.; Iniguez, C.; Ballester, F.; Ramon, R.; Vioque, J. Folic acid intake from diet and supplements in a population of pregnant women in Valencia, Spain. *Med. Clin. (Barc.)* **2010**, *135*, 637–643.

52. Martinez-Frias, M.L.; Grupo de trabajo del ECEMC. Folic acid dose in the prevention of congenital defects. *Med. Clin. (Barc.)* **2007**, *128*, 609–616.

53. Ministerio de Sanidad Servicios Sociales e Igualdad. Evaluación Nutricional de la Dieta Española. II. Micronutrientes. Available online: http://aesan.msssi. gob.es/AESAN/docs/docs/evaluacion_riesgos/estudios_evaluacion_nutricional/ Valoracion_nutricional_ENIDE_micronutrientes.pdf (accessed on 5 June 2014).
54. De-Regil, L.M.; Fernandez-Gaxiola, A.C.; Dowswell, T.; Pena-Rosas, J.P. Effects and safety of periconceptional folate supplementation for preventing birth defects. *Cochrane Database Syst. Rev.* **2010**, *10*, CD007950.
55. Ray, J.G.; Singh, G.; Burrows, R.F. Evidence for suboptimal use of periconceptional folic acid supplements globally. *BJOG* **2004**, *111*, 399–408.
56. Tort, J.; Lelong, N.; Prunet, C.; Khoshnood, B.; Blondel, B. Maternal and health care determinants of preconceptional use of folic acid supplementation in France: Results from the 2010 national perinatal survey. *BJOG* **2013**, *120*, 1661–1667.
57. Sicinska, E.; Wyka, J. Folate intake in Poland on the basis of literature from the last ten years (2000–2010). *Rocz. Panstw. Zakl. Hig.* **2011**, *62*, 247–256.
58. McNally, S.; Bourke, A. Periconceptional folic acid supplementation in a nationally representative sample of mothers. *Ir. Med. J.* **2012**, *105*, 236–238.
59. Silva-del Valle, M.A.; Sanchez-Villegas, A.; Serra-Majem, L. Association between the adherence to the Mediterranean diet and overweight and obesity in pregnant women in Gran Canaria. *Nutr. Hosp.* **2013**, *28*, 654–659.
60. Rodriguez-Bernal, C.L.; Ramon, R.; Quiles, J.; Murcia, M.; Navarrete-Munoz, E.M.; Vioque, J.; Ballester, F.; Rebagliato, M. Dietary intake in pregnant women in a Spanish Mediterranean area: As good as it is supposed to be? *Public Health Nutr.* **2013**, *16*, 1379–1389.
61. Dunlop, A.L.; Logue, K.M.; Thorne, C.; Badal, H.J. Change in women's knowledge of general and personal preconception health risks following targeted brief counseling in publicly funded primary care settings. *Am. J. Health Promot.* **2013**, *27*, S50–S57.
62. Juarez, S.; Revuelta-Eugercios, B.A.; Ramiro-Farinas, D.; Viciana-Fernandez, F. Maternal education and perinatal outcomes among Spanish women residing in southern Spain (2001–2011). *Matern. Child Health J.* **2013**, *18*, 1814–1822.
63. Zhou, S.J.; Anderson, A.J.; Gibson, R.A.; Makrides, M. Effect of iodine supplementation in pregnancy on child development and other clinical outcomes: A systematic review of randomized controlled trials. *Am. J. Clin. Nutr.* **2013**, *98*, 1241–1254.
64. Donnay, S.; Arena, J.; Lucas, A.; Velasco, I.; Ares, S.; Working Group on Disorders Related to Iodine Deficiency and Thyroid Dysfunction of the Spanish Society of Endocrinology and Nutrition. Iodine supplementation during pregnancy and lactation. Position statement of the working group on disorders related to iodine deficiency and thyroid dysfunction of the Spanish society of endocrinology and nutrition. *Endocrinol. Nutr.* **2014**, *61*, 27–34.
65. Sanchez, C.L.; Rodriguez, A.B.; Sanchez, J.; Gonzalez, R.; Rivero, M.; Barriga, C.; Cubero, J. Calcium intake nutritional status in breastfeeding women. *Arch. Latinoam. Nutr.* **2008**, *58*, 371–376.

66. Arija, V.; Cuco, G.; Vila, J.; Iranzo, R.; Fernandez-Ballart, J. Food consumption, dietary habits and nutritional status of the population of Reus: Follow-up from preconception throughout pregnancy and after birth. *Med. Clin. (Barc.)* **2004**, *123*, 5–11.
67. Anderson, A.S. Symposium on "nutritional adaptation to pregnancy and lactation". Pregnancy as a time for dietary change? *Proc. Nutr. Soc.* **2001**, *60*, 497–504.
68. Renfrew, M.J.; McFadden, A.; Bastos, M.H.; Campbell, J.; Channon, A.A.; Cheung, N.F.; Silva, D.R.; Downe, S.; Kennedy, H.P.; Malata, A.; *et al.* Midwifery and quality care: Findings from a new evidence-informed framework for maternal and newborn care. *Lancet* **2014**, *384*, 1129–1145.
69. Wallner, S.; Kendall, P.; Hillers, V.; Bradshaw, E.; Medeiros, L.C. Online continuing education course enhances nutrition and health professionals' knowledge of food safety issues of high-risk populations. *J. Am. Diet. Assoc.* **2007**, *107*, 1333–1338.
70. Suominen, M.H.; Kivisto, S.M.; Pitkala, K.H. The effects of nutrition education on professionals' practice and on the nutrition of aged residents in dementia wards. *Eur. J. Clin. Nutr.* **2007**, *61*, 1226–1232.

Sulphate in Pregnancy

Paul A. Dawson, Aoife Elliott and Francis G. Bowling

Abstract: Sulphate is an obligate nutrient for healthy growth and development. Sulphate conjugation (sulphonation) of proteoglycans maintains the structure and function of tissues. Sulphonation also regulates the bioactivity of steroids, thyroid hormone, bile acids, catecholamines and cholecystokinin, and detoxifies certain xenobiotics and pharmacological drugs. In adults and children, sulphate is obtained from the diet and from the intracellular metabolism of sulphur-containing amino acids. Dietary sulphate intake can vary greatly and is dependent on the type of food consumed and source of drinking water. Once ingested, sulphate is absorbed into circulation where its level is maintained at approximately 300 µmol/L, making sulphate the fourth most abundant anion in plasma. In pregnant women, circulating sulphate concentrations increase by twofold with levels peaking in late gestation. This increased sulphataemia, which is mediated by up-regulation of sulphate reabsorption in the maternal kidneys, provides a reservoir of sulphate to meet the gestational needs of the developing foetus. The foetus has negligible capacity to generate sulphate and thereby, is completely reliant on sulphate supply from the maternal circulation. Maternal hyposulphataemia leads to foetal sulphate deficiency and late gestational foetal death in mice. In humans, reduced sulphonation capacity has been linked to skeletal dysplasias, ranging from the mildest form, multiple epiphyseal dysplasia, to achondrogenesis Type IB, which results in severe skeletal underdevelopment and death *in utero* or shortly after birth. Despite being essential for numerous cellular and metabolic functions, the nutrient sulphate is largely unappreciated in clinical settings. This article will review the physiological roles and regulation of sulphate during pregnancy, with a particular focus on animal models of disturbed sulphate homeostasis and links to human pathophysiology.

Reprinted from *Nutrients*. Cite as: Dawson, P.A.; Elliott, A.; Bowling, F.G. Sulphate in Pregnancy. *Nutrients* **2015**, *7*, 1594–1606.

1. Introduction

Sulphate is an obligate nutrient for numerous metabolic and cellular processes, particularly in foetal growth and development [1]. The conjugation of sulphate (sulphonation) to certain endogenous molecules, including steroids (e.g., oestrogens) and thyroid hormone leads to their inactivation [2–4]. Importantly, the ratio of sulphonated (inactive) to unconjugated (active) hormones plays a role in modulating endocrine function, and therefore foetal and maternal physiology during pregnancy [3]. Additionally, sulphonation of structural components such as chondroitin sulphate, heparan sulphate and cerebroside sulphate is essential for the development and maintenance of tissue structure and function [5,6]. Furthermore, the foetal liver expresses abundant levels of sulphotransferases that mediate the sulphonation and clearance of xenobiotics and certain pharmacological drugs that are potentially detrimental to foetal development [7,8]. This latter role for sulphate is particularly important in human and animal gestation, as the developing foetus has negligible capacity to detoxify xenobiotics via the glucuronidation pathway that is largely inactive in the prenatal period [9,10]. Over the past few decades, numerous roles for sulphate have been described in human physiology (Figure 1A) [11]. However, despite these important physiological roles, sulphate is not routinely measured in clinical settings. Accordingly, this review highlights our current knowledge on sulphate nutrition with a particular focus on the roles and regulation of sulphate in human and animal gestation.

2. Sulphate is Obtained from the Diet

Sulphonation relies on a sufficient supply of sulphate, which is obtained from the diet as free inorganic sulphate (SO_4^{2-}) or generated from sulphonated compounds and the sulphur-containing amino acids, methionine and cysteine [5,12]. A well-balanced diet contributes approximately one third of estimated average body sulphate requirements (0.2–1.5 g SO_4^{2-}/day) [13–16]. Certain foods, including brassica vegetables and commercial breads contain a high sulphate content (>0.9 mg/g), whereas low sulphate levels (<0.1 mg/g) are found in some foods such as fresh apples and oranges [15]. In addition, the sulphate content of drinking water can vary greatly, from negligible levels in demineralised bottle water to >500 mg/L in water from spring-fed wells and dams [13–15]. Sulphate levels exceeding 500 mg/L of drinking water can result in an unpleasant taste, although some individuals are more sensitive to lower concentrations [16]. Inhalation of sulphate in air is estimated to contribute trace amounts (0.01–0.04 mg SO_4^{2-}/day) for adults [17]. In addition, certain prenatal multivitamin-multimineral supplements contain sulphate, primarily in the form of cupric sulphate anhydrous, zinc sulphate and manganese sulphate, with approximately 25–40 mg SO_4^{2-}/tablet.

Sulphate is one of the least toxic anions, with reported lethal doses being 45 g potassium sulphate or zinc sulphate for humans, and a minimal lethal dose of 200 mg/kg magnesium sulphate in mammals [18]. Osmotic diarrhoea has been reported in healthy adult males when they consumed 8 g of sodium sulphate (6.7 g sulphate) as a single dose, and in infants consuming sulphate concentrations >600 mg/L of water with an estimated sulphate intake of ≈66 mg/kg/day [19,20]. In addition, a self-reported laxative effect was reported in most adults consuming water with levels of sulphate 1000 to 2000 mg/L (approximately 14 to 29 mg/kg body weight) [16]. Similar findings of sulphate-induced osmotic diarrhoea have been reported in animal studies [21].

High concentrations of ingested magnesium sulphate have also been linked to osmotic diarrhoea but this is most likely due to the poor absorption of magnesium, as sulphate absorption is much higher [22,23]. Magnesium sulphate is also used for seizure prevention in preeclampsia or eclampsia, as well as a tocolytic agent, being administered i.v. to women shortly before preterm birth [24]. However, this treatment is rather unpleasant for some women with approximately 8% of women requiring cessation of treatment due to intolerable side-effects, including nausea, vomiting, flushing sweating and palpitations [24]. Oral supplements of ferrous sulphate (100 mg $FeSO_4$ per capsule per day, $\approx$63 mg sulphate per capsule) are prescribed to treat iron deficiency anaemia in pregnancy. However, ferrous sulphate can be irritating to the gastrointestinal tract [25], which is largely attributed to the ferrous ions [26]. Comparative data on the effects of different iron preparations have shown that ferrous sulphate may elicit stronger inflammatory processes in the pregnant rat and foetus, when compared to ferrous fumarate [27]. These findings warrant further investigations of ferrous sulphate and other iron preparations in human pregnancy. Whilst the above findings suggest that caution may be warranted in consuming sulphate levels significantly above that found in most foods, there are currently insufficient data to identify an upper intake level to cause adverse effects to human health. Nonetheless, both food ($\approx$0.85 g SO_4^{2-}/day) and drinking water ($\approx$0.78 g SO_4^{2-}/day) provide an important source of sulphate [16], particularly in late gestation when foetal sulphate demands are increasing.

The nutritional value of sulphate in bolstering the growth of laboratory rodents was first reported almost a century ago [28]. More recent animal studies have shown that restricting sulphate in both food and water can lead to sulphate deficiency and reduced growth, which can be reversed by sulphate supplementation [29–32]. In addition, high dietary sulphate intake and administration of sulphate salts ($MgSO_4$, Na_2SO_4 and $ZnSO_4$) can lead to increased circulating sulphataemia and enhanced sulphonation capacity [33–39]. However, there is currently no recommended dietary intake for inorganic sulphate in humans, mainly because sulphate can be generated from the sulphur-containing amino acids.

3. Generation of Sulphate from Intracellular Metabolism

Protein is comprised of approximately 4% of the sulphur-containing amino acids methionine and cysteine [40]. Considering that the recommended daily intake of protein for 19–50 year olds in pregnancy is 0.8–1.0 g/kg [41], then the estimated amount of sulphate generated from protein is approximately 1.7 g/day. Both adults and children have the capacity to metabolise methionine and cysteine to sulphate [1]. Methionine is converted to cysteine via the transsulphuration pathway, and cysteine is further oxidised to sulphate via 2 pathways: A minor pathway of sulphate generation via cystathionine γ-lyase (CTH) and cystathionine β-synthase (CBS);

and a major pathway via cysteine dioxygenase (CDO) (Figure 1B) [42]. Earlier studies reported the absence of CTH and CDO in human and rodent foetal liver, indicating that the developing foetus has a limited capacity to generate sulphate from the sulphur-containing amino acids [43,44]. This raises the question of which sources supply the high foetal demands for sulphate during pregnancy?

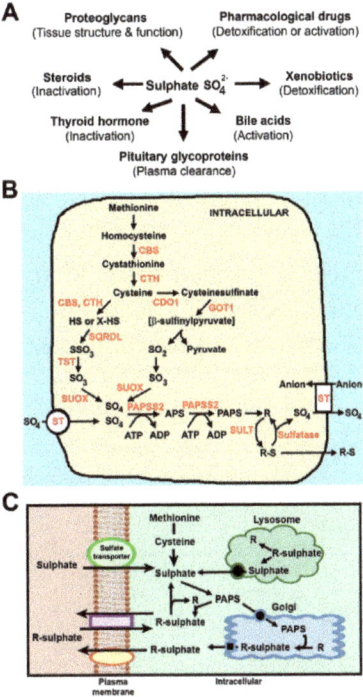

Figure 1. Biological roles of sulphate and pathways of sulphate homeostasis. (A) Sulphonation contributes to numerous cellular and metabolic functions in human physiology; (B) Pathways of intracellular sulphate generation and sulphonation. Methionine is converted to cysteine via the transsulphuration pathway involving cystathionine β-synthase (CBS) and cystathionine γ-lyase (CTH). Cysteine is converted to sulphate via two pathways: A minor pathway involving CBS, CTH, sulphide quinone reductase-like (SQRDL), thiosulphate sulphurtransferase (TST) and sulphite oxidase (SUOX); and a major pathway involving cysteine dioxygenase (CDO), glutamic-oxaloacetic transaminase 1 (GOT1) and SUOX. ST, Sulphate transporters; PAPSS2, PAPS synthetase; SULT, sulphotransferases; R represents those substrates shown in (A); (C) Flux of intracellular sulphate and sulphonated molecules. In adults and children, sulphate is obtained from: (i) extracellular sources via sulphate transporters; (ii) catabolism of methionine and cysteine; (iii) hydrolysis of proteoglycans in the lysosome; and (iv) sulphatase-mediated removal of sulphate from substrates in the cytosol.

113

In adults and children, circulating sulphate levels are influenced by absorption in the small intestine, reabsorption in the kidneys, and uptake into cells throughout the body (Figure 2A) [1]. Circulating sulphate is a major source of sulphate for supplying the intracellular sulphonation of substrates in the cytoplasm (steroids, hormones, xenobiotics and proteins) or golgi apparatus (proteoglycans) [45,46]. However, the overall flux of intracellular sulphate is maintained by four pathways (Figure 1C): (i) Extracellular sulphate from circulation is transported through the plasma membrane of cells via sulphate transporters; (ii) Methionine and cysteine are catabolised to sulphate; (iii) Sulphate is removed from proteoglycans via sulphatase enzymes in the lysosome and then transported into the cytoplasm; and (iv) Cytosolic sulphatases remove sulphate from sulphonated molecules. The latter three sources have negligible or low contributions to the foetal intracellular sulphate pool, which is therefore reliant on extracellular sources sulphate [1]. In addition, the developing foetus has immature renal reabsorption and intestinal absorption capacities, highlighting the obligate requirements for supplying sulphate from mother to foetus via the placenta throughout gestation.

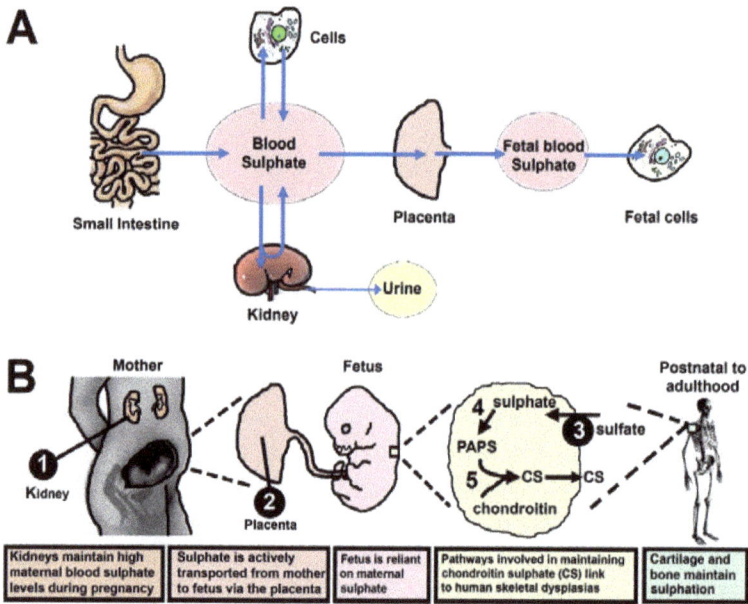

Figure 2. Fluxes of sulphate between tissues. (**A**) Contribution of the small intestine, kidneys and cells to sulphate homeostasis (**B**) Maternal, foetal and postnatal contributions to chondroitin sulphation. Disruption of pathways that maintain a sufficient supply of sulphate for chondrocytes (steps 1–3) or intracellular sulphonation of chondroitin (steps 4–5) lead to chondrodysplasias.

4. Sulphate Is Supplied from Mother to Foetus

During human and rodent pregnancy, maternal circulating sulphate levels increase by more than twofold to meet the gestational needs of the growing foetus [47,48], and this is remarkable because most plasma ion concentrations usually decrease slightly in pregnancy due to haemodilution [49] and speaks to its crucial role in foetal development. The increased maternal blood sulphate levels arise from increased sulphate reabsorption in the mother's kidneys (Figure 2B) [47,48], which is mediated by increased renal expression of the *SLC13A1* gene (aka NaS1, sodium sulphate transporter 1) [50]. Disruption of *SLC13A1* in humans and mice causes sulphate wasting into the urine [51,52], and this greatly reduces blood sulphate levels (hyposulphataemia). In mice, loss of the *Slc13a1* gene leads to behavioural abnormalities (reduced memory and olfactory function, and increased anxiety), reduced brain serotonin levels, growth retardation, impaired gastrointestinal mucin sulphonation and enhanced acetaminophen-induced liver toxicity [33,51–58]. In addition, pregnant female *Slc13a1* null mice exhibit hyposulphataemia throughout gestation, which leads to foetal sulphate deficiency and mid-gestational miscarriage [48].

A related gene *SLC13A4* (aka NaS2, sodium sulphate transporter 2) was recently found to be the most abundant sulphate transporter in the human and mouse placenta [50,59]. *SLC13A4* is localised to the syncytiotrophoblast layer of the placenta, the site of maternal-foetal nutrient exchange, where it is proposed to be supplying sulphate from mother to foetus [59]. Loss of placental SLC13A4 in mice leads to severe foetal developmental abnormalities and late gestational foetal death, highlighting the obligate requirement of sulphate for healthy foetal growth and development [60].

Over the past decade, interest in the roles and regulation of sulphate during pregnancy has expanded following the characterisation of growth restriction and foetal demise in animal models of reduced sulphonation capacity [11]. For example, mice lacking the Sult1e1 oestrogen sulphotransferase exhibit mid-gestational foetal loss [61]. Sult1e1 is expressed in the placenta where it is essential for generating the sulphonated forms of estrone sulphate, estradiol-3-sulphate and estriol sulphate. Foetal loss and impaired foetal growth have also been linked to several other sulphotransferases and sulphatases that maintain the required biological ratio of sulphonated to unconjugated proteins and proteoglycans [11]. Despite the evidence from animal studies that show the physiological importance for sulphate during pregnancy, there are no routine measurements of sulphate in clinical settings.

In humans, free inorganic sulphate (SO_4^{2-}) is the fourth most abundant anion in circulation (approximately 300 µmol/L) [62]. Early studies reported a twofold increase in plasma sulphate levels in pregnant women [35,63–65]. More recent studies used a validated ion chromatography method to establish reference ranges for maternal plasma sulphate levels in early (10–20 weeks) and late (30–37 weeks) gestation, as well as cord plasma sulphate levels from healthy term pregnancies [47]. These data will now enable clinical investigations into the outcomes of low plasma sulphate levels in mother and child, and will most likely expand our current knowledge into the consequences of sulphate deficiency, particularly skeletal development, which is sensitive to sulphate deficiency.

5. Reduced Sulphonation Capacity Perturbs Skeletal Growth and Development

In mammals, sulphonated proteoglycans are an essential component of extracellular matrices throughout the body, particularly in connective tissues [66,67]. The sulphate content of proteoglycans influences cell signalling function and the structural integrity of tissues [5]. Highly sulphonated glycoproteins, including chondroitin proteoglycan (CSPG), play important roles in the developing skeleton, with links to modulation of the Indian Hedgehog signalling pathway [68]. Importantly, sulphonation of CSPGs in chondrocytes is essential for normal skeletal growth and development, and several skeletal disorders have been attributed to genetic defects that lead to decreased sulphonation capacity [11].

Chondrocytes rely on an abundant supply of extracellular sulphate, to meet the intracellular demands for CSPG sulphonation (Figure 2B). Sulphate is transported into chondrocytes via the SLC26A2 sulphate transporter (step 3 of Figure 2B) [69]. More than 30 mutations in the human *SLC26A2* gene have been linked to chondrodysplasias [70], with the underlying metabolic defect being reduced sulphonation of chondroitin in chondrocytes [71]. Mutant *Slc26a2* mice also exhibit chondrodysplasias which mimics the biochemical and morphological phenotypes found in humans [71–73]. Treatment of the mutant *Slc26a2* mice with dietary *N*-acetyl cysteine, showed increased proteoglycan sulphonation and improved skeletal phenotypes [31], suggesting that thiol-containing compounds can bolster the intracellular sulphate levels needed for sulphonation of CSPGs.

Loss of PAPS (3'-phosphoadenosine 5'-phosphosulphate) synthetase has also been linked to impaired CSPG sulphonation and skeletal dysplasias [74]. PAPS is the universal sulphonate donor for all sulphonation reactions and its formation relies on a sufficient intracellular supply of sulphate (step 4 in Figure 2B) [75]. Mammalian genomes contain two PAPS synthetase genes, *PAPSS1* and *PAPSS2* [76–78]. *PAPSS2* has been linked to human pathophysiology, with similar skeletal phenotypes found in *Papss2* mutant mice [76,78]. In addition, disruption of the zebrafish PAPS transporter gene (*PAPST1*, aka *pinscher*) leads to cartilage defects [79]. Skeletal phenotypes are also found in patients with mutations in the chondroitin 6-*O*-sulphotransferase gene (step 5 in Figure 2B) [80], showing that chondroitin sulphonation is important for maintaining healthy skeletal development. These findings highlight the importance of pathways that lead to chondroitin sulphation for healthy development, growth and maintenance of the skeleton.

Currently, there is no cure for the most severe skeletal dysplasia forms, atelosteogenesis Type II and achondrogenesis Type IB, which result in skeletal underdevelopment and death *in utero* or in the neonatal period [70]. The mild (multiple epiphyseal) and moderate (diastrophic dysplasia) forms of the disease are treated with orthopaedic and pain management but these patients face a lifetime of disability. Other genes including *PAPSS2* have involvement with abnormal skeletal growth and development in humans [76], and the clinical spectrum associated with *PAPSS2* and *SLC26A2* has further expanded to include knee osteoarthritis [81], suggesting that sulphation disorders are likely to be more prevalent than the estimated 2% of all skeletal dysplasias which is based on live births [82]. This is also relevant to recent studies that have linked the renal *Slc13a1* sulphate transporter gene, which is important for maintaining circulating sulphate levels, to skeletal dysplasias in animals [83,84]. These findings are likely to be relevant for human skeletal growth and development. Collectively, the lack of curative treatments for the skeletal sulphonation disorders leads to significant burden on families and community [85].

The biochemical basis of under-sulphation in the skeletal sulphation disorders is well established [69,70,86] and warrants approaches to the development of therapies for increasing sulphation capacity. Prenatal diagnosis of babies with nonlethal sulphation disorders is helpful for clinical geneticists, neonatologists, obstetricians and anaesthesiologists to plan delivery and improve postnatal outcomes. However, many of these surviving babies face life-long physical impairments, placing a huge burden on affected families [85]. Currently, there is no cure for individuals with skeletal sulphonation disorders. Conventional treatments, including orthopaedic intervention and pain management for the non-lethal forms are inadequate and warrant develop of new therapeutic approaches. In humans, there is a dosage effect of sulphonation capacity on clinical outcomes, with negligible/low sulphonation leading to the lethal and severe skeletal dysplasias, whereas moderate reductions in sulphation give rise to milder clinical outcomes [70]. The dosage effect suggests that strategies which can increase sulphonation capacity in the skeleton should ameliorate the clinical presentations. This is relevant to the high foetal demands for sulphate in mid- to late-gestation [1], which provides a window in gestation when sulphate supplementation therapies may potentially provide the most benefit for foetuses affected by a skeletal sulphation disorder. If simple low cost maternal dietary interventions, using sulphonated compounds, could increase sulphonation capacity in the developing foetal skeleton, then this could potentially have enormous benefits for ameliorating the skeletal phenotypes in affected individuals.

6. Conclusion

Sulphate is an obligate nutrient for healthy growth and development. Despite being essential for numerous cellular and metabolic processes in foetal development, its importance is largely underappreciated in clinical settings. Animal models have shown the devastating physiological outcomes of reduced sulphonation capacity on foetal growth and development, which is relevant to the established link with human chondrodysplasias. A sufficient supply of sulphate, either from the diet or from the sulphur-containing amino acids, needs to be supplied from mother to foetus, particularly in late gestation when foetal demands for sulphate are high. The development of a validated method for sulphate quantitation, together with recent data for maternal plasma sulphate reference ranges, now warrants further investigations into the consequences of nutrient sulphate deficiency in mother and child.

Acknowledgments: This work was supported by the Mater Medical Research Institute, Mater Foundation and a Mater Foundation Research Fellowship to PAD.

Author Contributions: PAD conceived of the topic, participated in the design and coordination, and drafted the manuscript. AE and FGB participated in the design of the article, and helped draft the manuscript. All authors read and approved the final manuscript.

Conflicts of Interest: The authors declare no conflict of interest.

References

1. Dawson, P.A. Sulfate in fetal development. *Semin. Cell Dev. Biol.* **2011**, *22*, 653–659.
2. Darras, V.M.; Hume, R.; Visser, T.J. Regulation of thyroid hormone metabolism during fetal development. *Mol. Cell. Endocrinol.* **1999**, *151*, 37–47.
3. Dawson, P.A. The biological roles of steroid sulfonation. In *Steroids—From Physiology to Clinical Medicine*; Ostojic, S.M., Ed.; Intech: Rijeka, Croatia, 2012; pp. 45–64.
4. Richard, K.; Hume, R.; Kaptein, E.; Stanley, E.L.; Visser, T.J.; Coughtrie, M.W. Sulfation of thyroid hormone and dopamine during human development: Ontogeny of phenol sulfotransferases and arylsulfatase in liver, lung, and brain. *J. Clin. Endocrinol. Metab.* **2001**, *86*, 2734–2742.
5. Mulder, G.J.; Jakoby, W.B. Sulfation. In *Conjugation Reactions in Drug Metabolism: An Integrated Approach: Substrates, Co-substrates, Enzymes and Their Interactions in Vivo and in Vitro*; Mulder, G.J., Ed.; Taylor and Francis: London, UK, 1990; pp. 107–161.
6. Yamaguchi, Y. Heparan sulfate proteoglycans in the nervous system: Their diverse roles in neurogenesis, axon guidance, and synaptogenesis. *Semin. Cell Dev. Biol.* **2001**, *12*, 99–106.
7. Alnouti, Y.; Klaassen, C.D. Tissue distribution and ontogeny of sulfotransferase enzymes in mice. *Toxicol. Sci.* **2006**, *93*, 242–255.

8. Stanley, E.L.; Hume, R.; Coughtrie, M.W. Expression profiling of human fetal cytosolic sulfotransferases involved in steroid and thyroid hormone metabolism and in detoxification. *Mol. Cell. Endocrinol.* **2005**, *240*, 32–42.

9. Hines, R.N.; McCarver, D.G. The ontogeny of human drug-metabolizing enzymes: Phase I oxidative enzymes. *J. Pharmacol. Exp. Ther.* **2002**, *300*, 355–360.

10. McCarver, D.G.; Hines, R.N. The ontogeny of human drug-metabolizing enzymes: Phase II conjugation enzymes and regulatory mechanisms. *J. Pharmacol. Exp. Ther.* **2002**, *300*, 361–366.

11. Dawson, P.A. Role of sulphate in development. *Reproduction* **2013**, *146*, R81–R89.

12. Smith, J.T.; Acuff, R.V. An effect of dietary sulfur on liver inorganic sulfate in the rat. *Ann. Nutr. Metab.* **1983**, *27*, 345–348.

13. Allen, H.E.; Halley-Henderson, M.A.; Hass, C.N. Chemical composition of bottled mineral water. *Arch. Environ. Health* **1989**, *44*, 102–116.

14. Florin, T.; Neale, G.; Gibson, G.R.; Christl, S.U.; Cummings, J.H. Metabolism of dietary sulphate: Absorption and excretion in humans. *Gut* **1991**, *32*, 766–773.

15. Florin, T.H.J.; Neale, G.; Goretski, S.; Cummings, J.H. The sulfate content of foods and beverages. *J. Food Compos. Anal.* **1993**, *6*, 140–151.

16. National Research Council. Sulfate. In *Dietary Reference Intakes for Water, Potassium, Sodium, Chloride, and Sulfate*; The National Academies Press: Washington, DC, USA, 2005; pp. 424–448.

17. Health Canada. Sulphate. Available online: http://www.hc-sc.gc.ca/ewh-semt/pubs/water-eau/sulphate-sulfates/index-eng.php (accessed on 17 February 2015).

18. U.S. Environmental Protection Agency. Drinking Water Advisory: Consumer Acceptability Advice and Health Effects Analysis on Sulfate. 2003. Available online: http://water.epa.gov/action/advisories/drinking/upload/2008_01_10_support_cc1_sulfate_healtheffects.pdf (accessed on 17 February 2015).

19. Chien, L.; Robertson, H.; Gerrard, J.W. Infantile gastroenteritis due to water with high sulfate content. *Can. Med. Assoc. J.* **1968**, *99*, 102–104.

20. Cocchetto, D.M.; Levy, G. Absorption of orally administered sodium sulfate in humans. *J. Pharm. Sci.* **1981**, *70*, 331–333.

21. Paterson, D.W.; Wahlstrom, R.C.; Libal, G.W.; Olson, O.E. Effects of sulfate in water on swine reproduction and young pig performance. *J. Anim. Sci.* **1979**, *49*, 664–667.

22. Izzo, A.A.; Gaginella, T.S.; Capasso, F. The osmotic and intrinsic mechanisms of the pharmacological laxative action of oral high doses of magnesium sulphate. Importance of the release of digestive polypeptides and nitric oxide. *Magnes. Res.* **1996**, *9*, 133–138.

23. Morris, M.E.; LeRoy, S.; Sutton, S.C. Absorption of magnesium from orally administered magnesium sulfate in man. *J. Toxicol. Clin. Toxicol.* **1987**, *25*, 371–382.

24. Doyle, L.W.; Crowther, C.A.; Middleton, P.; Marret, S.; Rouse, D. Magnesium sulphate for women at risk of preterm birth for neuroprotection of the fetus. *Cochrane Database Syst. Rev.* **2007**, *18*, CD004661.

25. Panarelli, N.C. Drug-induced injury in the gastrointestinal tract. *Semin. Diagn. Pathol.* **2014**, *31*, 165–175.

26. Proudfoot, A.T.; Simpson, D.; Dyson, E.H. Management of acute iron poisoning. *Med. Toxicol.* **1986**, *1*, 83–100.

27. Toblli, J.E.; Cao, G.; Oliveri, L.; Angerosa, M. Effects of iron polymaltose complex, ferrous fumarate and ferrous sulfate treatments in anemic pregnant rats, their fetuses and placentas. *Inflamm. Allergy Drug Targets* **2013**, *12*, 190–198.

28. Daniels, A.L.; Rich, J.K. The role of inorganic sulfates in nutrition. *J. Biol. Chem.* **1918**, *36*, 27–32.

29. Hou, C.; Wykes, L.J.; Hoffer, L.J. Urinary sulfur excretion and the nitrogen/sulfur balance ratio reveal nonprotein sulfur amino acid retention in piglets. *J. Nutr.* **2003**, *133*, 766–772.

30. McGarry, P.C.; Roe, D.A. Development of sulfur depletion in pregnant and fetal rats: Interaction of protein restriction and indole or salicylamide administration. *J. Nutr.* **1973**, *103*, 1279–1290.

31. Pecora, F.; Gualeni, B.; Forlino, A.; Superti-Furga, A.; Tenni, R.; Cetta, G.; Rossi, A. *In vivo* contribution of amino acid sulfur to cartilage proteoglycan sulfation. *Biochem. J.* **2006**, *398*, 509–514.

32. Price, V.F.; Jollow, D.J. Effects of sulfur-amino acid-deficient diets on acetaminophen metabolism and hepatotoxicity in rats. *Toxicol. Appl. Pharmacol.* **1989**, *101*, 356–369.

33. Dawson, P.A.; Gardiner, B.; Lee, S.; Grimmond, S.; Markovich, D. Kidney transcriptome reveals altered steroid homeostasis in NaS1 sulfate transporter null mice. *J. Steroid Biochem. Mol. Biol.* **2008**, *112*, 55–62.

34. Hindmarsh, K.W.; Mayers, D.J.; Wallace, S.M.; Danilkewich, A.; Ernst, A. Increased serum sulfate concentrations in man due to environmental factors: Effects on acetaminophen metabolism. *Vet. Hum. Toxicol.* **1991**, *33*, 441–445.

35. Morris, M.E.; Levy, G. Serum concentration and renal excretion by normal adults of inorganic sulfate after acetaminophen, ascorbic acid, or sodium sulfate. *Clin. Pharmacol. Ther.* **1983**, *33*, 529–536.

36. Ricci, J.; Oster, J.R.; Gutierrez, R.; Schlessinger, F.B.; Rietberg, B.; O'Sullivan, M.J.; Clerch, A.R.; Vaamonde, C.A. Influence of magnesium sulfate-induced hypermagnesemia on the anion gap: Role of hypersulfatemia. *Am. J. Nephrol.* **1990**, *10*, 409–411.

37. Slattery, J.T.; Levy, G. Reduction of acetaminophen toxicity by sodium sulfate in mice. *Res. Commun. Chem. Pathol. Pharmacol.* **1977**, *18*, 167–170.

38. Waring, R.; Klovrza, L.V. Sulphur metabolism in autism. *J. Nutr. Environ. Med.* **2000**, *10*, 25–32.

39. Wu, Y.; Zhang, X.; Bardag-Gorce, F.; Robel, R.C.; Aguilo, J.; Chen, L.; Zeng, Y.; Hwang, K.; French, S.W.; Lu, S.C.; *et al.* Retinoid X receptor alpha regulates glutathione homeostasis and xenobiotic detoxification processes in mouse liver. *Mol. Pharmacol.* **2004**, *65*, 550–557.

40. Brand, E. Amino acid composition of simple proteins. *Ann. NY Acad. Sci.* **1946**, *47*, 187–228.

41. Australian Government. *Nutrient Reference Values for Australia and New Zealand*; NHMRC: Canberra, Australia, 2014.

42. Ueki, I.; Roman, H.B.; Valli, A.; Fieselmann, K.; Lam, J.; Peters, R.; Hirschberger, L.L.; Stipanuk, M.H. Knockout of the murine cysteine dioxygenase gene results in severe impairment in ability to synthesize taurine and an increased catabolism of cysteine to hydrogen sulfide. *Am. J. Physiol. Endocrinol. Metab.* **2011**, *301*, E668–E684.

43. Gaull, G.; Sturman, J.A.; Raiha, N.C. Development of mammalian sulfur metabolism: Absence of cystathionase in human fetal tissues. *Pediatr. Res.* **1972**, *6*, 538–547.

44. Loriette, C.; Chatagner, F. Cysteine oxidase and cysteine sulfinic acid decarboxylase in developing rat liver. *Experientia* **1978**, *34*, 981–982.

45. Strott, C.A. Steroid sulfotransferases. *Endocr. Rev.* **1996**, *17*, 670–697.

46. Strott, C.A. Sulfonation and molecular action. *Endocr. Rev.* **2002**, *23*, 703–732.

47. Dawson, P.A.; McIntyre, H.D.; Petersen, S.; Gibbons, K.; Bowling, F.G.; Hurrion, E. Sulfate in human pregnancy and preterm babies: What we ought to know. *J. Paed. Child Health* **2014**, *50*, 46.

48. Dawson, P.A.; Sim, P.; Simmons, D.G.; Markovich, D. Fetal loss and hyposulfataemia in pregnant NaS1 transporter null mice. *J. Reprod. Dev.* **2011**, *57*, 444–449.

49. Lind, T. Clinical chemistry of pregnancy. *Adv. Clin. Chem.* **1980**, *21*, 1–24.

50. Dawson, P.A.; Rakoczy, J.; Simmons, D.G. Placental, renal, and ileal sulfate transporter gene expression in mouse gestation. *Biol. Reprod.* **2012**, *87*, 1–9.

51. Bowling, F.G.; Heussler, H.S.; McWhinney, A.; Dawson, P.A. Plasma and urinary sulfate determination in a cohort with autism. *Biochem. Genet.* **2012**, *51*, 147–153.

52. Dawson, P.A.; Beck, L.; Markovich, D. Hyposulfatemia, growth retardation, reduced fertility and seizures in mice lacking a functional NaS_i-1 gene. *Proc. Natl. Acad. Sci. USA* **2003**, *100*, 13704–13709.

53. Dawson, P.A.; Gardiner, B.; Grimmond, S.; Markovich, D. Transcriptional profile reveals altered hepatic lipid and cholesterol metabolism in hyposulfatemic NaS1 null mice. *Physiol. Genomics* **2006**, *26*, 116–124.

54. Dawson, P.A.; Huxley, S.; Gardiner, B.; Tran, T.; McAuley, J.L.; Grimmond, S.; McGuckin, M.A.; Markovich, D. Reduced mucin sulfonation and impaired intestinal barrier function in the hyposulfataemic NaS1 null mouse. *Gut* **2009**, *58*, 910–919.

55. Dawson, P.A.; Steane, S.E.; Markovich, D. Behavioural abnormalities of the hyposulfataemic Nas1 knock-out mouse. *Behav. Brain Res.* **2004**, *154*, 457–463.

56. Dawson, P.A.; Steane, S.E.; Markovich, D. Impaired memory and olfactory performance in NaSi-1 sulphate transporter deficient mice. *Behav. Brain Res.* **2005**, *159*, 15–20.

57. Lee, S.; Dawson, P.A.; Hewavitharana, A.K.; Shaw, P.N.; Markovich, D. Disruption of NaS1 sulfate transport function in mice leads to enhanced acetaminophen-induced hepatotoxicity. *Hepatology* **2006**, *43*, 1241–7124.

58. Lee, S.; Kesby, J.P.; Muslim, M.D.; Steane, S.E.; Eyles, D.W.; Dawson, P.A.; Markovich, D. Hyperserotonaemia and reduced brain serotonin levels in NaS1 sulphate transporter null mice. *Neuroreport* **2007**, *18*, 1981–1985.

59. Simmons, D.G.; Rakoczy, J.; Jefferis, J.; Lourie, R.; McIntyre, H.D.; Dawson, P.A. Human placental sulfate transporter mRNA profiling identifies abundant SLC13A4 in syncytiotrophoblasts and SLC26A2 in cytotrophoblasts. *Placenta* **2013**, *34*, 381–384.

60. Rakoczy, J.; Dawson, P.A.; Simmons, D.G. Loss of placental sulphate transporter SLC13A4 causes severe developmental defects and embryonic lethality. *Placenta* **2014**, *35*, A96–A97.

61. Tong, M.H.; Jiang, H.; Liu, P.; Lawson, J.A.; Brass, L.F.; Song, W.C. Spontaneous fetal loss caused by placental thrombosis in estrogen sulfotransferase-deficient mice. *Nat. Med.* **2005**, *11*, 153–159.

62. Cole, D.E.; Evrovski, J. The clinical chemistry of inorganic sulfate. *Crit. Rev. Clin. Lab. Sci.* **2000**, *37*, 299–344.

63. Cole, D.E.; Baldwin, L.S.; Stirk, L.J. Increased inorganic sulfate in mother and fetus at parturition: Evidence for a fetal-to-maternal gradient. *Am. J. Obstet. Gynecol.* **1984**, *148*, 596–599.

64. Cole, D.E.; Baldwin, L.S.; Stirk, L.J. Increased serum sulfate in pregnancy: Relationship to gestational age. *Clin. Chem.* **1985**, *31*, 866–867.

65. Tallgren, L.G. Inorganic sulphate in relation to the serum thyroxine level and in renal failure. *Acta Med. Scand.* **1980**, *640*, 1–100.

66. Habuchi, H.; Habuchi, O.; Kimata, K. Sulfation pattern in glycosaminoglycan: Does it have a code? *Glycoconj. J.* **2004**, *21*, 47–52.

67. Klüppel, M. The roles of chondroitin-4-sulfotransferase-1 in development and disease. *Prog. Mol. Biol. Transl. Sci.* **2010**, *93*, 113–132.

68. Cortes, M.; Baria, A.T.; Schwartz, N.B. Sulfation of chondroitin sulfate proteoglycans is necessary for proper Indian hedgehog signaling in the developing growth plate. *Development* **2009**, *136*, 1697–1706.

69. Rossi, A.; Bonaventure, J.; Delezoide, A.L.; Superti-Furga, A.; Cetta, G. Undersulfation of cartilage proteoglycans *ex vivo* and increased contribution of amino acid sulfur to sulfation *in vitro* in McAlister dysplasia/atelosteogenesis type 2. *Eur. J. Biochem.* **1997**, *248*, 741–747.

70. Dawson, P.A.; Markovich, D. Pathogenetics of the human SLC26 transporters. *Curr. Med. Chem.* **2005**, *12*, 385–396.

71. Cornaglia, A.I.; Casasco, A.; Casasco, M.; Riva, F.; Necchi, V. Dysplastic histogenesis of cartilage growth plate by alteration of sulphation pathway: A transgenic model. *Connect. Tissue Res.* **2009**, *50*, 232–242.

72. Forlino, A.; Piazza, R.; Tiveron, C.; Della Torre, S.; Tatangelo, L.; Bonafe, L.; Gualeni, B.; Romano, A.; Pecora, F.; Superti-Furga, A.; *et al.* A diastrophic dysplasia sulfate transporter (SLC26A2) mutant mouse: Morphological and biochemical characterization of the resulting chondrodysplasia phenotype. *Hum. Mol. Genet.* **2005**, *14*, 859–871.

73. Hästbacka, J.; de la Chapelle, A.; Mahtani, M.; Clines, G.; Reeve-Daly, M.P.; Daly, M.; Hamilton, B.A.; Kusumi, K.; Trivedi, B.; Weaver, A.; *et al.* The diastrophic dysplasia gene encodes a novel sulfate transporter: Positional cloning by fine-structure linkage disequilibrium mapping. *Cell* **1994**, *78*, 1073–1087.

74. Sugahara, K.; Schwartz, N.B. Defect in 3'-phosphoadenosine 5'-phosphosulfate synthesis in brachymorphic mice. I. Characterization of the defect. *Arch. Biochem. Biophys.* **1982**, *214*, 589–601.

75. Klassen, C.D.; Boles, J. The importance of 3'-phosphoadenosine 5'-phosphosulfate (PAPS) in the regulation of sulfation. *FASEB J.* **1997**, *11*, 404–418.

76. Faiyaz ul Haque, M.; King, L.M.; Krakow, D.; Cantor, R.M.; Rusiniak, M.E.; Swank, R.T.; Superti-Furga, A.; Haque, S.; Abbas, H.; Ahmad, W.; *et al.* Mutations in orthologous genes in human spondyloepimetaphyseal dysplasia and the brachymorphic mouse. *Nat. Genet.* **1998**, *20*, 157–162.

77. Kurima, K.; Warman, M.L.; Krishnan, S.; Domowicz, M.; Krueger, R.C., Jr.; Deyrup, A.; Schwartz, N.B. A member of a family of sulfate-activating enzymes causes murine brachymorphism. *Proc. Natl. Acad. Sci. USA* **1998**, *95*, 8681–8685.

78. Xu, Z.H.; Otterness, D.M.; Freimuth, R.R.; Carlini, E.J.; Wood, T.C.; Mitchell, S.; Moon, E.; Kim, U.J.; Xu, J.P.; Siciliano, M.J.; *et al.* Human 3'-phosphoadenosine 5'-phosphosulfate synthetase 1 (PAPSS1) and PAPSS2: Gene cloning, characterization and chromosomal localization. *Biochem. Biophys. Res. Commun.* **2000**, *268*, 437–444.

79. Clément, A.; Wiweger, M.; von der Hardt, S.; Rusch, M.A.; Selleck, S.B.; Chien, C.B.; Roehl, H.H. Regulation of zebrafish skeletogenesis by ext2/dackel and papst1/pinscher. *PLoS Genet.* **2008**, *4*, e1000136.

80. Thiele, H.; Sakano, M.; Kitagawa, H.; Sugahara, K.; Rajab, A.; Höhne, W.; Ritter, H.; Leschik, G.; Nürnberg, P.; Mundlos, S. Loss of chondroitin 6-O-sulfotransferase-1 function results in severe human chondrodysplasia with progressive spinal involvement. *Proc. Natl. Acad. Sci. USA* **2004**, *101*, 10155–10160.

81. Ikeda, T.; Mabuchi, A.; Fukuda, A.; Hiraoka, H.; Kawakami, A.; Yamamoto, S.; Machida, H.; Takatori, Y.; Kawaguchi, H.; Nakamura, K.; Ikegawa, S. Identification of sequence polymorphisms in two sulfation-related genes, PAPSS2 and SLC26A2, and an association analysis with knee osteoarthritis. *J. Hum. Genet.* **2001**, *46*, 538–543.

82. Stevenson, D.A.; Carey, J.C.; Byrne, J.L.; Srisukhumbowornchai, S.; Feldkamp, M.L. Analysis of skeletal dysplasias in the Utah population. *Am. J. Med. Genet. A* **2012**, *158A*, 1046–1054.

83. Neff, M.W.; Beck, J.S.; Koeman, J.M.; Boguslawski, E.; Kefene, L.; Borgman, A.; Ruhe, A.L. Partial deletion of the sulfate transporter SLC13A1 is associated with an osteochondrodysplasia in the Miniature Poodle breed. *PLoS One* **2012**, *7*, e51917.

84. Zhao, X.; Onteru, S.K.; Piripi, S.; Thompson, K.G.; Blair, H.T.; Garrick, D.J.; Rothschild, M.F. In a shake of a lamb's tail: Using genomics to unravel a cause of chondrodysplasia in Texel sheep. *Anim. Genet.* **2012**, *43*, 9–18.

85. Orenius, T.; Krüger, L.; Kautiainen, H.; Hurri, H.; Pohjolainen, T. The sense of coherence and its relation to health factors among patients with diastrophic dysplasia. *J. Pub. Health Epidem.* **2012**, *4*, 305–310.

86. Rossi, A.; Kaitila, I.; Wilcox, W.R.; Rimoin, D.L.; Steinmann, B.; Cetta, G.; Superti-Furga, A. Proteoglycan sulfation in cartilage and cell cultures from patients with sulfate transporter chondrodysplasias: Relationship to clinical severity and indications on the role of intracellular sulfate production. *Matrix Biol.* **1998**, *17*, 361–369.

Maternal Consumption of Non-Staple Food in the First Trimester and Risk of Neural Tube Defects in Offspring

Meng Wang, Zhi-Ping Wang, Li-Jie Gao, Hui Yang and Zhong-Tang Zhao

Abstract: To study the associations between maternal consumption of non-staple food in the first trimester and risk of neural tube defects (NTDs) in offspring. Data collected from a hospital-based case-control study conducted between 2006 and 2008 in Shandong/Shanxi provinces including 459 mothers with NTDs-affected births and 459 mothers without NTDs-affected births. Logistic regression models were used to examine the associations between maternal consumption of non-staple food in the first trimester and risk of NTDs in offspring. The effects were evaluated by odds ratio (OR) and 95% confidence intervals (95% CIs) with SAS9.1.3.software. Maternal consumption of milk, fresh fruits and nuts in the first trimester were protective factors for total NTDs. Compared with consumption frequency of <1 meal/week, the ORs for milk consumption frequency of 1–2, 3–6, ≥7 meals/week were 0.50 (95% CI: 0.28–0.88), 0.56 (0.32–0.99), and 0.59 (0.38–0.90), respectively; the ORs for fresh fruits consumption frequency of 1–2, 3–6, ≥7 meals/week were 0.29 (95% CI: 0.12–0.72), 0.22 (0.09–0.53), and 0.32 (0.14–0.71), respectively; the ORs for nuts consumption frequency of 1–2, 3–6, ≥7 meals/week were 0.60 (95% CI: 0.38–0.94), 0.49 (0.31–0.79), and 0.63 (0.36–1.08), respectively. Different effects of above factors on NTDs were found for subtypes of anencephaly and spina bifida. Maternal non-staple food consumption of milk, fresh fruits and nuts in the first trimester was associated with reducing NTDs risk in offspring.

Reprinted from *Nutrients*. Cite as: Wang, M.; Wang, Z.-P.; Gao, L.-J.; Yang, H.; Zhao, Z.-T. Maternal Consumption of Non-Staple Food in the First Trimester and Risk of Neural Tube Defects in Offspring. *Nutrients* **2015**, 7, 3067–3077.

1. Introduction

Neural tube defects (NTDs) are a group of severe human congenital malformations caused by the incomplete closure of neural tube within about 28 days following conception [1]. NTDs are complex disorders and appear to be affected by multiple factors, with both genetic and environmental contributions. Folic acid and vitamin B12, as crucial factors for metabolic pathways, have been extensively studied and demonstrated the important roles in development of NTDs [2,3]. Since the introduction of folic acid fortification in staple food, many countries have reported declines in NTDs incidence overall [4–9]. However, a large number of NTDs cases still occur and the cause remains unclear. Thus, there is a need to research additional dietary factors, such as maternal non-staple food consumption in first trimester. In recent decades, studies have reported that intake of fresh fruits or vegetables, unpasteurized milk, pickled vegetables and caffeine during pregnancy may be associated with NTDs risk in offspring [10–13]. However, due to the different populations and food intake frequency in each study, the findings are not completely consistent without providing a clear conclusion. A previous study conducted by Piirainen *et al.* indicates that women may be more open to dietary change during pregnancy than at other times [14]. Considering the first trimester includes the critical window of neural tube closure, evaluating the effects of non-staple food consumption and proposing beneficial adjustment in maternal diets in the first trimester may have great public health implications.

Beginning in 2008, we performed a hospital-based case-control study in Shanxi and Shandong provinces to explore the risk factors of NTDs. In this study, we solicited the maternal non-staple food consumption information in the first trimester to investigate the potential associations with NTDs in offspring.

2. Methods

2.1. Participants

A hospital-based case-control study was conducted in Shandong and Shanxi provinces in China. According to differences of NTDs incidence, 18 counties in Shandong Province and 6 counties in Shanxi Province were randomly selected to serve as research sites. As eligible cases, we selected 459 mothers who gave birth to NTDs infants or whose NTDs-affected pregnancies were terminated based on the ultrasonic diagnosis within two years from January 2006 to December 2007. Then, from March to December 2008, we interviewed the participants to collect the relevant information face-to-face with the structured questionnaire. Based on ICD-10, in this study, NTDs included anencephaly (Q00.0), spina bifida (Q05) and encephalocele (Q01) complying with related defining features and diagnostic criteria specified in "Birth Defects Monitoring Manual of China". The diagnosis was confirmed and the case was classified by full-time doctors. A total of 459 control mothers who gave birth to healthy infants in the same area, same hospital and within a week in the same year were enrolled. In particular, our study abided by the "Declaration of Helsinki" and the informed consents were obtained from the case and control mothers. This study was reviewed by research institutional review board of Shandong University and approved by the ethics committee (2006BA105A01).

2.2. Questionnaire

With the designed questionnaire, the interviewer solicited all the relevant information during the six months before until 3 months after conception of the participants face-to-face. The questionnaire design went through literature review, panel discussion, check and approval by experts, and revisions after pilot study. The same structured questionnaire was administered to each pair of mothers by the same one trained interviewer. Questionnaires were used to collect the information about mothers' demographic characteristics, reproductive history and illness history, lifestyle behaviors, environmental hazardous substances exposure, nutritional status, diet adjustment, specific food consumption and the consumption frequency in the first trimester, use of folic acid from six months before until 3 months after conception. The contents of questionnaire have been described fully elsewhere [10]. Notably, the food frequency questionnaire has been tested and proved to be validated and tailored for a Chinese diet in the pilot study.

2.3. The Definition of Study Variables

During the interview, mothers were asked to report what they ate in the first trimester. In order to standardize the answers, the mothers were asked to read an enclosed list of food as a memory aid before replying. In this study, the non-staple food included meat, animal giblets, eggs, milk, legume, fresh vegetables, fresh fruits, nuts, pickled vegetable, alcohol and coffee. To access the above food consumption frequency in the first trimester, women were asked to estimate the food consumption frequency ($\leq$1 meal per month, 2–3 meals per month, 1–2 meals per week, 3–6 meals per week, $\geq$7 meals per week).

In order to adjust the potential confounding factors, the following covariates were taken into consideration: maternal periconceptional occupation (farmer, factory worker, and business/officer/solider/technologist), annual per capita income ($\leq$3600 ¥, 3600–7200 ¥, >7200 ¥), maternal education level (<middle school graduate, middle school graduate, >middle school graduate), maternal prepregnancy BMI (underweight, normal weight, overweight, and obesity), history of abortion or induced labor (yes, no), history of chronic disease before conception (yes, no), family history of birth defects (yes, no), maternal diet adjustment (yes, no), folic acid intake (never intake, periconceptional intake, within three months before conception intake, and within three months after conception intake.)

2.4. Statistical Analysis

Descriptive statistics were used to describe the demographic characteristics of subjects with frequency and proportion. Univariate conditional logistic regression analyses were carried out to evaluate effects of the covariates on the NTDs risk.

Univariate conditional logistic regression analyses were carried out to preliminarily determine which of the non-staple food consumption were associated with the risk of NTDs. In this part, the food consumption frequency was divided into two grades: <1 meal per week and ≥1 meal per week.

A multivariate conditional logistic regression model was constructed by adding all the significant factors from the univariate conditional logistic regression analyses and finally determined the food significantly associated with the risk of NTDs.

In order to further analyze each grade effect of the food on NTDs risk, a multivariate conditional logistic regression model was conducted. In this part, the food consumption frequency was divided into four grades: <1 meal per week, 1–2 meals per week, 3–6 meals per week and ≥7 meals per week. In addition, we constructed another three multivariate conditional logistic regression analyses to determine whether there were differences in the three major NTDs subtypes (anencephaly, spina bifida and encephalocele).

The effect values were reported by odds ratio (OR), with their 95% confidence intervals (95% CIs). The database was set up through EpiData3.1 and the data went through statistical process adopting analysis software SAS9.1.3.

3. Results

3.1. Social-Economic Characteristics of the Participants

A total of 459 pairs of participants were identified in the study. Among them, 259 pairs were from Shandong Province and 200 pairs were from Shanxi Province. Among total NTDs cases, there were 194 anencephaly cases (42.3%), 200 spina bifida cases (43.6%) and 65 encephalocele cases (14.1%), and there were no difference in NTDs types between the two provinces. Frequencies and proportions of social-economic characteristics among case and control mothers were shown in Table 1. Compared to control mothers, case mothers were more likely to be farmers, more likely to have lower annual per capita, education level, obese and more likely to have an abortion or induced labor, family history of birth defects, chronic disease before conception, not more likely to adjust diet in the first trimester and take folic acid supplementation periconceptionally.

Table 2 showed univariate analysis of the associations between weekly food consumption and NTDs risk. Compared to food consumption frequency <1 meal, the significant factors were meat consumption ≥1 meal, animal giblets consumption ≥1 meal, eggs consumption ≥1 meal, legume consumption ≥1 meal, milk consumption ≥1 meal, fresh vegetables consumption ≥1 meal, fresh fruits consumption ≥1 meal, nuts consumption ≥1 meal, picked vegetables consumption ≥1 meal.

Table 3 showed multivariate analysis of the associations between weekly food consumption and NTDs risk. Finally, food consumption of milk, fresh fruits and nuts entered the model. Compared to the food consumption frequency <1 meal per weekly, ORs for mothers who consumed milk, fresh fruits and nuts with the frequency ≥1 meal were 0.62 (95% CI = 0.42–0.93), 0.31 (95% CI = 0.14–0.70), and 0.62 (95% CI = 0.43–0.89).

Table 1. Demographic and obstetric characteristics of subjects and their relationship with neural tube defects (NTDs).

Factors	Cases (N = 459; %)	Controls (N = 459; %)	OR	95% CI
Maternal periconceptional occupation				
Farmer	349 (76.0)	329 (71.7)	Ref.	
Factory worker	57 (12.4)	35 (7.6)	1.46	0.91–2.33
Business/officer/soldier/technologist	53 (11.5)	95 (20.7)	0.46	0.30–0.70
Annual per capita income (¥)				
≤3600	232 (50.5)	175 (38.1)	Ref.	
3600–7200	159 (34.6)	164 (35.7)	0.64	0.46–0.89
>7200	68 (14.8)	120 (26.1)	0.35	0.24–0.53
Maternal education level				
<Middle school graduate	119 (25.9)	46 (10.0)	Ref.	
Middle school graduate	298 (64.9)	312 (68.0)	0.33	0.22–0.51
>Middle school graduate	42 (9.2)	101 (22.0)	0.14	0.08–0.24
Body mass index(BMI of mother)				
Normal	20 (4.4)	34 (7.4)	Ref.	
Underweight	313 (68.2)	334 (72.8)	1.64	0.92–2.95
Overweight	94 (20.5)	81 (17.6)	2.03	1.06–3.88
Obese	25 (5.4)	8 (1.7)	5.11	1.93–13.49
Family history of birth defects				
No	432 (94.1)	449 (98.0)	Ref.	
Yes	27 (5.9)	9 (2.0)	2.89	1.35–6.17
Abortion or induced labor				
No	244 (53.2)	280 (61.0)	Ref.	
Yes	215 (46.8)	179 (39.0)	1.38	1.06–1.80
Chronic disease before conception				
No	429 (93.5)	445 (96.9)	Ref.	
Yes	30 (6.5)	14 (3.1)	2.33	1.19–4.59
Diet adjustment in the first trimester				
No	251 (54.7)	131 (28.5)	Ref.	
Yes	208 (45.3)	328 (71.5)	0.27	0.20–0.38
Folic acid intake				
Never	326 (71.0)	243 (52.9)	Ref.	
Periconceptional folic acid intake [a]	22 (4.8)	77 (16.8)	0.22	0.22–0.36
Within three months before conception folic acid intake [b]	17 (3.7)	28 (6.1)	0.48	0.25–0.90
Within three months after conception folic acid intake [c]	94 (20.5)	111 (24.2)	0.61	0.44–0.87

OR odds ratio, CI confidence interval, Ref reference; Percentages of each variable may not equal 100 because of missing data or rounding; [a]: Take 0.4 mg of folic acid tablet daily and used across the time of 3 months before and 3 months after conception and continued for at least 1 month; [b]: Take 0.4 mg of folic acid tablet daily and used 3 months before conception and continued for at least 1 month; [c]: Take 0.4 mg of folic acid tablet daily and used 3 months after conception and continued for at least 1 month.

Table 2. Univariate analysis of the association between weekly food consumption and NTDs risk.

Weekly Food Consumption	Cases *N*	Controls *N*	OR	95% CI
Meat consumption				
<1 meal	201 (43.8)	131 (28.5)	*Ref.*	
≥1 meal	257 (56.0)	328 (71.5)	0.43	0.31–0.60
Animal giblets consumption				
<1 meal	378 (82.4)	321 (69.9)	*Ref.*	
≥1 meal	81 (17.6)	137 (29.8)	0.50	0.36–0.69
Eggs consumption				
<1 meal	68 (14.8)	49 (10.7)	*Ref.*	
≥1 meal	391 (85.2)	410 (89.3)	0.65	0.42–0.99
Legume consumption				
<1 meal	142 (30.9)	110 (24.0)	*Ref.*	
≥1 meal	115 (25.1)	92 (20.0)	0.70	0.52–0.94
Milk consumption				
<1 meal	234 (51.0)	151 (32.9)	*Ref.*	
≥1 meal	224 (48.8)	308 (67.1)	0.41	0.30–0.55
Fresh vegetables consumption				
<1 meal	15 (3.3)	2(0.4)	*Ref.*	
≥1 meal	444 (96.7)	457 (99.6)	0.13	0.03–0.58
Fresh fruits consumption				
<1 meal	58 (12.6)	12 (2.6)	*Ref.*	
≥1 meal	401 (87.4)	446 (97.2)	0.16	0.08–0.33
Nuts consumption				
<1 meal	266 (58.0)	184 (40.1)	*Ref.*	
≥1 meal	193 (43.0)	274 (59.7)	0.46	0.35–0.62
Picked vegetables consumption				
<1 meal	267 (58.2)	323 (70.4)	*Ref.*	
≥1 meal	192 (41.8)	136 (29.6)	1.76	1.32–2.34

OR odds ratio; CI confidence interval; *Ref.* reference group.

Table 4 further showed the specific effects of different food consumption frequency on the risk of NTDs, anencephaly and spina bifida respectively. For total NTDs, a 41%–50% reduction in risk of NTDs was observed at all levels of milk consumption (ORs ranged from 0.50 to 0.59 and the 95% CIs did not include the null). A 68%–78% reduction in risk of NTDs was observed at all levels of fresh fruits consumption (ORs ranged from 0.22 to 0.32 and the 95% CIs did not include the null). For anencephaly, a 94%–95% reduction in risk of NTDs was observed at all levels of fresh fruits consumption (ORs ranged from 0.05 to 0.06 and the 95% CIs did not include the null). For spina bifida, a 57%–83% reduction in risk of NTDs was observed at all levels of fresh fruits consumption (ORs ranged from 0.17 to 0.43 and the 95% CIs did not include the null).

Table 3. Multivariate analysis of association between weekly food consumption and NTDs risk.

Weekly Food Consumption	Case N	Control N	OR *	95% CI
Milk consumption				
<1 meal	234 (51.0)	151 (32.9)	Ref.	
≥1 meal	224 (48.8)	308 (67.1)	0.62	0.42–0.93
Fresh fruits consumption				
<1 meal	58 (12.6)	12 (2.6)	Ref.	
≥1 meal	401 (87.4)	446 (97.2)	0.31	0.14–0.70
Nuts consumption				
<1 meal	266 (58.0)	184 (40.1)	Ref.	
≥1 meal	193 (42.0)	274 (59.7)	0.62	0.43–0.89

OR odds ratio; CI confidence interval; Ref. reference group; * ORs were adjusted for all variables listed in Tables 2 and 2.

Table 4. Effects of food consumption frequency on all NTDs, anencephaly, spina bifida and encephalocele.

Food Consumption Frequency	Case N	Control N	NTDs		Anencephaly		Spina Bifida	
			OR *	95% CI	OR *	95% CI	OR *	95% CI
Milk consumption								
<1 meal per week	234 (51.0)	151 (32.9)	Ref.		Ref.		Ref.	
1–2 meals per week	48 (10.5)	57 (12.4)	0.50	0.28–0.88	1.64	0.63–4.26	0.17	0.07–0.43
3–6 meals per week	53 (11.5)	60 (13.1)	0.56	0.32–0.99	1.54	0.62–3.86	0.26	0.11–0.63
≥7 meals per week	123 (26.8)	191 (41.6)	0.59	0.38–0.90	1.20	0.58–2.48	0.43	0.21–0.88
Fresh fruits consumption								
<1 meal per week	58 (12.6)	12 (2.6)	Ref.		Ref.		Ref.	
1–2 meals per week	54 (11.8)	44 (9.6)	0.29	0.12–0.72	0.06	0.01–0.49	0.46	0.11–1.86
3–6 meals per week	56 (12.2)	75 (16.4)	0.22	0.09–0.53	0.05	0.01–0.34	0.32	0.09–1.14
≥7 meals per week	291(63.4)	327 (71.2)	0.32	0.14–0.71	0.06	0.01–0.37	0.57	0.17–1.95
Nuts consumption								
<1 meal per week	266 (58.0)	184 (40.1)	Ref.		Ref.		Ref.	
1–2 meals per week	73 (15.9)	95 (20.7)	0.60	0.38–0.94	0.94	0.44–2.00	0.31	0.14–0.69
3–6 meals per week	63 (13.7)	99 (21.6)	0.49	0.31–0.79	0.50	0.22–1.12	0.58	0.28–1.19
≥7 meals per week	57 (12.4)	80 (17.4)	0.63	0.36–1.08	0.29	0.11–0.81	0.94	0.42–2.10

OR odds ratio; CI confidence interval; Ref. reference group; * ORs were adjusted for all variables listed in Table 2 and consumption of milk, fresh fruits and nuts (≥1 meal and <1 meal).

4. Discussion

In this study, we found that maternal non-staple food consumption of milk, fresh fruits and nuts in the first trimester were associated with NTDs risk in offspring. Among them, maternal consumption of milk in the first trimester was associated with reducing the risk for total NTDs and spina bifida, but not for anencephaly. Fresh fruits consumption in the first trimester was associated with decreasing the risk for total NTDs and anencephaly, but not for spina bifida. With specific consumption frequency, nuts were associated with reducing risk of total NTDs (1–6 meals per week), subtypes of anencephaly (≥7 meals per week) and spina bifida (1–2 meals per week). In addition, our study also indicated that the preventive effect of milk weakened with the increased consumption frequency, both on total NTDs and spina bifida; moderate amount of fresh fruits consumption with frequency of 3–6 meals per week showed the strongest effects on total NTDs and anencephaly.

Milk contained many potentially NTDs-related nutrients, and vitamin B12 was one of them. Recently, studies have showed that low maternal vitamin B12 was a risk factor for NTDs [3,15,16]. Tucker *et al.* [17] first observed the vitamin B12 from milk was better absorbed than from meat. Naik *et al.* [18] further demonstrated that regular intake of milk could improve the vitamin B12 status among vegetarians with vitamin B12 deficient. In addition, studies suggested that dietary choline and betaine might help to prevent NTDs [19,20], and milk was one of the major food contributors [20,21]. However, due to the production methods, modern cow milk might have a high content of estrogen [22], which was reported associated with reducing serum folate availability [23]. In our study, the negative effects might partly explain why the preventive effect of milk on NTDs weakened with the increased consumption frequency in our study.

Preventive effects of fresh fruits for NTDs have been identified in many studies [24,25]. Consistent with previous studies, our results showed that fresh fruits consumption in the first trimester was associated with reducing risk of total NTDs and anencephaly. Regarding the effect of fresh fruits on spina bifida, our results indicated that fresh fruits were not associated with the risk of spina bifida. A previous study conducted by Yin *et al.* [26] confirmed our findings and reported no association between fresh fruits and spina bifida, although the population and consumption frequency were varied. However, a case-control study in Italy found that occasional consumption (less than 3 times a week) of fruits and vegetables was a risk factor for spina bifida [27]. In addition, our study presented that too much amount of fresh fruits consumption (≥7 meals per week) would weaken the NTDs preventive effect, which was never mentioned in other studies. An assumption we proposed was that too much fruits consumption might reduce other food intakes, such as meat, eggs or milk, by which affected the maternal diet quality during pregnancy eventually.

There were few studies on the association between nuts consumption in the first trimester and NTDs risk in offspring. In this study, we found that mothers consuming nuts with specific weekly frequency had a lower risk for total NTDs, subtypes of anencephaly and spina bifida. Although the biological mechanisms underlying the NTDs preventive effects of nuts were complicated and still remained unclear, our findings might be partly explained by the components of nuts. First, folate, a most important vitamin in preventing NTDs, was found to be abundant in

131

nuts [28]. Second, nuts were good source of dietary myo-inositol, which had been observed associated with NTDs risk in offspring [29,30]. A study even proposed that myo-inositol soft gelatin capsules should be considered for the preventive treatment of NTDs in folate-resistant subjects [31].

Our study had several strengths. Good validity of cases classified by full time doctors with specified diagnostic criteria was helpful to minimize the misclassification of the participants. Besides, we evaluated the related factors for the three major NTDs subtypes, which would not obscure the potential associations that may be interfered by etiological heterogeneity.

Our study also had some limits. Firstly, with a retrospective design, our collected information from mothers up to 2 years after pregnancy, and recall bias could be a concern in our study. Secondly, in our study, the relatively small sample sizes limited our ability to study the association between non-staple food consumption in the first trimester and risk of the NTDs subtype of encephalocele. Thirdly, we did not collect the further information of non-staple food in study, such as milk type (unpasteurized milk or packet milk), the specific kind of fruits *et al*, which may affect the final results more or less. Fourthly, the short period of neural tube closure and diet adjustment after a mother realized she was pregnant might lead to exposure misclassification in our study. Finally, as there was bias resulted from some non-response mothers, the representative of the controls also could be a concern in this study.

In conclusion, the findings of the present study demonstrated that non-staple food of milk, fresh fruits, and nuts were associated with decreasing NTDs risk in offspring. Although the associations needed to be confirmed by further studies, we suggested that adequate intake of milk, fresh fruits and nuts were necessary for pregnant women in the first trimester.

Acknowledgments: We were grateful to the local doctors and health care workers at local CDC and hospitals in Shanxi and Shandong provinces for their assistance with the investigation and data collection in this study. The study was sponsored by a grant of the effectiveness evaluation of hospital-based comprehensive birth defects intervention methods, Ministry of Science and Technology of China (2006BA105A01).

Author Contributions: Meng Wang planned the study and collected, analyzed the data with Li-Jie Gao and Hui Yang. Zhong-Tang Zhao and Zhi-Ping Wang gave much advice and directions in both study design and preparing of the manuscript. All the authors have read and approved the final submitted version.

Conflicts of Interest: The authors report no conflict of interest.

References

1. Blencowe, H.; Cousens, S.; Modell, B.; Lawn, J. Folic acid to reduce neonatal mortality from neural tube disorders. *Int. J. Epidemiol.* **2010**, *39*, i110–i121.
2. Botto, L.D.; Moore, C.A.; Khoury, M.J.; Erickson, J.D. Neural-tube defects. *N. Engl. J. Med.* **1999**, *341*, 1509–1519.

3. Wang, Z.P.; Shang, X.X.; Zhao, Z.T. Low maternal vitamin B12 is a risk factor for neural tube defects: A meta-analysis. *J. Matern. Fetal Neonatal Med.* **2012**, *25*, 389–394.

4. Sayed, A.R.; Bourne, D.; Pattinson, R.; Nixon, J.; Henderson, B. Decline in the prevalence of neural tube defects following folic acid fortification and its cost-benefit in South Africa. *Birth Defects Res. A Clin. Mol. Teratol.* **2008**, *82*, 211–216.

5. Williams, L.J.; Mai, C.T.; Edmonds, L.D.; Shaw, G.M.; Kirby, R.S.; Hobbs, C.A.; Sever, L.E.; Miller, L.A.; Meaney, F.J.; Levitt, M. Prevalence of spina bifida and anencephaly during the transition to mandatory folic acid fortification in the United States. *Teratology* **2002**, *66*, 33–39.

6. Boulet, S.L.; Yang, Q.; Mai, C.; Kirby, R.S.; Collins, J.S.; Robbins, J.M.; Meyer, R.; Canfield, M.A.; Mulinare, J. National Birth defects Prevention Network. Trends in the postfortification prevalence of spina bifida and anencephaly in the United States. *Birth Defects Res. A Clin. Mol. Teratol.* **2008**, *82*, 527–532.

7. Ray, J.G.; Meier, C.; Vermeulen, M.J.; Boss, S.; Wyatt, P.R.; Cole, D.E. Association of neural tube defects and folic acid food fortification in Canada. *Lancet* **2002**, *360*, 2047–2048.

8. De Wals, P.; Tairou, F.; van Allen, M.I.; Uh, S.H.; Lowry, R.B.; Sibbald, B.; Evans, J.A.; van den Hof, M.C.; Zimmer, P.; Crowley, M.; *et al.* Reduction in neural-tube defects after folic acid fortification in Canada. *N. Engl. J. Med.* **2007**, *357*, 135–142.

9. López-Camelo, J.S.; Castilla, E.E.; Orioli, I.M.; INAGEMP (Instituto Nacional de Genética Médica Populacional); ECLAMC (Estudio Colaborativo Latino Americano de Malformaciones Congénitas). Folic acid flour fortification: Impact on the frequencies of 52 congenital anomaly types in three South American countries. *Am. J. Med. Genet. A* **2010**, *152*, 2444–2458.

10. Wang, M.; Wang, Z.P.; Gao, L.J.; Gong, R.; Zhang, M.; Lu, Q.B.; Zhao, Z.T. Periconceptional factors affect the risk of neural tube defects in offspring: A hospital-based case-control study in China. *J. Matern. Fetal Neonatal Med.* **2013**, *26*, 1132–1138.

11. Li, Z.; Ren, A.; Zhang, L.; Guo, Z.; Li, Z. A population-based case-control study of risk factors for neural tube defects in four high-prevalence areas of Shanxi province, China. *Paediatr. Perinat. Epidemiol.* **2006**, *20*, 43–53.

12. Deb, R.; Arora, J.; Saraswathy, K.N.; Kalla, A.K. Association of sociodemographic and nutritional factors with risk of neural tube defects in the North Indian population: A case-control study. *Public Health Nutr.* **2014**, *17*, 376–382.

13. Schmidt, R.J.; Romitti, P.A.; Burns, T.L.; Browne, M.L.; Druschel, C.M.; Olney, R.S. National Birth Defects Prevention Study. Maternal caffeine consumption and risk of neural tube defects. *Birth Defects Res. A Clin. Mol. Teratol.* **2009**, *85*, 879–889.

14. Piirainen, T.; Isolauri, E.; Lagström, H.; Laitinen, K. Impact of dietary counseling on nutrient intake during pregnancy: A prospective cohort study. *Br. J. Nutr.* **2006**, *96*, 1095–1104.

15. Suarez, L.; Hendricks, K.; Felkner, M.; Gunter, E. Maternal serum B12 levels and risk for neural tube defects in a Texas-Mexico border population. *Ann. Epidemiol.* **2003**, *13*, 81–88.

16. Molloy, A.M.; Kirke, P.N.; Troendle, J.F.; Burke, H.; Sutton, M.; Brody, L.C.; Scott, J.M.; Mills, J.L. Maternal vitamin B12 status and risk of neural tube defects in a population with high neural tube defect prevalence and no folic acid fortification. *Pediatrics* **2009**, *123*, 917–923.

17. Tucker, K.L.; Rich, S.; Rosenberg, I.; Jacques, P.; Dallal, G.; Wilson, P.W.; Selhub, J. Plasma vitamin B-12 concentrations relate to intake source in the Framingham Offsprings study. *Am. J. Clin. Nutr.* **2000**, *71*, 514–522.

18. Naik, S.; Bhide, V.; Babhulkar, A.; Mahalle, N.; Parab, S.; Thakre, R.; Kulkarni, M. Daily milk intake improves vitamin B-12 status in young vegetarian Indians: An intervention trial. *Nutr. J.* **2013**, *12*, 136.

19. Lavery, A.M.; Brender, J.D.; Zhao, H.; Sweeney, A.; Felkner, M.; Suarez, L.; Canfield, M.A. Dietary intake of choline and neural tube defects in Mexican Americans. *Birth Defects Res A Clin. Mol. Teratol.* **2014**, *100*, 463–471.

20. Shaw, G.M.; Carmichael, S.L.; Yang, W.; Selvin, S.; Schaffer, D.M. Periconceptional dietary intake of choline and betaine and neural tube defects in offspring. *Am. J. Epidemiol.* **2004**, *160*, 102–109.

21. Mygind, V.L.; Evans, S.E.; Peddie, M.C.; Miller, J.C.; Houghton, L.A. Estimation of usual intake and food sources of choline and betaine in New Zealand reproductive age women. *Asia Pac. J. Clin. Nutr.* **2013**, *22*, 319–324.

22. Ganmaa, D.; Wang, P.Y.; Qin, L.Q.; Hoshi, K.; Sato, A. Is milk responsible for male reproductive disorders? *Med. Hypotheses* **2001**, *57*, 510–514.

23. Butterworth, C.E., Jr.; Hatch, K.D.; Macaluso, M.; Cole, P.; Sauberlich, H.E.; Soong, S.J.; Borst, M.; Baker, W. Folate deficiency and cervical dysplasia. *JAMA* **1992**, *267*, 528–533.

24. Zhang, T.; Xin, R.; Gu, X.; Wang, F.; Pei, L.; Lin, L.; Chen, G.; Wu, J.; Zheng, X. Maternal serum vitamin B12, folate and homocysteine and the risk of neural tube defects in the offspring in a high-risk area of China. *Public Health Nutr.* **2009**, *12*, 680–686.

25. Li, Z.W.; Zhang, L.; Ye, R.W.; Liu, J.M.; Pei, L.J.; Zheng, X.Y.; Ren, A.G. Maternal periconceptional consumption of pickled vegetables and risk of neural tube defects in offspring. *Chin. Med. J. (Engl.)* **2011**, *124*, 1629–1633.

26. Yin, Z.; Xu, W.; Xu, C.; Zhang, S.; Zheng, Y.; Wang, W.; Zhou, B. A population-based case-control study of risk factors for neural tube defects in Shenyang, China. *Childs Nerv. Syst.* **2011**, *27*, 149–154.

27. De Marco, P.; Merello, E.; Calevo, M.G.; Mascelli, S.; Pastorino, D.; Crocetti, L.; de Biasio, P.; Piatelli, G.; Cama, A.; Capra, V. Maternal periconceptional factors affect the risk of spina bifida-affected pregnancies: An Italian case-control study. *Childs Nerv. Syst.* **2011**, *27*, 1073–1081.

28. Simpson, J.L.; Bailey, L.B.; Pietrzik, K.; Shane, B.; Holzgreve, W. Micronutrients and women of reproductive potential: Required dietary intake and consequences of dietary deficiency or excess. Part I-Folate, Vitamin B12, Vitamin B6. *J. Matern. Fetal Neonatal Med.* **2010**, *23*, 1323–1343.

29. Groenen, P.M.; Peer, P.G.; Wevers, R.A.; Swinkels, D.W.; Franke, B.; Mariman, E.C.; Steeqers-Theunissen, R.P. Maternal myo-inositol, glucose, and zinc status is associated with the risk of offspring with spina bifida. *Am. J. Obstet. Gynecol.* **2003**, *189*, 1713–1719.
30. Reece, E.A.; Khandelwal, M.; Wu, Y.K.; Borenstein, M. Dietary intake of myo-inositol and neural tube defects in offspring of diabetic rats. *Am. J. Obstet. Gynecol.* **1997**, *176*, 536–539.
31. De Grazia, S.; Carlomagno, G.; Unfer, V.; Cavalli, P. Myo-inositol soft gel capsules may prevent the risk of coffee-induced neural tube defects. *Expert Opin. Drug Deliv.* **2012**, *9*, 1033–1039.

Low Maternal Vitamin B12 Status Is Associated with Lower Cord Blood HDL Cholesterol in White Caucasians Living in the UK

Antonysunil Adaikalakoteswari, Manu Vatish, Alexander Lawson,
Catherine Wood, Kavitha Sivakumar, Philip G. McTernan, Craig Webster,
Neil Anderson, Chittaranjan S. Yajnik, Gyanendra Tripathi and
Ponnusamy Saravanan

Abstract: Background and Aims: Studies in South Asian population show that low maternal vitamin B12 associates with insulin resistance and small for gestational age in the offspring. Low vitamin B12 status is attributed to vegetarianism in these populations. It is not known whether low B12 status is associated with metabolic risk of the offspring in whites, where the childhood metabolic disorders are increasing rapidly. Here, we studied whether maternal B12 levels associate with metabolic risk of the offspring at birth. Methods: This is a cross-sectional study of 91 mother-infant pairs (n = 182), of white Caucasian origin living in the UK. Blood samples were collected from white pregnant women at delivery and their newborns (cord blood). Serum vitamin B12, folate, homocysteine as well as the relevant metabolic risk factors were measured. Results: The prevalence of low serum vitamin B12 (<191 ng/L) and folate (<4.6 µg/L) were 40% and 11%, respectively. Maternal B12 was inversely associated with offspring's Homeostasis Model Assessment 2-Insulin Resistance (HOMA-IR), triglycerides, homocysteine and positively with HDL-cholesterol after adjusting for age and BMI. In regression analysis, after adjusting for likely confounders, maternal B12 is independently associated with neonatal HDL-cholesterol and homocysteine but not triglycerides or HOMA-IR. Conclusions: Our study shows that low B12 status is common in white women and is independently associated with adverse cord blood cholesterol.

Reprinted from *Nutrients*. Cite as: Adaikalakoteswari, A.; Vatish, M.; Lawson, A.; Wood, C.; Sivakumar, K.; McTernan, P.G.; Webster, C.; Anderson, N.; Yajnik, C.S.; Tripathi, G.; Saravanan, P. Low Maternal Vitamin B12 Status Is Associated with Lower Cord Blood HDL Cholesterol in White Caucasians Living in the UK. *Nutrients* **2015**, *7*, 2401–2414.

1. Introduction

The prevalence of childhood obesity is increasing rapidly [1,2]. Recently, the Early Childhood Longitudinal Study demonstrated that 27.3% of children were either overweight or obese by the time they enter kindergarten in the United States [1]. Higher rate of childhood obesity is a likely contributor for the increasing incidence of type 2 diabetes (T2D) earlier in life as well as pre-gestational and gestational diabetes (GDM) in women [3]. It is known that childhood obesity independently predicts obesity and metabolic disorders in the adulthood [4]. Children born with lower HDL and higher triglyceride levels were small for gestational age (SGA) and had higher abdominal circumference [5]. It is known that both higher abdominal circumference and SGA are associated with future development of T2D and GDM [6,7] in many populations.

Although current adverse lifestyle (nutrition and physical inactivity) contributes to obesity, a growing body of evidence links nutrient imbalance in early life to the development of metabolic disorders in childhood and in adults [8]. Many studies support this link including the Dutch-famine study. Individuals exposed to nutritional imbalance during pregnancy are likely to be obese, have early onset of coronary artery disease, T2D and worse cognitive performances as adults [9]. Emerging evidence from clinical studies show that key maternal micronutrients involved in the one-carbon metabolism (1-C) can cause adverse metabolic programming. Independent studies from South Asia have demonstrated that children born to mothers with low vitamin B12 [10,11] and higher folate [12] have greater insulin resistance. In addition, low maternal B12 levels independently contributed to the risk of small for gestational age (SGA), which has been shown to increase the metabolic risk of the offspring [13]. Vegetarianism is the likely cause of high prevalence of low B12 levels in these population [14]. In a Brazilian pregnancy cohort, low maternal B12 was associated with lower levels of the methyl donor (*S*-adenosyl methionine—SAM) in the cord blood [15]. A study in a Chinese population demonstrated that low maternal B12 is common during pregnancy and is associated with an altered methylation pattern of the insulin growth factor 2 (IGF2) promoter region in the cord blood [16], highlighting a potential role of B12 on fetal growth. Further, animal studies showed that maternal vitamin B12 deficiency resulted in higher adiposity, insulin resistance, blood pressure [17] and adverse lipid profile in the offspring [18,19]. These investigations provide evidence that low maternal B12 could be an independent determinant of adverse metabolic phenotypes in the offspring.

Recently, we demonstrated in Europeans and Indians with T2D that vitamin B12 deficiency is associated with adverse lipid profile [20]. Re-analysis of the UK National Diet and Nutrition Survey data showed that low vitamin B12 levels (<191 ng/L) is common in the adult population (10%) and in women of reproductive age (14%) [21]. Our preliminary study of white pregnant women showed that the rate of low B12 status was as high as 20% at 16–18 weeks of gestation [22].

Despite the evidence that vitamin B12 deficiency is a potential contributor for adverse offspring metabolic phenotypes and the prevalence of low B12 status is increasing in White Caucasian population, the link between maternal B12 status and metabolic risk at birth is unexplored in the White Caucasian population. Therefore, the objective of our study was to investigate whether maternal B12 levels in white women independently associate with the metabolic risk at birth.

2. Methods

2.1. Study Population

The study was conducted in University Hospital Coventry Warwickshire (UHCW), Coventry, UK. All study participants were pregnant women delivering at 39–40 weeks of gestation. The Coventry local research ethics committee approved the study, and all patients gave written informed consent (Research Ethics Committees 07/H1210/141). Women with known chronic diseases were excluded. Maternal data including parity, smoking, BMI and birth weight were collected from pregnancy records. Folic acid supplement use collected but detailed dietary history was not recorded. Maternal BMI measured routinely at the first pregnancy visit (before 10 weeks of gestation). We collected 182 maternal venous and cord blood samples (91 mother-newborn pairs) at the time of delivery. Extrapolating from our preliminary studies [21,22], we anticipated around 20%–25% of the mothers to have low levels of vitamin B12 (<191 ng/L). To detect a similar proportion of low B12 status a sample size of 100–120 was required. The samples were collected in the fasting state, in tubes without anticoagulant and centrifuged at 2000 rpm/10 min. Serum was separated, aliquoted and stored at $-80\,^{\circ}$C until analysis.

2.2. Analytical Determinations

Serum glucose, cholesterol, triglycerides, HDL cholesterol were determined using an auto analyser Synchron CX7 (Beckman Coulter, Fullerton, CA, USA) based on enzymatic colorimetric assays. Insulin was measured using Invitrogen ELISA kit (Camarillo, CA, USA) according to manufacturer's instructions. LDL cholesterol was calculated using Friedewald formula. Insulin resistance (HOMA-IR) was calculated by the Homeostasis Model Assessment 2 computer model (HOMA2) using fasting insulin and glucose levels [10]. Serum B12 and folate were determined by electrochemiluminescent immunoassay using a Roche Cobas immunoassay analyzer (Roche Diagnostics UK, Burgess Hill, UK). Similar to other studies [20,23,24], we have used 191–663 ng/L for serum Vitamin B12 and 4.6–18.7 µg/L for serum folate as normal range, respectively. The inter-assay coefficient of variations for B12 and folate were 3.9% and 3.7%, respectively. To avoid potential bias, all the biochemical analyses were conducted in a single batch to minimise assay variation. All the laboratory personnel were blinded and did not have any access to the clinical data. Serum homocysteine was determined by stable isotopic dilution analysis liquid chromatography (LC-MS/MS) [25] using a Waters Equity UPLC system (Waters, Milford, CT, USA) coupled to an API 4000 tandem mass spectrometer (Applied Biosystems, Warrington, UK). Due to the uncertainty of defining deficiencies of serum vitamin B12 and folate levels during pregnancy and cord blood, the terms "low B12 status" and "low folate status" were used throughout the manuscript if the levels were below 191 ng/L and 4.6 µg/L, respectively.

2.3. Statistical Analysis

Continuous data are reported either as mean $\pm$ standard deviation (SD) or geometric mean with 95% confidence intervals (CI). Categorical data are reported in numbers (percentages). The distributions of the maternal and neonatal parameters such as vitamin B12, folate, cholesterol, triglycerides, HDL, LDL, glucose, insulin, HOMA-IR and homocysteine concentrations were skewed; these data were log-transformed before analyses. Student's t-test was used for comparison of groups. Bivariate correlations were done using Pearson test. Variables that showed significant associations with dependent variable (neonatal metabolic risk factors) were included as independent variables in the multiple linear regression analyses. To facilitate comparison, dependent and independent variables were converted into standard deviation scores (SDS). The data are presented as SD change in offspring outcome per SD change in maternal vitamin B12, folate and homocysteine. Associations between maternal vitamin B12, folate and homocysteine concentrations and offspring outcomes were examined in multivariate linear regression using 3 models. Model 1: unadjusted; Model 2: adjusted for maternal age, BMI, glucose, insulin, parity, folic acid supplement use, smoking, vitamin B12, folate and homocysteine; Model 3: Model 2 + respective maternal variable. All tests were two-sided, and p values of <0.05 were considered to be statistically significant. All analyses were performed using SPSS Statistics version 21 (IBM Corp, Armonk, NY, USA).

3. Results

3.1. B12, Folate and Homocysteine Status

The clinical characteristics of mothers and neonates are shown in Table 1. The prevalence of serum low vitamin B12 and folate status in women during pregnancy were 40% and 11% in mothers and 29% and 0% in neonates, respectively (Table 1). In cord blood, all the biochemical parameters were significantly lower than in maternal serum, except for the B12 and folate levels (Table 1). Children born to mothers with low B12 status had significantly lower B12 levels compared to those born to mothers with normal levels (Table 2). Mothers with higher parity and smoking had lower B12 levels. Those with self-reported folic acid supplement use had higher

139

B12 and lower homocysteine levels (Table 3). Maternal B12, folate and homocysteine showed strong positive correlation with the respective offspring indices (B12: $r = 0.648$, folate: $r = 0.706$, homocysteine: $r = 0.756$, all $p < 0.0001$) (Supplementary Figure S1a–c). Neonatal homocysteine showed negative correlation with maternal B12 and folate (B12: $r = -0.409$, $p < 0.0001$; folate: $r = -0.346$, $p < 0.001$; Supplementary Figure S2a,b).

Table 1. Clinical characteristics of mothers and neonate.

	Mother	Neonate
	$n = 91$	$n = 91$
Age (years)	32.7 ± 5.9 [a]	-
Weight (Kg)	77.7 ± 18.1	3.57 ± 0.26
Height (m)	1.62 ± 0.09	-
BMI (early pregnancy) (kg/m^2)	29.4 ± 6.2	-
Glucose (mmol/L)	4.37 ± 0.42	3.88 ± 0.52
Insulin (mIU/L)	11.6 (12.9, 17.4) [b]	8.01 (8.62, 11.9)
Triglycerides (mmol/L)	2.69 (2.62, 3.06)	0.23 (0.22, 0.26)
Cholesterol (mmol/L)	6.48 (6.31, 6.89)	1.68 (1.63, 1.84)
LDL cholesterol (mmol/L)	3.53 (3.46, 3.95)	0.82 (0.79, 0.95)
HDL cholesterol (mmol/L)	1.56 (1.53, 1.72)	0.74 (0.72, 0.83)
HOMA-IR	1.37 (1.55, 2.09)	0.99 (1.04, 1.41)
Vitamin B12 (ng/L)	218 (213, 289)	290 (292, 418)
Low B12 status (%)	36 (40) [c]	26 (29)
Folate (µg/L)	10.5 (10.9, 13.2)	16.8 (16.4, 17.7)
Low folate status (%)	10 (11)	0
Homocysteine (µmol/L)	6.23 (6.02, 7.54)	5.76 (5.64, 6.85)

[a] Mean ± SD (all such values); [b] Geometric mean (95% CI) (all such values); [c] Numbers (percentages) (all such values).

Table 2. Clinical characteristics of mothers and neonate according to maternal B12 levels.

	Mothers		Neonate	
	Maternal B12 ≥191 (ng/L)	Maternal B12 <191 (ng/L)	Maternal B12 ≥191 (ng/L)	Maternal B12 <191 (ng/L)
	$n = 55$	$n = 36$	$n = 55$	$n = 36$
Age (years)	33.0 ± 6.2 [a]	32.3 ± 5.6	-	-
Weight (Kg)	74.3 ± 15.8	82.9 ± 20.8 *	3.58 ± 0.31	3.57 ± 0.18
Height (m)	1.62 ± 0.07	1.61 ± 0.11	-	-
BMI (early pregnancy) (kg/m^2)	28.4 ± 6.1	30.8 ± 6.4 *	-	-
Glucose (mmol/L)	4.40 ± 0.46	4.36 ± 0.34	3.85 ± 0.52	3.94 ± 0.52
Insulin (mIU/L)	10.4 (11.7, 18.0) [b]	13.7 (12.7, 18.6)	8.27 (8.33, 12.75)	7.64 (7.30, 12.40)
Triglycerides (mmol/L)	2.49 (2.37, 2.93)	3.04 (2.82, 3.48) *	0.21 (0.20, 0.24)	0.26 (0.23, 0.32) **
Cholesterol (mmol/L)	6.23 (5.99, 6.72)	6.86 (6.51, 7.43) *	1.72 (1.64, 1.92)	1.62 (1.51, 1.83)
LDL cholesterol (mmol/L)	3.29 (3.16, 3.82)	3.91 (3.67, 4.38) *	0.79 (0.76, 0.90)	0.87 (0.77, 1.09)
HDL cholesterol (mmol/L)	1.61 (1.54, 1.80)	1.49 (1.42, 1.70)	0.79 (0.76, 0.91)	0.67 (0.62, 0.77) *
HOMA-IR	1.18 (1.37, 2.14)	1.68 (1.57, 2.27)	0.94 (0.95, 1.41)	1.08 (0.98, 1.63)
Vitamin B12 (ng/L)	288 (265, 378)	146 (139, 155) ***	367 (354, 544)	202 (187, 234) ***
Low B12 status (%)	0	36 (40) [c]	8 (14.5)	18 (50)
Folate (µg/L)	11.7 (11.5, 14.6)	9.0 (8.5, 12.4) *	17.6 (17.0, 18.5)	15.7 (14.9, 17.2) **
Low folate status (%)	3 (5.5)	7 (19.4)	0	0
Homocysteine (µmol/L)	5.50 (5.26, 6.18)	7.53 (6.69, 10.1) ***	4.97 (4.74, 5.59)	7.09 (6.58, 8.96) ***

[a] Mean ± SD (all such values); [b] Geometric mean (95% CI) (all such values); [c] Numbers (percentages) (all such values); * p-value compared to maternal B12 (≥191 ng/L) group; * $p < 0.05$; ** $p < 0.01$; *** $p < 0.001$.

Table 3. Vitamin B12, folate and homocysteine in mothers and neonate according to maternal smoking status, parity and folate supplement use.

	Smoking	$n = 91$	Vitamin B12 (ng/L)	Folate (µg/L)	Homocysteine (µmol/L)
Maternal	No (%)	55	245 (227, 357)	10.7 (10.6, 13.9)	6.15 (5.61, 8.08)
	Yes (%)	45	189 (176, 224) **	10.1 (9.7, 13.3)	6.33 (5.90, 7.45)
Neonate	No (%)	55	327 (305, 502)	16.9 (16.4, 18.2)	5.42 (5.06, 6.58)
	Yes (%)	45	252 (232, 364) *	16.5 (15.8, 17.7)	6.21 (5.80, 7.68)
	Parity				
Maternal	Para 0 (%)	18	248 (203, 332)	13.7 (11.8, 17.9)	6.25 (5.21, 8.03)
	Para 1 (%)	48	224 (201, 347)	11.1 (10.8, 14.1)	6.12 (5.73, 7.43)
	Para ≥2 (%)	34	195 (179, 239) *	8.2 (7.6, 11.6) **	6.4 (5.31, 8.97)
Neonate	Para 0 (%)	18	327 (264, 479)	17.9 (16.6, 19.6)	5.61 (4.50, 7.59)
	Para 1 (%)	48	284 (258, 487)	16.9 (16.3, 18.1)	5.91 (5.53, 7.30)
	Para ≥2 (%)	34	283 (250, 396)	16.0 (15.2, 17.4) *	5.67 (5.08, 7.15)
	Folate supplement users				
Maternal	Yes (%)	85	224 (216, 305)	11.1 (11.3, 14.0)	6.06 (5.77, 7.44)
	No (%)	15	187 (154, 245)	6.8 (5.5, 9.3) ***	7.42 (6.02, 9.61) *
Neonate	Yes (%)	85	311 (306, 445)	17.4 (17.0, 18.2)	5.57 (5.40, 6.53)
	No (%)	15	213 (134, 391)	13.5 (12.0, 15.6) ***	7.01 (5.34, 10.33) *

Data are geometric mean (95% CI); * p-value compared to geometric mean in the respective group(s); * $p < 0.05$; ** $p < 0.01$; *** $p < 0.001$.

3.2. Maternal B12 and Metabolic Risk of Offspring

Maternal B12 adjusted for age and BMI was inversely associated with metabolic risk factors such as triglycerides ($r = -0.219$; $p = 0.047$), HOMA-IR ($r = -0.232$; $p = 0.041$), homocysteine ($r = -0.423$; $p = 0.0001$) and positively with HDL-cholesterol ($r = 0.315$; $p = 0.004$) (Figure 1a–d) in the offspring. Despite similar birth weight, offspring of low B12 mothers had significantly lower HDL-cholesterol, higher triglycerides and homocysteine than those of normal B12 mothers (Table 2). Multiple regression analysis was carried out to assess whether maternal B12 independently associated with these metabolic risk factors in the offspring by adjusting for likely confounders. The model included maternal age, parity, smoking, folic acid supplement use, BMI, glucose, insulin, folate and homocysteine as independent variables. In addition, for offspring's lipid parameters, respective maternal variable was also included in the model (maternal triglycerides for offspring's triglycerides, *etc.*). After all these adjustments, maternal B12 was independently associated with the offspring's HDL and homocysteine. Though similar trends were seen for the triglycerides and HOMA-IR, these were not statistically significant. No sex-specific changes were seen in any of these analyses (data not shown). Maternal B12 explained 5.1% of the variation in offspring's HDL and 10.6% in homocysteine (Table 4).

Table 4. Association of maternal B12, folate and homocysteine with neonate metabolic risk factors.

Maternal Variable (SDS)	Triglycerides * β	95% CI	p	Cholesterol * β	95% CI	p	HDL * β	95% CI	p	LDL * β	95% CI	p	Insulin * β	95% CI	p	Glucose * β	95% CI	p	Homocysteine * β	95% CI	p
Maternal B12 *																					
Model 1	−0.148	(−0.38, 0.09)	0.210	0.109	(−0.11, 0.33)	0.317	0.296	(0.07, 0.52)	0.010	−0.044	(−0.26, 0.17)	0.691	0.070	(−0.21, 0.21)	0.516	−0.005	(−0.22, −0.21)	0.960	−0.381	(−0.58, −0.18)	<0.001
Model 2	−0.086	(−0.38, 0.21)	0.562	0.178	(−0.08, 0.44)	0.173	0.294	(0.05, 0.54)	0.018	0.070	(−0.26, 0.39)	0.672	−0.063	(−0.17, 0.29)	0.593	−0.088	(−0.14, −0.31)	0.438	−0.200	(−0.35, −0.05)	0.009
Model 3	−0.079	(−0.39, 0.23)	0.609	0.170	(−0.09, 0.43)	0.198	0.295	(0.08, 0.51)	0.009	0.056	(−0.28, 0.39)	0.736	−0.062	(−0.17, 0.29)	0.602	−0.093	(−0.12, 0.30)	0.378			
Maternal Folate *																					
Model 1	−0.109	(−0.33, 0.11)	0.326	−0.210	(−0.42, 0.001)	0.051	−0.025	(−0.25, 0.19)	0.825	−0.173	(−0.38, 0.04)	0.111	0.040	(−0.17, 0.25)	0.705	−0.124	(−0.33, 0.09)	0.243	−0.327	(−0.53, −0.13)	0.002
Model 2	−0.084	(−0.43, 0.26)	0.625	−0.204	(−0.49, 0.08)	0.160	−0.236	(−0.51, 0.04)	0.091	−0.079	(−0.40, 0.24)	0.625	0.133	(−0.15, 0.42)	0.357	−0.035	(−0.31, 0.24)	0.799	−0.004	(−0.19, 0.18)	0.966
Model 3	−0.093	(−0.45, 0.26)	0.600	−0.200	(−0.49, 0.09)	0.169	−0.209	(−0.46, 0.04)	0.099	−0.082	(−0.41, 0.24)	0.616	0.136	(−0.15, 0.43)	0.353	−0.039	(−0.29, 0.22)	0.763			
Maternal Homocysteine *																					
Model 1	0.218	(−0.00, 0.44)	0.050	0.290	(−0.07, 0.51)	0.009	0.119	(−0.13, 0.36)	0.336	0.265	(0.06, 0.47)	0.013	0.001	(−0.21, 0.21)	0.993	0.121	(−0.09, 0.34)	0.269	0.752	(0.62, 0.89)	<0.001
Model 2	0.137	(−0.19, 0.47)	0.473	0.206	(−0.08, 0.49)	0.156	0.093	(−0.23, 0.41)	0.556	0.224	(−0.09, 0.54)	0.160	0.037	(−0.23, 0.31)	0.785	0.057	(−0.21, 0.32)	0.669	0.696	(0.52, 0.87)	<0.001
Model 3	0.126	(−0.23, 0.48)	0.474	0.230	(−0.07, 0.53)	0.129	0.158	(−0.13, 0.45)	0.278	0.248	(−0.08, 0.57)	0.130	0.043	(−0.24, 0.32)	0.759	0.089	(−0.16, 0.34)	0.469			

Neonate's Metabolic Risk Factors (SDS)

* Log transformed for statistical comparisons. β represents SDS change in the dependent variable per SDS change in the independent variable. Model 1: unadjusted; Model 2: Maternal age, BMI, glucose, insulin, parity, folic acid supplement use, smoking, vitamin B12, folate and homocysteine; Model 3: Model 2 + respective maternal variable such as a—Model 2 + maternal triglycerides, b—Model 2 + maternal cholesterol, c—Model 2 + maternal HDL, d—Model 2 + maternal LDL, e—Model 2 + maternal insulin, f—Model 2 + maternal glucose, g—Model 2 + maternal homocysteine.

142

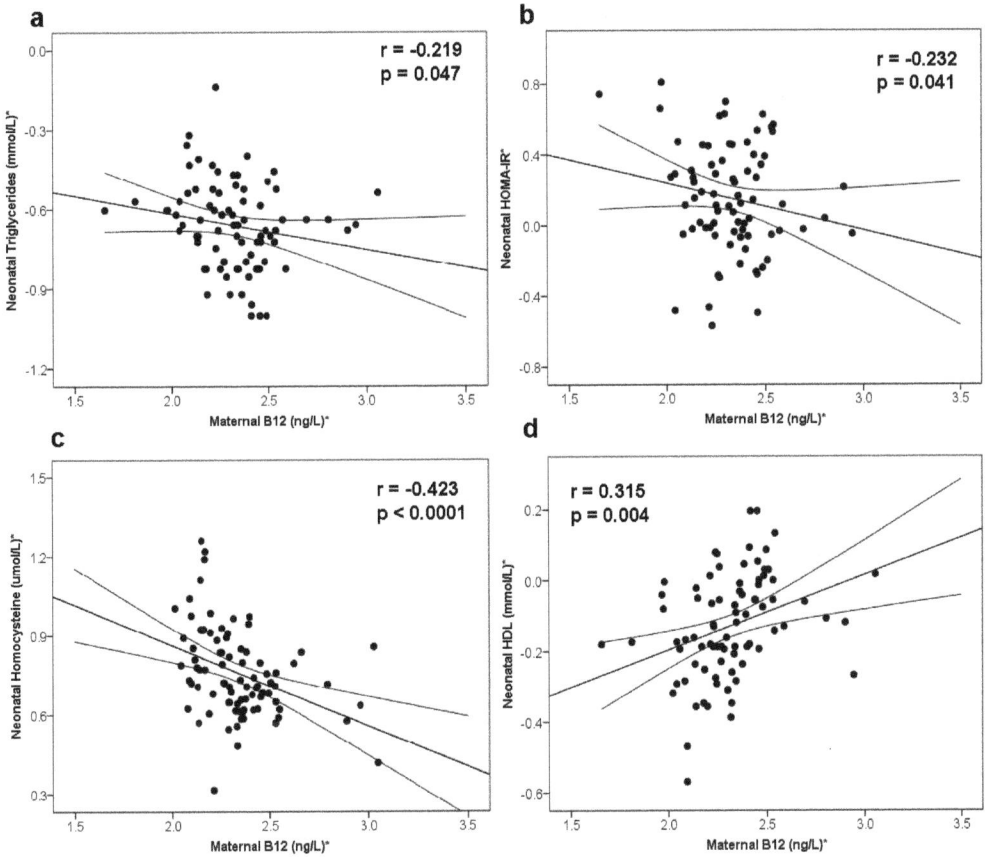

Figure 1. Correlation between maternal B12 (adjusted for age and BMI) and metabolic risk factors of neonates. (**a**) Maternal B12 and neonatal triglycerides, (**b**) Maternal B12 and neonatal Homeostasis Model Assessment 2-Insulin Resistance (HOMA-IR), (**c**) Maternal B12 and neonatal homocysteine, (**d**) Maternal B12 and neonatal HDL. * Log-transformed for statistical comparisons.

3.3. Maternal Folate and Homocysteine and Metabolic Risk of Offspring

Maternal folate negatively associated with offspring's cholesterol ($r = -0.214$; $p = 0.045$), LDL ($r = -0.233$; $p = 0.030$) and homocysteine ($r = -0.346$; $p = 0.001$). Maternal homocysteine positively associated with offspring's triglycerides ($r = 0.239$; $p = 0.030$), cholesterol ($r = 0.247$; $p = 0.022$) and LDL ($r = 0.244$; $p = 0.026$), however, these associations diminished after adjusting for all likely confounders (Table 4).

4. Discussion

Our study is the first to show that maternal vitamin B12 levels adversely associated with markers of metabolic risk at birth, in particular lipid profiles. Our observed rates of low B12 status in mothers (40%) is common at the time of delivery though it is not as high as in the South Asian population [10,11,26]. Haemodilution and increased nutrient demand by the growing fetus [27] are known contributors to low B12 levels during pregnancy. In addition, consumption of processed foods, improving hygiene and reheating of cooked food, all known to reduce the bioavailable B12 in food products, could have contributed to lower B12 levels in this population [20,28]. The presence of higher homocysteine in the low B12 group suggest that these low levels are clinically significant and represent true insufficiency at the tissue level.

Our findings show that low maternal B12 status was associated with offspring's insulin resistance, lower HDL and higher triglycerides (Figure 1a,b,d). However, when multivariate analysis was used to assess the effect of B12 across the spectrum, only HDL was statistically significant after adjusting for the possible confounders (Table 4). In support of this, adverse lipid profile (higher total cholesterol and triglycerides) was noticed in rats born to vitamin B12 restricted dams [18,19]. In addition, we have recently demonstrated that adipocytes cultured in low B12 condition showed increased cholesterol levels and was due to hypomethylation of cholesterol transcription factor (SREBF1 and LDLR) [29]. The clinical findings observed in this study thus add evidence that low maternal B12 status adversely affects lipid profile in the offspring. We did not see any significant association between maternal and neonatal lipids (data not shown). While this was surprising, it was similar to other observations, where only lipids from GDM mothers associated with foetal lipids and not from non-GDM mothers [30,31].

Our study also showed that maternal B12 showed a stronger inverse association with neonatal homocysteine than folate (Supplementary Figure S2a,b). In multiple regression analysis, after adjusting for the possible confounders, only maternal B12 and not folate, was independently associated with neonatal homocysteine (Table 4). The association between maternal folate and neonatal homocysteine became insignificant, when maternal homocysteine was added in the stepwise regression model (Table 4). This suggests that the effect of folate on neonatal homocysteine is likely to be mediated through maternal homocysteine while the effect of B12 could be partly independent of maternal homocysteine. Similar to our findings, Molloy *et al.* showed in an Irish population that low maternal B12 levels predicted hyperhomocysteinemia in both the newborns and the mothers [32]. Thus, our findings confirm that in folate replete populations, B12 is the strongest driver of homocysteine [10], an established metabolic risk factor [33]. Our study also showed that the BMI was higher in the low B12 group (Table 2). Similar observations were

144

seen other studies [29–31]. The cause and effect of this relationship is not known. Theoretically this could have contributed to higher maternal lipids and in turn higher lipids in cord blood. However, we did not see any correlation between maternal and cord lipids and our regression analysis adjusted for maternal lipids (Table 4).

The plausible biochemical reasons that low maternal B12 status increase the metabolic risk in the offspring might be, firstly, in the cytoplasm, vitamin B12 acts as a cofactor for conversion of homocysteine to methionine, the direct precursor of S-adenosylmethionine (SAM) which is the common donor required for methylation of DNA, protein and lipids [10,26,34]. Secondly, in mitochondria, vitamin B12 also acts a cofactor for the conversion of methylmalonyl Co-A (MM-CoA) to succinyl Co-A. Thus, low vitamin B12 causes higher MM-CoA levels. This in turn can inhibit carnitine palmitoyl transferase-1 (CPT-1), the rate-limiting enzyme for fatty acid β-oxidation, thereby increasing lipogenesis [10,35]. As these mechanisms involve methylation of DNA, this might lead to higher metabolic risk in the offspring by adverse epigenetic programming in addition to directly affecting β-oxidation of fatty acids. *In vivo* and interventional studies are required to identify the exact mechanisms and prove the causality.

Similar to B12, low maternal folate levels also showed adverse correlations with the metabolic risk markers of the offspring but these differences disappeared in regression models. Women with highest B12 and folate levels gave birth to children with lowest homocysteine levels compared to those with lowest B12 and folate levels (7.80 *vs.* 4.85 µmol/L, $p < 0.001$; Supplementary Table S1). Taken together, these findings suggest that optimising the circulating levels of these two B vitamins during pregnancy, is likely to be beneficial to the offspring.

Strengths and limitations: Our study is cross sectional and from a single-centre. However, this is the first study to report the associations between maternal B12 and lipid profiles in the offspring. A prospective cohort of women from before or early pregnancy would have been a better model. As the pathophysiological link, if any, between maternal nutrient status and offspring metabolic risk seem to happen earlier in pregnancy, such longitudinal study would have strengthened our findings [9,10]. Our findings call for such studies to be conducted urgently. Studies have reported that B12 levels progressively decline during pregnancy [36]. Therefore, the effect size we observed during late pregnancy might have been an overestimate if early pregnancy samples were tested. We did not use the microbiological assay for B12 measurements, which is known to be more sensitive at the lower levels of B12. This may have underestimated the rate of low B12 status [37] and in turn, the association with the metabolic risk factors in the offspring. We did not have a detailed socioeconomic status of the participants. It is known that lower socioeconomic status is an important confounder of adverse lipid profiles and BMI but the link between socioeconomic status and B12 is not known. Therefore, this is also a limitation of our observation and future studies should collect detailed socioeconomic status. Finally, although our sample size was adequate to demonstrate the low B12 status, it was probably too small to demonstrate the independent associations between maternal folate and homocysteine status and cord blood lipids.

In summary, our study shows that maternal vitamin B12 plays an important role in lipid metabolism in the offspring and that their restriction *in utero* may predispose them to the increased metabolic risk. However, these findings need to be replicated, ideally in a larger cohort of pregnant women from early pregnancy. In addition, *in vivo* and interventional studies are required to prove the exact mechanisms and the potential causal link. If proven, optimizing B12 levels of young women around the peri-conceptional period, could offer novel opportunities to reduce the burden of obesity and related metabolic disorders of the next generation.

Acknowledgments: The authors acknowledge all the clinic staffs including the labour ward at University Hospital Coventry Warwickshire (UHCW) and George Eliot Hospital (GEH), the assistance of clinical research nurses (Selvin Selvamoni and Jackie Farmer) and research coordinators (Amitha Gopinath and Karen Rouault) in supporting the recruitment of the women. The funding body did not have any input on the design, objectives or the analysis of the results. The study was supported by Diabetes Research Fund, George Eliot NHS trust, Nuneaton, UK and RCUK block grant (funding open access publication charges).

Author Contributions: Adaikala Antonysunil performed the statistical analysis, interpreted the data and drafted the initial manuscript. Manu Vatish contributed to patient recruitment, study design and reviewed the manuscript for intellectual content. Alexander Lawson & Craig Webster involved in the measurement of homocysteine by LC-MS and data collection of all the samples in Heartlands Hospital, Birmingham. Catherine Wood & Neil Anderson involved in the measurement of vitamin B12, folate and data collection of all the samples at George Eliot Hospital, Nuneaton. Kavitha Sivakumar contributed to patient recruitment, sample collection, storage and data collection. Philip G. McTernan co-ordinated and supported the data collection, contributed to the other biochemical analysis and made important contributions to the design of the study and reviewed the manuscript for important intellectual content. Chittaranjan S. Yajnik made important contributions to the design of the study, revised and reviewed the manuscript for important intellectual content. Ponnusamy Saravanan & Gyanendra Tripathi conceived the research question, designed the study, contributed to data interpretation, critically reviewed the manuscript, and approved the final manuscript as submitted. Ponnusamy Saravanan is the guarantor of this work and had full access to all the data presented in the study and takes full responsibility for the integrity and the accuracy of the data analysis. All authors approved the final manuscript as submitted.

Conflicts of Interest: The authors declare no conflict of interest.

References

1. Cunningham, S.A.; Kramer, M.R.; Narayan, K.M. Incidence of childhood obesity in the united states. *N. Engl. J. Med.* **2014**, *370*, 403–411.
2. Weiss, R.; Kaufman, F.R. Metabolic complications of childhood obesity: Identifying and mitigating the risk. *Diabetes Care* **2008**, *31*, S310–S316.

3. Ignell, C.; Claesson, R.; Anderberg, E.; Berntorp, K. Trends in the prevalence of gestational diabetes mellitus in southern sweden, 2003–2012. *Acta Obstet. Gynecol. Scand.* **2014**, *93*, 420–424.

4. Lawlor, D.A.; Benfield, L.; Logue, J.; Tilling, K.; Howe, L.D.; Fraser, A.; Cherry, L.; Watt, P.; Ness, A.R.; Davey Smith, G.; *et al.* Association between general and central adiposity in childhood, and change in these, with cardiovascular risk factors in adolescence: Prospective cohort study. *BMJ* **2010**, *341*.

5. Nayak, C.D.; Agarwal, V.; Nayak, D.M. Correlation of cord blood lipid heterogeneity in neonates with their anthropometry at birth. *Indian J. Clin. Biochem. IJCB* **2013**, *28*, 152–157.

6. Whincup, P.H.; Kaye, S.J.; Owen, C.G.; Huxley, R.; Cook, D.G.; Anazawa, S.; Barrett-Connor, E.; Bhargava, S.K.; Birgisdottir, B.E.; Carlsson, S.; *et al.* Birth weight and risk of type 2 diabetes: A systematic review. *JAMA* **2008**, *300*, 2886–2897.

7. Pettitt, D.J.; Jovanovic, L. Low birth weight as a risk factor for gestational diabetes, diabetes, and impaired glucose tolerance during pregnancy. *Diabetes Care* **2007**, *30* (Suppl. 2), S147–S149.

8. Barker, D.J.; Osmond, C.; Kajantie, E.; Eriksson, J.G. Growth and chronic disease: Findings in the Helsinki birth cohort. *Ann. Hum. Biol.* **2009**, *36*, 445–458.

9. Roseboom, T.J.; Painter, R.C.; van Abeelen, A.F.; Veenendaal, M.V.; de Rooij, S.R. Hungry in the womb: What are the consequences? Lessons from the dutch famine. *Maturitas* **2011**, *70*, 141–145.

10. Yajnik, C.S.; Deshpande, S.S.; Jackson, A.A.; Refsum, H.; Rao, S.; Fisher, D.J.; Bhat, D.S.; Naik, S.S.; Coyaji, K.J.; Joglekar, C.V.; *et al.* Vitamin B12 and folate concentrations during pregnancy and insulin resistance in the offspring: The pune maternal nutrition study. *Diabetologia* **2008**, *51*, 29–38.

11. Stewart, C.P.; Christian, P.; Schulze, K.J.; Arguello, M.; LeClerq, S.C.; Khatry, S.K.; West, K.P. Low maternal vitamin B-12 status is associated with offspring insulin resistance regardless of antenatal micronutrient supplementation in rural Nepal. *J. Nutr.* **2011**, *141*, 1912–1917.

12. Krishnaveni, G.V.; Veena, S.R.; Karat, S.C.; Yajnik, C.S.; Fall, C.H. Association between maternal folate concentrations during pregnancy and insulin resistance in Indian children. *Diabetologia* **2014**, *57*, 110–121.

13. Dwarkanath, P.; Barzilay, J.R.; Thomas, T.; Thomas, A.; Bhat, S.; Kurpad, A.V. High folate and low vitamin B-12 intakes during pregnancy are associated with small-for-gestational age infants in South Indian women: A prospective observational cohort study. *Am. J. Clin. Nutr.* **2013**, *98*, 1450–1458.

14. Saravanan, P.; Yajnik, C.S. Role of maternal vitamin B12 on the metabolic health of the offspring: A contributor to the diabetes epidemic? *Br. J. Diabetes Vasc. Disease* **2010**, *10*, 109–114.

15. Guerra-Shinohara, E.M.; Morita, O.E.; Peres, S.; Pagliusi, R.A.; Sampaio Neto, L.F.; D'Almeida, V.; Irazusta, S.P.; Allen, R.H.; Stabler, S.P. Low ratio of *S*-adenosylmethionine to *S*-adenosylhomocysteine is associated with vitamin deficiency in Brazilian pregnant women and newborns. *Am. J. Clin. Nutr.* **2004**, *80*, 1312–1321.

16. Ba, Y.; Yu, H.; Liu, F.; Geng, X.; Zhu, C.; Zhu, Q.; Zheng, T.; Ma, S.; Wang, G.; Li, Z.; *et al.* Relationship of folate, vitamin B12 and methylation of insulin-like growth factor-II in maternal and cord blood. *Eur. J. Clin. Nutr.* **2011**, *65*, 480–485.

17. Sinclair, K.D.; Allegrucci, C.; Singh, R.; Gardner, D.S.; Sebastian, S.; Bispham, J.; Thurston, A.; Huntley, J.F.; Rees, W.D.; Maloney, C.A.; *et al.* DNA methylation, insulin resistance, and blood pressure in offspring determined by maternal periconceptional B vitamin and methionine status. *Proc. Natl. Acad. Sci. USA* **2007**, *104*, 19351–19356.

18. Garcia, M.M.; Gueant-Rodriguez, R.M.; Pooya, S.; Brachet, P.; Alberto, J.M.; Jeannesson, E.; Maskali, F.; Gueguen, N.; Marie, P.Y.; Lacolley, P.; *et al.* Methyl donor deficiency induces cardiomyopathy through altered methylation/acetylation of PGC-1alpha by PRMT1 and SIRT1. *J. Pathol.* **2011**, *225*, 324–335.

19. Kumar, K.A.; Lalitha, A.; Pavithra, D.; Padmavathi, I.J.; Ganeshan, M.; Rao, K.R.; Venu, L.; Balakrishna, N.; Shanker, N.H.; Reddy, S.U.; *et al.* Maternal dietary folate and/or vitamin B12 restrictions alter body composition (adiposity) and lipid metabolism in Wistar rat offspring. *J. Nutr. Biochem.* **2013**, *24*, 25–31.

20. Adaikalakoteswari, A.; Jayashri, R.; Sukumar, N.; Venkataraman, H.; Pradeepa, R.; Gokulakrishnan, K.; Anjana, R.; McTernan, P.G.; Tripathi, G.; Patel, V.; *et al.* Vitamin B12 deficiency is associated with adverse lipid profile in Europeans and Indians with type 2 diabetes. *Cardiovasc. Diabetol.* **2014**, *13*.

21. Saravanan, P.; Maheshwaran, H.; Stranges, S.; Thorogood, M. Population levels of B12 and folic acid: Do we need to consider B12 fortification to prevent gestational diabetes and cardiovascular risk? *Diabet. Med.* **2010**, *27* (Suppl. 1), 37–188.

22. Saravanan, P.; Wood, C.; Andersen, N. B12 deficiency is more common than folate deficiency in early pregnancy: Do we need to consider B12 fortification? *Diabetologia* **2010**, *53*, S151–S152.

23. Milman, N.; Byg, K.E.; Bergholt, T.; Eriksen, L.; Hvas, A.M. Cobalamin status during normal pregnancy and postpartum: A longitudinal study comprising 406 Danish women. *Eur. J. Haematol.* **2006**, *76*, 521–525.

24. Milman, N.; Byg, K.E.; Hvas, A.M.; Bergholt, T.; Eriksen, L. Erythrocyte folate, plasma folate and plasma homocysteine during normal pregnancy and postpartum: A longitudinal study comprising 404 Danish women. *Eur. J. Haematol.* **2006**, *76*, 200–205.

25. Magera, M.J.; Lacey, J.M.; Casetta, B.; Rinaldo, P. Method for the determination of total homocysteine in plasma and urine by stable isotope dilution and electrospray tandem mass spectrometry. *Clin. Chem.* **1999**, *45*, 1517–1522.

26. Finer, S.; Saravanan, P.; Hitman, G.; Yajnik, C. The role of the one-carbon cycle in the developmental origins of type 2 diabetes and obesity. *Diabet. Med.* **2014**, *31*, 263–272.

27. Wallace, J.M.; Bonham, M.P.; Strain, J.; Duffy, E.M.; Robson, P.J.; Ward, M.; McNulty, H.; Davidson, P.W.; Myers, G.J.; Shamlaye, C.F.; *et al.* Homocysteine concentration, related B vitamins, and betaine in pregnant women recruited to the Seychelles child development study. *Am. J. Clin. Nutr.* **2008**, *87*, 391–397.

28. United States Department of Agriculture. USDA Table of Nutrient Retention Factors, Release 5. 2003. Available online: http://www.ars.usda.gov/Main/docs.htm?docid= 9448 (accessed on 27 March 2015).

29. Adaikalakoteswari, A.; Finer, S.; Voyias, P.D.; McCarthy, C.M.; Vatish, M.; Moore, J.; Smart-Halajko, M.; Bawazeer, N.; Al-Daghri, N.M.; McTernan, P.G.; *et al.* Vitamin B12 insufficiency induces cholesterol biosynthesis by limiting S-adenosylmethionine and modulating the methylation of SREBF1 and LDLR genes. *Clin. Epigenetics* **2015**, *7*.

30. Schaefer-Graf, U.M.; Graf, K.; Kulbacka, I.; Kjos, S.L.; Dudenhausen, J.; Vetter, K.; Herrera, E. Maternal lipids as strong determinants of fetal environment and growth in pregnancies with gestational diabetes mellitus. *Diabetes Care* **2008**, *31*, 1858–1863.

31. Schaefer-Graf, U.M.; Meitzner, K.; Ortega-Senovilla, H.; Graf, K.; Vetter, K.; Abou-Dakn, M.; Herrera, E. Differences in the implications of maternal lipids on fetal metabolism and growth between gestational diabetes mellitus and control pregnancies. *Diabet. Med.* **2011**, *28*, 1053–1059.

32. Molloy, A.M.; Mills, J.L.; Cox, C.; Daly, S.F.; Conley, M.; Brody, L.C.; Kirke, P.N.; Scott, J.M.; Ueland, P.M. Choline and homocysteine interrelations in umbilical cord and maternal plasma at delivery. *Am. J. Clin. Nutr.* **2005**, *82*, 836–842.

33. Wald, D.S.; Law, M.; Morris, J.K. Homocysteine and cardiovascular disease: Evidence on causality from a meta-analysis. *BMJ* **2002**, *325*, 1202.

34. Dominguez-Salas, P.; Cox, S.E.; Prentice, A.M.; Hennig, B.J.; Moore, S.E. Maternal nutritional status, C(1) metabolism and offspring DNA methylation: A review of current evidence in human subjects. *Proc. Nutr. Soc.* **2012**, *71*, 154–165.

35. Brindle, N.P.; Zammit, V.A.; Pogson, C.I. Regulation of carnitine palmitoyltransferase activity by malonyl-CoA in mitochondria from sheep liver, a tissue with a low capacity for fatty acid synthesis. *Biochem. J.* **1985**, *232*, 177–182.

36. Cikot, R.J.; Steegers-Theunissen, R.P.; Thomas, C.M.; de Boo, T.M.; Merkus, H.M.; Steegers, E.A. Longitudinal vitamin and homocysteine levels in normal pregnancy. *Br. J. Nutr.* **2001**, *85*, 49–58.

37. Carmel, R.; Agrawal, Y.P. Failures of cobalamin assays in pernicious anemia. *N. Engl. J. Med.* **2012**, *367*, 385–386.

Folate Deficiency Could Restrain Decidual Angiogenesis in Pregnant Mice

Yanli Li, Rufei Gao, Xueqing Liu, Xuemei Chen, Xinggui Liao, Yanqing Geng, Yubin Ding, Yingxiong Wang and Junlin He

Abstract: The mechanism of birth defects induced by folate deficiency was focused on mainly in fetal development. Little is known about the effect of folate deficiency on the maternal uterus, especially on decidual angiogenesis after implantation which establishes vessel networks to support embryo development. The aim of this study was to investigate the effects of folate deficiency on decidual angiogenesis. Serum folate levels were measured by electrochemiluminescence. The status of decidual angiogenesis was examined by cluster designation 34 (CD34) immunohistochemistry and the expression of angiogenic factors, including vascular endothelial growth factor A (VEGFA), placental growth factor (PLGF), and VEGF receptor 2 (VEGFR2) were also tested. Serum levels of homocysteine (Hcy), follicle stimulating hormone (FSH), luteinizing hormone (LH), prolactin (PRL), progesterone (P4), and estradiol (E2) were detected by Enzyme-linked immunosorbent assay. The folate-deficient mice had a lower folate level and a higher Hcy level. Folate deficiency restrained decidual angiogenesis with significant abnormalities in vascular density and the enlargement and elongation of the vascular sinus. It also showed a reduction in the expressions of VEGFA, VEGFR2, and PLGF. In addition, the serum levels of P4, E2, LH, and PRL were reduced in folate-deficient mice, and the expression of progesterone receptor (PR) and estrogen receptor α (ERα) were abnormal. These results indicated that folate deficiency could impaire decidual angiogenesis and it may be related to the vasculotoxic properties of Hcy and the imbalance of the reproductive hormone.

Reprinted from *Nutrients*. Cite as: Li, Y.; Gao, R.; Liu, X.; Chen, X.; Liao, X.; Geng, Y.; Ding, Y.; Wang, Y.; He, J. Folate Deficiency Could Restrain Decidual Angiogenesis in Pregnant Mice. *Nutrients* **2015**, *7*, 6425–6445.

1. Introduction

Birth defects or congenital anomalies are one of the major causes of disability in developed and developing countries [1]. The March of Dimes estimated that 7.4 million infants are born each year with a serious birth defect. Of these births, 94% occur in middle- and low-income countries [2]. Birth defects are also a population health problem affecting the quality of the birth population in China. In high-prevalence areas of China, the prevalence of birth defects was 537.2 per 10,000 births and the first five main birth defects were anencephaly, congenital heart

150

diseases, spina bifida, hydrocephaly, and encephalocele [3]. The causes of birth defects can be grouped into three main categories: (1) genetic, (2) environmental, and (3) complex genetic and unknown. Environmental causes are estimated to be responsible for approximately 5%–10% of the total amount of birth defects. Environmental causes include nutritional deficiencies, maternal illnesses, infectious agents, and teratogenic drugs [2].

Folate is one of the B vitamins and it plays a crucial role in one-carbon metabolism for physiological DNA synthesis and cell division, as well as in the conversion of homocysteine (Hcy) to methionine and so on. The influence of folate nutritional status on pregnancy outcomes has long been recognized [4]. Folate supplementation has been shown to reduce the occurrence of neural tube defects [5]. A preventive effect of folate on heart defects in newborns has also been proposed [6]. Folate deficiency or attendant elevated levels of homocysteine have been associated with orofacial clefts [7], down syndrome [8], placental abruptions [9], pre-eclampsia [10], spontaneous abortion [11], intrauterine growth retardation, and pre-term birth [12]. However, less is known about the mechanism of how folate deficiency induces birth defects. Our previous study showed that folate deficiency did not influence embryo implantation in mice [13]. It suggested that the pregnancy abnormalities, including lower female fertility, lower embryo number, and lower fetal viability, caused by folate deficiency may occur mainly after embryo implantation. Endometrial decidualization, placentation, and the development of the embryo itself are all important for normal pregnancy outcomes after embryo implantation. There have been many studies focused on the effect of folate deficiency on placentation and the development of the embryo itself, whereas little is known about the role of folate deficiency on maternal decidualization [7–12]. Angiogenesis, which establishes a network of vessels and sinusoids to support embryo development, is essential for endometrial decidualization [14]. Decidual angiogenesis forms a new vascular network that serves as the first exchange apparatus between the maternal circulation and the developing embryo and thus is a crucial and fundamental process for embryonic survival and a successful pregnancy [15]. Vascular endothelial growth factor A (VEGFA), placental growth factor (PLGF), and vascular endothelial growth factor (VEGF) receptor 2 (VEGFR2) are key molecules regulating decidual angiogenesis and maternal spiral artery remodeling. They are expressed in the endometrium, decidua, and placenta and play an important role in ensuring a successful pregnancy [16,17]. However, it is not known whether the establishment of the decidual vascular network is influenced by folate deficiency.

Here, we investigated the effect of folate deficiency on decidual angiogenesis after implantation with a folate-deficient pregnant mouse model. This study will help to elucidate the mechanisms of pregnancy abnormalities induced by folate deficiency.

2. Experimental Section

2.1. Animals

A folate-deficient pregnant mouse model was established as described by Gao *et al.* [13]. Six-to-eight-week-old National Institutes of Health female mice (mean ± standard error of the mean (SEM): 22 ± 1.8 g) were purchased from the Animal Facility of Chongqing Medical University, China (Certificate No.: SCXK (YU) 20070001) and caged in a specific pathogen-free animal room under a controlled environment (12 h light/12 h darkness). Mice in the folate-deficient group were fed a diet containing no folate (Research Diets, New Brunswick, USA) for five weeks before mating, and mice in the normal group were fed a normal diet. The estrus mice were mated with fertile males of the same strain (E1 = the day a vaginal plug was found). All animal procedures were approved by the Ethics Committee of Chongqing Medical University (NO. 20110016). Pregnant dams were sacrificed on Embryonic day 6 (E6), Embryonic day 7 (E7), and Embryonic day 8 (E8) at 9–10 a.m and decidual tissue was collected for the subsequent experiments. There were at least 15 mice sacrificed every day in every group.

2.2. Detection of Serum Folate, Hcy, P4, E2, FSH, LH, and PRL

Blood samples were collected from the eye socket and placed at room temperature for 3 h to obtain the serum. To verify the utility of the mouse model, serum folate levels of mice were measured using an electrochemiluminescence before mating [18]. The serum levels of Hcy, progesterone (P4), estradiol (E2), follicle stimulating hormone (FSH), luteinizing hormone (LH), and prolactin (PRL) were detected using an enzyme-linked immunosorbent assay (ELISA) (Yan Hui Biological Technology, Shanghai, China) according to the manufacturer's recommended instructions.

2.3. Hematoxylin-Eosin (H&E) Staining

The uterus was extracted and fixed in 4% paraformaldehyde (PFA) solution overnight at 4 °C and then embedded in paraffin. Tissue sections (4 μm) were mounted on glass slides. H&E staining was performed using standard protocols on the paraffin sections. The sections were mounted and stained with hematoxylin-eosin. A minimum of 10 histological sections from the uteri were assessed using 10× or 40× magnification and photographed using an Olympus B × 50 (Olympus) photomicroscope.

2.4. Immunohistochemistry

The uterus was extracted and fixed in 4% PFA solution overnight at 4 °C and then embedded in paraffin. Tissue sections were deparaffinized in xylene and rehydrated in descending concentrations of ethanol, followed by antigen retrieval in an Ethylene Diamine Tetraacetic Acid Antigen Retrieval Solution (pH 8.0, Beyotim, Shanghai, China) for 20 min in a microwave oven at 95 °C. Endogenous peroxidase was inhibited by incubation with 3% H_2O_2 for 10 min at room temperature. The tissue sections were blocked in 10% normal goat serum for 30 min. The sections were incubated with a rabbit monoclonal anti-cluster designation 34 (CD34) (ab81289, Abcam, Shanghai, China) antibody at a 1:100 dilution, a rabbit monoclonal anti-VEGFA (ab52917, Shanghai, China) antibody at a 1:50 dilution, a rabbit polyclonal anti-VEGFR2 (07-158, Millipore, Billerica, USA) antibody at a 1:100 dilution, and a goat polyclonal anti-PLGF (sc-1882, Santa Cruz, California, USA) antibody at a 1:30 dilution at 4 °C overnight. After incubation with the primary antibody, the tissue sections were incubated with corresponding biotinylated secondary antibodies. The chromogenic reaction was conducted with diaminobenzidine (Zhongshan Biosciences, Beijing, China) for 3 to 5 min and terminated by rinsing with water. The sections were subsequently stained with hematoxylin. Immunohistochemistry was performed on four-to-five pregnant mice from each group and each sample was assayed three times. The VEGFA, VEGFR2, and PLGF protein localization was analyzed and quantified using Medical Image Analysis Software (Beihang University, Beijing, China) and a yellowish-brown stain was determined as positive.

2.5. Western Blotting

Proteins were extracted from 40 mg decidual tissue collected at various time points during the post-implantation period from the two groups using a cell lysis buffer for western blotting and immunoprecipitation (Beyotim, Shanghai, China). Protein concentration was determined using the bicinchoninic acid Protein Assay kit (Beyotim, Shanghai, China). Samples were boiled in 5× sodium dodecylsulfate (SDS) sample loading buffer for 10 min and then loaded onto a 10% SDS-polyacrylamide gel (Beyotim, Shanghai, China). Following electrophoresis, proteins were transferred onto polyvinylidene difluoride membranes (Bio-Rad, California, USA). The membranes were blocked for 80 min at room temperature in a Tris Buffered Saline with Tween (TBST) buffer (20 mM Tris (pH 7.6), 137 mM NaCl, and 0.05% (w/v) Tween 20) containing 5% non-fat milk. Immunoblotting was performed by incubating the membranes in 5% milk-TBST overnight at 4 °C with a rabbit monoclonal anti-VEGFA (ab52917, Abcam, Shanghai, China) antibody at a 1:500 dilution, a rabbit polyclonal anti-VEGFR2 (07-158, Abcam, Millipore, Billerica,

USA) antibody at a 1:500 dilution, a rat monoclonal anti-PLGF (ab51654, Abcam, Shanghai, China) antibody at a 1:500 dilution, a mouse monoclonal anti-β-actin (ab8226, Abcam, Shanghai, China) antibody at a 1:1000 dilution, a rabbit monoclonal anti-estrogen receptor α (ERα) (04-227, Millipore, Billerica, USA) antibody at a 1:500 dilution, and a mouse monoclonal anti-progesterone receptor (PR) (ab2765, Abcam, Shanghai, China) antibody at a 1:500 dilution. Membranes were washed three times with TBST followed by incubation with the corresponding secondary antibody at room temperature for 80 min. After washing three times with TBST, positive bands were detected by enhanced chemiluminescence reagents (Beyotim, Shanghai, China) and quantified by densitometry using Quantity One version 4.4.0 software. Western blotting was performed on four-to-five pregnant mice from each group, and each sample was assayed three times.

2.6. Real-Time polymerase chain reaction (RT-PCR)

Total RNA was extracted from 30 mg decidual tissue using Trizol reagent (Invitrogen, Carlsbad, USA) according to the manufacturer's instructions. cDNA synthesis was performed with 1 μg total RNA treated with DNase I in a 20 mL reaction system using the First Strand synthesis for RT-PCR kit (Takara, Dalian, China). cDNA was stored at $-20\,°C$ until real-time RT-PCR analysis. Specific primers for VEGFA, VEGFR2, PLGF, and β-actin were designed and produced by Sangon Biotech (Shanghai, China). The sequences of the primers used are shown in Table 1. To compare transcript levels of VEGFA, VEGFR2, and PLGF between the normal group and the folate-deficient group, real-time RT-PCR was carried out using SYBR Premix Ex Taq kits (Takara, Dalian, China) and a Bio-Rad CFX96 Real-Time System (Bio-Rad, California, USA). The real time RT-PCR master mixture (15 uL) consisted of 7.5 μL of 2× SYBR Premix Ex Taq, 0.6 μL of 10 pmol/mL primers, 1.2 μL of cDNA, and 5.1 μL of double-distilled H_2O according to the manufacturer's recommendations. The PCR conditions were as follows: initial denaturation at $94\,°C$ for 30 s; 40 cycles of 10 s at $94\,°C$ (denaturation), and 30 s at corresponding primer melting temperature (Tm). Relative gene expression levels were calculated with the $2^{-\Delta\Delta Ct}$ method [19]. Real time RT-PCR was performed on six pregnant mice from each group and each sample was assayed three times.

2.7. Statistical Analysis

Data were analyzed using the Statistical Package for the Social Sciences (SPSS) statistical software (version 16.0, SPSS, Chicago, USA). Values are given as the mean $\pm$ SEM. The differences between groups in serum levels of folate, Hcy, P4, and E2 and the expression of VEGFA, VEGFR2, PLGF, and PR were analyzed with Student's t-test. Bonferroni correction was used for multiple testing, while the differences between groups in serum levels of FSH, LH, and PRL were analyzed with two-way analysis of variance. A $p < 0.05$ was considered statistically significant.

Table 1. Sequences of forward and reverse primers used in real-time RT-PCR ($5' \rightarrow 3'$).

Gene	Forward	Reverse
VEGFA	GTCCAACTTCTGGGCTCTTCT	CCCTCTCCTCTTCCTTCTCTTC
VEGFR2	TGGCAAATACAACCCTTCAGAT	GTCACCAATACCCTTTCCTCAG
PLGF	GCCGATAAAGACAGCCAACA	CATTCACAGAGCACATCCTGA
β-actin	CCTGAGGCTCTTTTCCAGCC	TAGAGGTCTTTACGGATGTCAACGT

VEGFA, vascular endothelial growth factor A; VEGFR2, vascular endothelial growth factor receptor 2; PLGF, placental growth factor.

3. Results

3.1. Validation of the Folate-Deficient Pregnant Mouse Model

The electro-chemiluminescence immunoassay was used to measure the serum folate levels to verify the validity of the pregnant mouse model. As shown in Table 2, serum folate levels were significantly decreased in the folate-deficient group ($p < 0.01$), which was consistent with our previous study [20]. In addition, Hcy, the intermediate product in folate metabolism and one of the factors influencing the biological functions of the vascular endothelium, serum levels were also determined with ELISA. As shown in Table 3, serum Hcy levels were significantly increased in the folate-deficient group ($p < 0.01$).

Table 2. Serum folate levels (ng/mL) in the pregnant mice (mean ± standard error of the mean (SEM)).

	Normal (*n*)	Folate-deficient (*n*)	*p*
Serum folate	>20 (*10*)	4.83 ± 0.48 (*19*)	<0.01

Table 3. Serum Hcy levels (μmol/L) in the pregnant mice (mean ± standard error of the mean (SEM)).

	Normal (*n*)	Folate-deficient (*n*)	*p*
E6	7.50 ± 0.24 (*5*)	11.06 ± 0.40 (*5*)	<0.01
E7	6.75 ± 0.41 (*5*)	12.05 ± 0.57 (*5*)	<0.01
E8	8.26 ± 0.32 (*5*)	12.46 ± 0.61 (*5*)	<0.01

E6, Embryonic day 6; E7, Embryonic day 7; E8, Embryonic day 8.

3.2. Decidual Angiogenesis Was Restrained in Folate-Deficient Pregnant Mice

To determine whether there was any abnormal angiogenesis in the folate-deficient group, the structural changes in blood vessels, the molecular regulation of angiogenesis, and the vascular remodeling in the uterus were analyzed from E6 to E8, which was after implantation (E4–5) but prior to initial placenta establishment (E9–10). As illustrated in the H&E staining, no obvious abnormalities could be seen in the folate-deficient group (Figure 1). With the development of the process of pregnancy, there was no significant difference in morphology and structure in the two groups. In the folate-deficient mice, the blastocyst could implant in the mesangial contralateral visibly. Stroma cell decidulization occurred around the blastocyst continuously and formed the primary decidual zone and secondary decidual zone gradually. The development of the blastocyst was normal as well. However, the significant abnormalities were observed in the vascular density and the enlargement and elongation of vascular sinus folding in folate-deficient pregnant mice, as evidenced with CD34 staining from E6 to E8 (Figure 2). Normally, variable-sized vascular sinus foldings [21] are distributed symmetrically in the central region of the uterus and are enlarged and elongated over time, whereas fine mesh-like blood vessels are arrayed in the anti-mesometrial region, which was similar to our findings (Figure 2). Closer observation of the central region revealed that the sprouting process was most active at E6 (Figure 2A), whereas enlargement and elongation of vascular sinus folding and intussusception of blood vessels [22] were dominant from E7 to E8. Time-series analyses indicated that, compared with E6, the number of large-sized vascular sinus foldings in the central region as well as blood vessel densities in the anti-mesometrial region were markedly increased at E7 and E8 (Figure 2B,C). A significant decrease in vascular density was observed in the folate-deficient group from E6 to E8 as compared with the normal group (Figure 2). The vascular sinus foldings, which predominantly extend into the intermediate zone from the mesometrial to the anti-mesometrial region of the decidua, appeared to be diminished in the folate-deficient group as compared with the normal group, especially at E7 and E8 (Figure 2B,C).

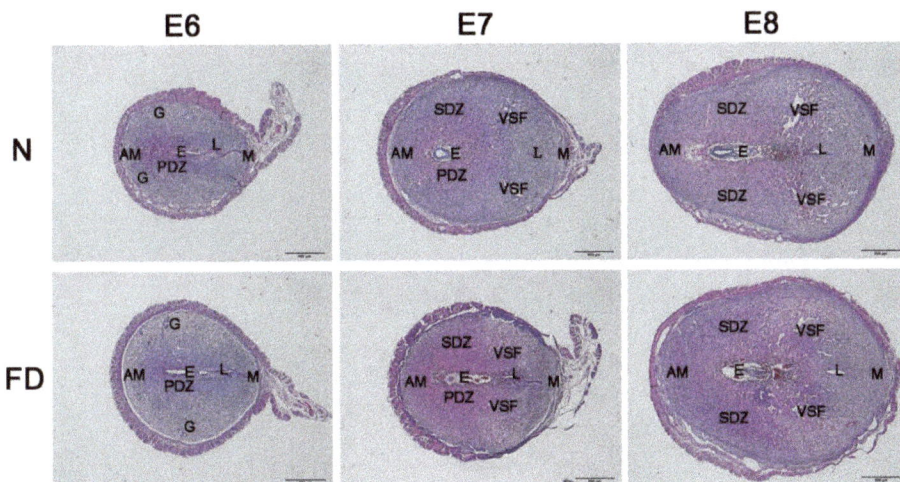

Figure 1. Uterine section's hematoxylin-eosin staining from E6 to E8. No significant abnormal decidualization or embryonic development occurred in the folate-deficient group. N: normal group; FD: folate-deficient group; E: embryo; L: luminal epithelium; G: glandular epithelium; PDZ: primary decidual zone; SDZ: secondary decidual zone; M: mesometrial; AM: anti-mesometrial; VSF: vascular sinus folding; Scale bar: 500 μm; E6, Embryonic day 6; E7, Embryonic day 7; E8, Embryonic day 8.

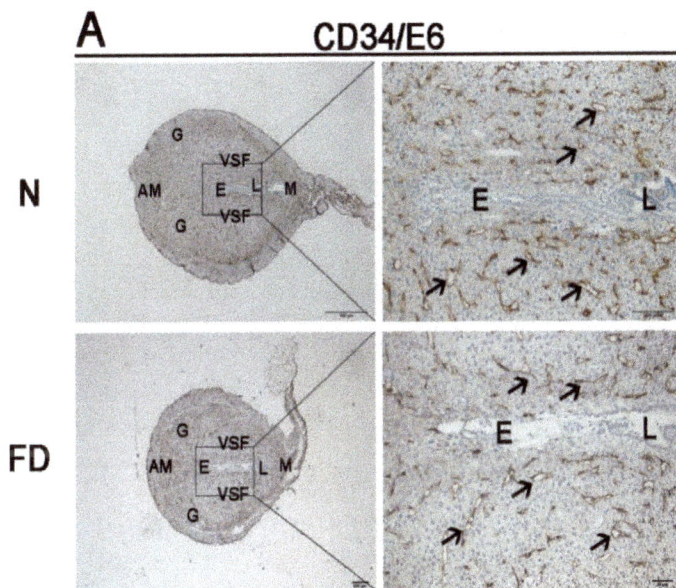

Figure 2. *Cont.*

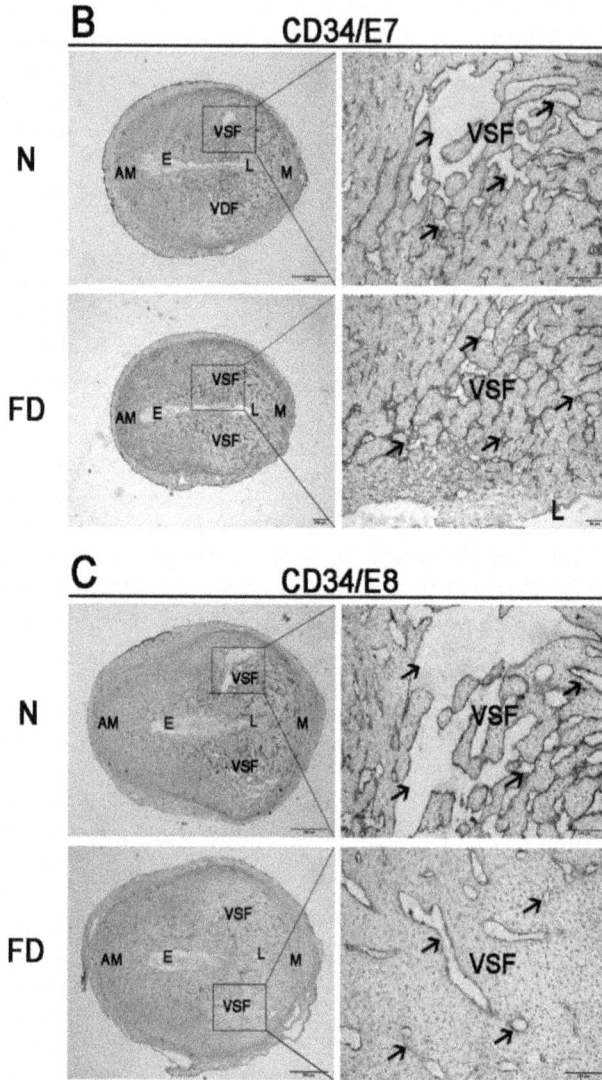

Figure 2. Immunohistochemistry staining with cluster designation 34 (CD34) from Embryonic day 6 (E6) to Embryonic day 8 (E8). Impaired formation of decidual angiogenesis was detected in the folate-deficient group. The pictures in the right column are the higher magnification images of the black boxes in the left column. (**A**) The magnified area was the central region around the embryo in uterus at E6. (**B, C**) The magnified area was one side of VSF at E7 and E8. Arrow indicates the variable-sized blood vessels. N: normal group; FD: folate-deficient group; E: embryo; L: luminal epithelium; G: glandular epithelium; M: mesometrial; AM: anti-mesometrial; VSF: vascular sinus folding. Scale bar: 500 μm (left), 100 μm (right).

3.3. The Expression of VEGFA, VEGFR2, and PLGF Was Reduced in Folate-Deficient Decidual Tissue

Immunohistochemical staining for VEGFA, PLGF, and VEGFR2 in the decidual tissue on E8 is shown in Figure 3. VEGFA was distributed mainly in a wide area of the secondary decidual zone (PDZ) and embryo in both normal and folate-deficient mice, but the expression of VEGFA in folate-deficient mice was depressed (Figure 3A). VEGFR2 was localized mainly in the vascular sinus folding close to the anti-mesometrial region in normal mice, whereas VEGFR2 surrounded the embryo mainly in folate-deficient mice (Figure 3B). The localization of PLGF was similar to VEGFA in normal mice, but it did not distribute in the embryo. However, PLGF was mainly located in the central region of the uterus instead of the PDZ in folate-deficient mice (Figure 3C). The relative amounts of VEGFA, PLGF, and VEGFR2 mRNAs detected by real-time RT-PCR are shown in Figure 4A. The relative fold change of VEGFA, PLGF, and VEGFR2 mRNA in the folate-deficient mice was decreased compared with the levels in normal mice from E6 to E8 ($p < 0.01$). The protein expression levels of VEGFA, PLGF, and VEGFR2 analyzed by Western blotting were correlated with the level of mRNAs (Figure 4B).

3.4. Folate-Deficient Mice Showed Disordered Reproductive Hormone Levels

Correct steroid hormone levels characterize a successful pregnancy, including decidualization, angiogenesis, and placentation. Angiogenesis could be impaired by abnormal steroid hormone levels [23]. To further assess the effect of folate deficiency on steroid hormone levels, we measured the serum levels of P4 and E2 from E6 to E8 by ELISA. As shown in Table 4, folate-deficient mice presented a decreasing trend in serum levels of P4 and E2 compared with normal mice. Western blotting demonstrated that the protein expression of PR in decidual tissue was decreased from E6 to E8, whereas the protein expression of ERα was increased in the folate-deficient group compared with the normal group (Figure 5). Because the secretion of P4 and E2 is regulated by gonadotropins, including FSH, LH and PRL, we also detected these three gonadotropins at the same time. The results showed that folate-deficient mice had aberrant gonadotropin levels (Table 5, Figure 6). Although there was no significant difference in the serum FSH levels between the two groups ($F = 0.791$, $p = 0.384$), the folate-deficient mice had a relatively lower serum level of LH ($F = 22.905$, $p < 0.001$) and PRL ($F = 17.465$, $p < 0.001$) compared with the normal mice (Figure 6).

159

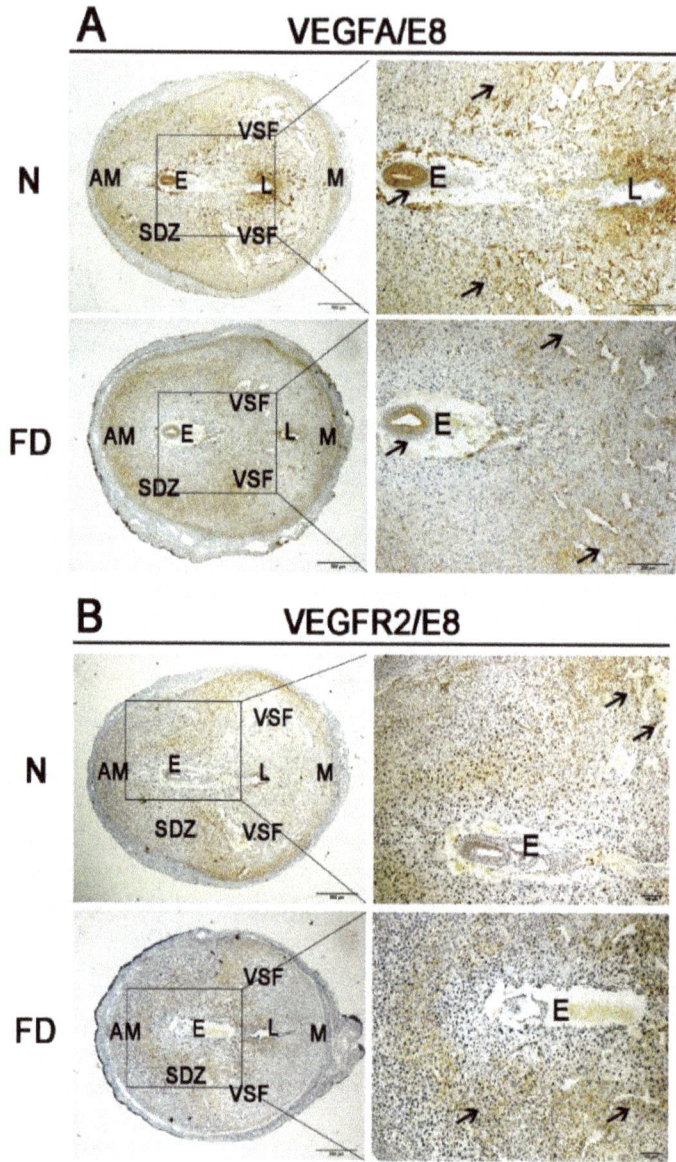

Figure 3. *Cont.*

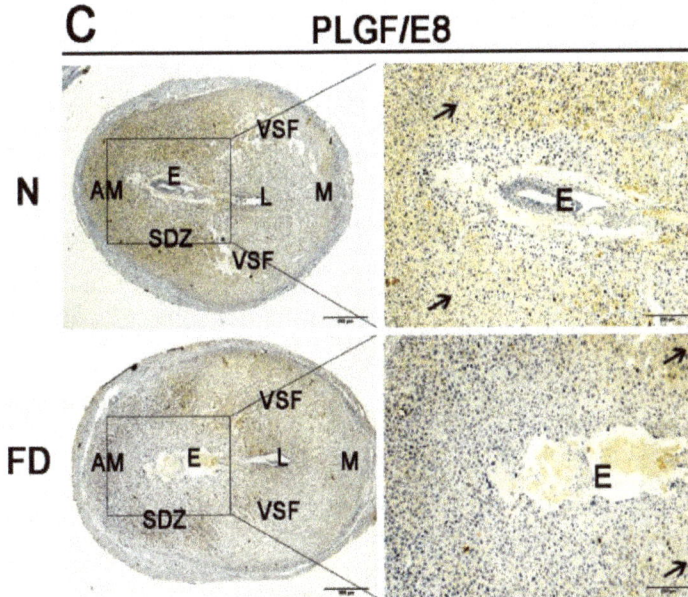

Figure 3. Immunohistochemistry staining with vascular endothelial growth factor A (VEGFA), vascular endothelial growth factor receptor 2 (VEGFR2), and placental growth factor (PLGF). Decreased expression of VEGFA, VEGFR2, and PLGF was detected in the folate-deficient group. The pictures in the right column are the higher magnification images of the black boxes in the left column. Additionally, the black boxes were the uterus's central region around the embryo. Arrow indicates each factor's different expression and distribution between two groups. (**A**) VEGFA was localized to a wide area of the secondary decidual zone (PDZ) and the embryo in both normal and folate-deficient mice, but there was decreased expression in the folate-deficient group. (**B**) VEGFR2 was localized mainly to the VSF close to the AM region in normal mice, whereas VEGFR2 was localized mainly to part of the PDZ in folate-deficient mice. (**C**) PLGF had a similar localization pattern as VEGFA in normal mice but was not expressed in the embryo. However, PLGF was expressed mainly in the central region of the uterus instead of in the PDZ in folate-deficient mice. N: normal group; FD: folate-deficient group; E: embryo; L: luminal epithelium; SDZ: secondary decidual zone; M: mesometrial; AM: anti-mesometrial; VSF: vascular sinus folding. Scale bar: 500 μm (left), 200 μm (right).

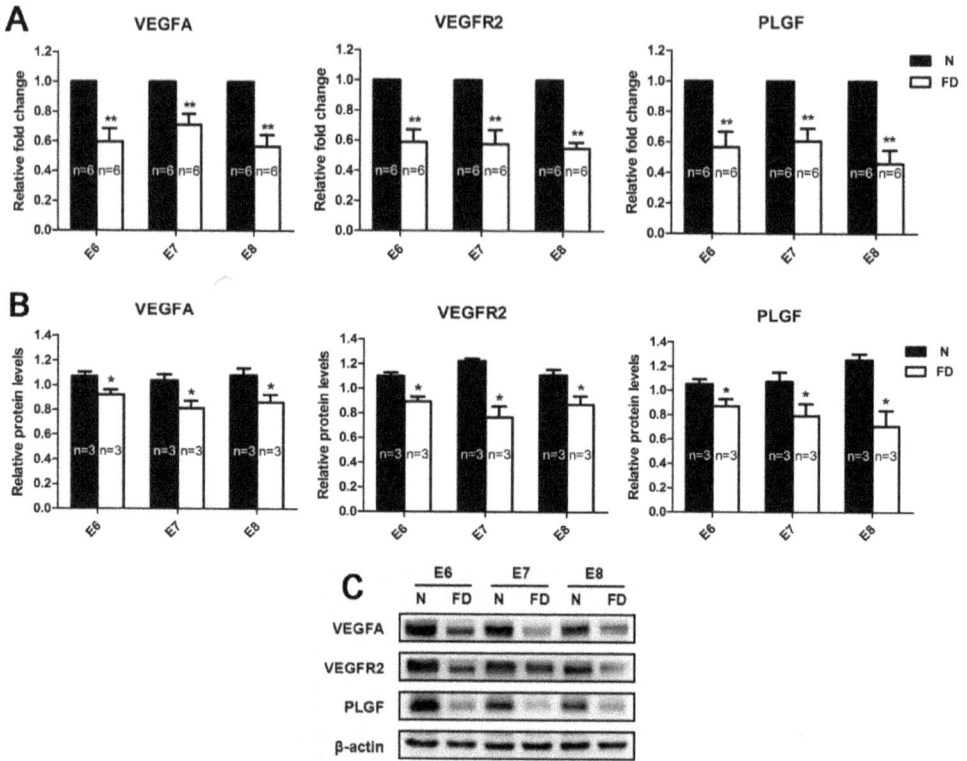

Figure 4. Real-time polymerase chain reaction (RT-PCR) and western blot analysis of the expression of vascular endothelial growth factor A (VEGFA), vascular endothelial growth factor receptor 2 (VEGFR2), and placental growth factor (PLGF) from Embryonic day 6 (E6) to Embryonic day 8 (E8). (**A**) The mRNA levels of VEGFA, VEGFR2, and PLGF in folate-deficient mice were significantly decreased compared with normal mice from E6 to E8 (** $p < 0.01$). Data are presented as the mean ± standard error of the mean (SEM). (**B**) Protein levels in folate-deficient mice were compared with normal mice. Statistical analysis of protein expression was from three independent experiments (* $p < 0.05$). Data are presented as the mean ± SEM. (**C**) Western blot analysis of three angiogenic growth factors. β-actin was used as a loading control. The protein levels of VEGFA, VEGFR2, and PLGF showed similar trends to the mRNAs levels. N: normal group, FD: folate-deficient group.

Table 4. Serum P4 and E2 levels in the pregnant mice (mean $\pm$ standard error of the mean (SEM)).

| | P4 (ng/mL) | | | E2 (pmol/L) | | |
	Normal (*n*)	Folate-deficient (*n*)	*p*	Normal (*n*)	Folate-deficient (*n*)	*p*
E6	11.02 $\pm$ 0.44 (4)	8.79 $\pm$ 0.17 (4)	0.009	42.39 $\pm$ 0.82 (3)	29.97 $\pm$ 0.60 (4)	<0.001
E7	10.02 $\pm$ 0.21 (4)	7.56 $\pm$ 0.18 (4)	<0.001	38.01 $\pm$ 0.77 (3)	26.50 $\pm$ 0.65 (4)	<0.001
E8	10.24 $\pm$ 0.16 (4)	6.20 $\pm$ 0.26 (4)	<0.001	38.76 $\pm$ 0.71 (3)	23.26 $\pm$ 0.71 (4)	<0.001

P4, progesterone; E2, estradiol.

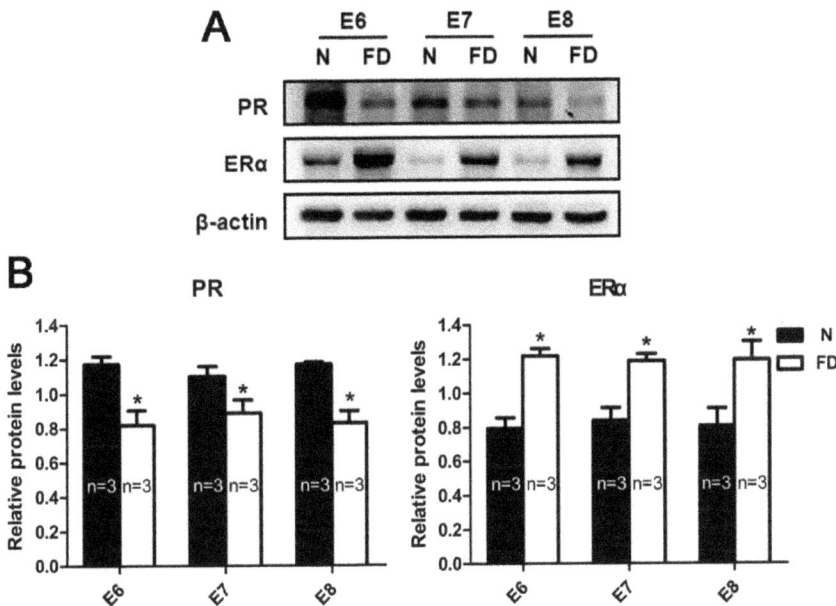

Figure 5. Western blot analysis of the expression of progesterone receptor (PR) and estrogen receptor α (ERα) from Embryonic day 6 (E6) to Embryonic day 8 (E8). (**A**) Protein levels are expressed relative to the normal group and β-actin was used as a loading control. (**B**) Statistical analysis of protein expression from three independent experiments. (* $p < 0.05$). PR was significantly decreased in the folate-deficient group compared with the normal group, whereas ERα was elevated significantly in folate-deficient mice. β-actin was used as a loading control. N: normal group; FD: folate-deficient group.

Table 5. Serum FSH, LH, and PRL levels in the pregnant mice (mean ± standard error of the mean (SEM)).

	FSH (mIU/mL)		LH (mIU/mL)		PRL (ng/mL)	
	Normal (*n*)	Folate-deficient (*n*)	Normal (*n*)	Folate-deficient (*n*)	Normal (*n*)	Folate-deficient (*n*)
E6	47.38 ± 4.02 (3)	45.50 ± 2.23 (5)	3.72 ± 0.51 (3)	2.66 ± 0.15 (5)	31.74 ± 3.23 (3)	24.21 ± 1.76 (5)
E7	53.49 ± 4.43 (3)	51.07 ± 2.46 (5)	4.52 ± 0.60 (3)	3.28 ± 0.20 (5)	32.94 ± 3.53 (3)	25.21 ± 1.42 (5)
E8	48.36 ± 3.62 (3)	46.45 ± 2.19 (5)	3.88 ± 0.45 (3)	2.95 ± 0.21 (5)	31.46 ± 1.70 (3)	24.78 ± 1.55 (5)

FSH, follicle stimulating hormone; LH, luteinizing hormone; PRL, prolactin.

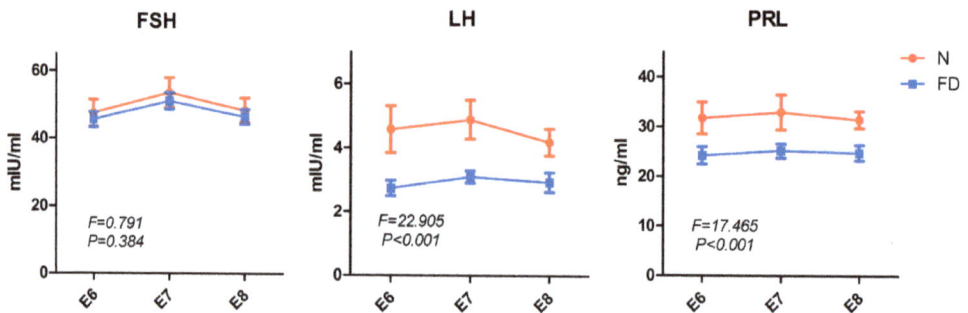

Figure 6. Serum follicle stimulating hormone (FSH), luteinizing hormone (LH) and prolactin (PRL) levels in the pregnant mice. Serum LH ($F = 22.905$, $p < 0.001$) and PRL ($F = 17.465$, $p < 0.001$) levels were decreased in the folate-deficient group significantly, but the level of FSH ($F = 0.791$, $p = 0.384$) was not significantly different between the two groups. Data are presented as the mean ± standard error of the mean (SEM). N: normal group; FD: folate-deficient group.

4. Discussion

In humans, the influence of folate nutritional status on various outcomes of a pregnancy has long been recognized. Although fetuses are known to concentrate folate from the maternal circulation to fulfill their nutrient requirements, it has been demonstrated in several animal models, including rat [24], monkey [25], golden hamster [26], and mouse [27], that severe maternal folate deficiency in the preconception and gestational periods may hamper female fertility and embryo and fetal viability. These animal findings emphasize that folate is indispensable during mammalian folliculogenesis and fetal development. However, much less is known about the mechanism of the folate deficiency on reproduction. Our previous study showed that a five-week folate deficiency status did not influence embryo implantation, and the methylation and expression of two molecules (cadherin 1 and progesterone receptor) essential for uterine receptivity were not altered either [13]. However, the outcome of the folate-deficient pregnant mice was not favorable (supplementary information). It is well known that successful implantation does not necessarily mean a successful pregnancy. After implantation, the normal uterine decidualization, placentation, and a healthy embryo are all crucial for pregnancy. Decidual angiogenesis forms a new vascular network that serves as the first exchange apparatus between the maternal circulation and the embryo that is necessary for embryonic survival and a successful pregnancy. Therefore, in this study, we focused on decidual angiogenesis, which occurs shortly after interstitial implantation.

In rodents and humans, the implanting conceptus stimulates decidualization in a specific spatial-temporal pattern [28]. The decidual reaction occurs during early pregnancy when the fibroblast-like endometrial stromal cells transiently proliferate and then differentiate into large, polyploid decidual cells. However, no significant abnormalities could be seen in the folate-deficient group as evidenced by the hematoxylin-eosin staining in our study. In response to the implanting blastocyst, neoangiogenesis establishes a network of vessels and sinusoids within the compact decidual tissue to serve as the first exchange apparatus between the maternal circulation and the developing embryo [29]. In the normal group, closer observations of the central region revealed that the sprouting process was most active at E6, and enlargement and elongation of vascular sinus folding and intussusception of blood vessels were dominant from E7 to E8. However, compared with the normal group, a significant decrease in vascular density was observed in the folate-deficient group from E6 to E8. The vascular sinus foldings, which predominantly extend into the intermediate zone from the mesometrial to the anti-mesometrial region of the decidua, also appeared to be diminished at E7 and E8 in the folate-deficient group. Taken together, these results indicate that folate deficiency could restrain decidual angiogenesis in pregnant mice.

The VEGF family is important in regulating decidual angiogenesis and maternal spiral artery remodeling [29]. The endometrium, decidua, and placenta are rich sources of angiogenic growth factors [30]. Several studies have reported the expression of VEGFA and its receptors in first-trimester human decidua, including in endothelial cells, epithelial cells, macrophages, and trophoblasts [31,32]. Therefore, VEGFA seems to play an active role in trophoblast invasion and angiogenesis during implantation. Though VEGFA can play several roles with different receptors, some researchers [15,33] demonstrated that mouse decidual angiogenesis could be blocked by interference with the vascular endothelial growth factor VEGFA/VEGFR2 pathway, the main player in initiating sprouting angiogenesis. PLGF is abundantly expressed in the human placenta, with expression increasing from the first trimester to the late second trimester and subsequently declining until delivery [34]. It is expressed in villous and extravillous trophoblast cells, vascular endothelium, and decidual stromal cells, and may act as a mediator of trophoblast function and angiogenesis during early pregnancy [35]. PLGF is known to mediate the formation of a mature and stable vessel network, which is an important feature in facilitating and resisting the dramatic increase in blood supply at the implantation site to serve the growing demands of the fetus [36]. PLGF and VEGFA have synergistic effects in the induction of angiogenesis, but PLGF-induced vessels are more mature and stable than VEGF-induced vessels [37,38]. In our study, a reduction of these three factors (VEGFA, VEGFR2, and PLGF) was accompanied by the damage of decidual angiogenesis in pregnant mice during the post-implantation period. It revealed that the abnormal expression and distribution of VEGFA, VEGFR2, and PLGF resulted in abnormal decidual angiogenesis in folate-deficient pregnant mice.

Previous studies have found that Hcy has vasculotoxic properties, causing endothelial cell damage and dysfunction [39,40]. Hcy is also known to induce oxidative stress responses [39] and to decrease the cellular antioxidant potential [40], which can damage all components of the endothelial cell. To explore why the decidual angiogenesis was impaired in folate-deficient mice, we tested the serum Hcy levels during the post-implantation period. It is known that dietary or genetically determined folate deficiency leads to Hcy accumulation [41] because both the remethylation and transsulfuration [42] pathways are inhibited in folate deficiency. We found a significant increase in the serum Hcy levels in the folate-deficient group compared with the normal group. When endothelial cells are exposed to Hcy *in vitro*, protein misfolding may be induced in the endoplasmic reticulum by altering local redox potential and interfering with disulfide bond formation [43]. Accumulation of misfolded proteins in the endoplasmic reticulum can trigger an unfolded protein response [44], which may cause cellular growth arrest [40] and apoptosis [45] if the endoplasmic reticulum stress is prolonged. In addition, Hcy exposure causes impaired early extra-embryonic vascular development, as evidenced by the altered composition of the vascular beds as well as the reduced expression of VEGFA and VEGFR2 [46] and even reduced the expression of VEGFA in a dose-dependent manner *in vitro* [47]. These findings were in accordance with our results, which showed that the reduced expression of VEGFA, VEGFR2, and PLGF in folate-deficient pregnant mice impacts decidual angiogenesis and may be associated with the increased serum Hcy levels.

Ovarian steroid hormones play a pivotal role in directing early uterine events during pregnancy, including make the uterus competent to attach to the blastocyst and initiate the process of implantation [48,49]. Subsequently, ovarian steroid hormones regulate a series of complex interactions at the interface between the developing embryo and the cells in the stromal compartment, leading to the formation of decidua, which supports embryo growth and maintains early pregnancy [50]. The cellular actions of these hormones are mediated through intracellular estrogen receptor and progesterone receptor proteins, which are hormone-inducible transcription factors [51]. The receptors were known to bind their respective hormone, to bind to DNA, and to regulate specific gene transcription. These genomic actions trigger the expression of specific gene networks in different cell types within the uterus, and the products of these genes in turn mediate the pregnancy. Angiogenesis also could be impaired by abnormal ovarian steroid hormone levels. Two decades ago, Keshet *et al.* first suggested that high VEGFA expression in decidual stromal cells could be regulated by ovarian steroid hormones [52]. Since then, the roles of P4, E2, and their receptors in decidual angiogenesis have been studied. Both P4 and E2 have been shown to induce VEGF expression in human uterine stromal cells [53,54]. In this study, the folate-deficient mice presented disordered ovarian steroid hormone levels and their receptors' expression was also abnormal compared with normal mice. Western blotting showed significant down-regulation of PR and up-regulation of ERα in folate-deficient groups, respectively. We detected a low level of E2 in folate deficiency in pregnant mice during E6 to E8, but there was a significant increase in ERα expression compared with the control group. The inconsistency between levels of this hormone and its receptor has been noted in several *in vivo* studies involving drug treatments or others [55]. The strength of the effect of hormones is related to the number of the hormone-receptor complex, so keeping the appropriate number of this complex is necessary to maintain the organism's normal functions. Either serum hormone level or the hormone receptor has a quantitative/qualitative change that could result in endometrial lesions. Hormone-activated receptors exert a feedback regulatory effect on the transcription of their own parent genes. Thus, the decreased downstream products may be responsible for the increased expression of ERα. Certainly we need to research it further to verify this hypothesis. In addition, Gao's research showed that the ERα promoter was significantly less methylated in the folate-deficient tissues compared with the normal ones [13]. The increased expression of ERα in decidual tissue may be due to the low level of methylation of ERα. However, no matter which reason led to increased expression of ERα, the E2-activated ERα complex was reduced authentically in folate-deficient pregnant mice and the complex's function was getting weak. Therefore, we speculated that folate deficiency may disturb the balance between P4 and E2, as well as their respective receptors. Additionally, the reduction of VEGFA, VEGFR2, and PLGF may be connected with this disordered balance.

In addition, it is known that reproductive fecundity depends on the coordinated functions of organs and glands along the hypothalamic-pituitary-gonadal axis. Gonadoptropin are synthesized in the pituitary gland and induce the ovaries to produce P4 and E2. The main function of FSH is to stimulate ovarian growth and promote follicular development [56]. LH participates in ovarian regulation, plays a critical role in follicular maturation, ovulation, and corpus luteum development, and intervenes in the synthesis of steroid hormones [57]. PRL secretion induced by mating leads to increased endothelial cell proliferation in the corpus luteum of pregnant rodents and plays a critical role in corpus luteum maintenance, which promotes progesterone production and the maintenance of gestation [58]. To investigate whether disruption of the pituitary regulation of the ovary might be responsible for the reduction in steroid hormone levels, we also measured serum gonadotropins, including FSH, LH, and PRL. There was no significant difference in serum FSH levels between the two groups; however, folate-deficient mice had lower serum levels of LH and PRL compared with normal mice in our study, indicating that the effect of folate deficiency on hypothalamic-pituitary-gonadal axis function was likely to be causal in the disordered steroid hormone levels. Moreover, P4 and E2 are cholesterol-derived, phylogenetically old steroid hormones [59]. They are synthesized during steroid hormone metabolization within several cell types such as the corpus luteum and placenta [60]. In a recent review [61], a novel insight into the interactions between folate and the lipid metabolism was put forward. The folate-deficient diet led to steatosis by altering the balance of phospholipids, including phosphatidylcholine, phosphatidylethanolamine, sphingomyelin, and components of very low-density lipoprotein (VLDL) that transport lipids from the liver. In addition, Hcy and the lipid metabolism are interrelated, at least partly, via methyl group metabolism [62]. It was found that lipid metabolism-related genes and associated metabolic pathways were regulated extensively by folate deficiency. These findings may explain our results of disordered steroid hormone levels in folate-deficient mice but still leave much to be explored in future efforts.

In conclusion, folate deficiency could impair decidual angiogenesis via the down-regulation of pro-angiogenic factors including VEGFA, VEGFR2, and PLGF, which results in a poor vascular network. In addition, the vasculotoxic properties of Hcy and abnormal reproductive hormone levels may contribute to the impaired decidual angiogenesis. Our previous published study had enriched the awareness that folate deficiency disrupts the proliferation-apoptosis balance and that the mitochondrial apoptosis pathway of endometrial decidual cells was inhibited in folate-deficient pregnant mice. Additionally, the marker genes' expression of endometrium decidualization in mice, including bone morphogenetic protein 2 (BMP2), homeobox A 10 (Hoxa10), matrix metalloproteinase 2 (MMP2), and matrix metalloproteinase 9 (MMP9) proteins was markedly reduced in folate-deficient mice. Combining all the evidence, we reach the final conclusion that folate deficiency could effect the uterine decidualization and decidual angiogenesis of pregnant mice. This research may provide some theories and evidence for investigating the mechanism underlying poor reproduction in females that have poor folate intake and absorption.

5. Conclusions

Folate deficiency could impair decidual angiogenesis via the down-regulation of pro-angiogenic factors including VEGFA, VEGFR2, and PLGF, which results in a poor vascular network. In addition, the vasculotoxic properties of Hcy and abnormal reproductive hormone levels may contribute to the impaired decidual angiogenesis.

Acknowledgments: This study was supported by grants from the National Nature Science Foundation of China (No.31271246).

Author Contributions: Junlin He and Rufei Gao designed the study; Yanli Li carried out the laboratory experiments, prepared figures, and wrote the manuscript; Rufei Gao revised the manuscript; Xinggui Liao helped to collect the tissue; Yanqing Geng helped to carry out the laboratory experiments; Xueqing Liu, Xuemei Chen, Yubin Ding, and Yingxiong Wang assisted to analyze the data and interpret the results.

Conflicts of Interest: The authors declare that there are no conflicts of interest that could be perceived as prejudicing the impartiality of the research reported.

References

1. Mathers, C.D.; Loncar, D. Projections of global mortality and burden of disease from 2002 to 2030. *PLoS Med.* **2006**, *3*, e442.
2. Castillo, T.S. Services for the care and prevention of birth defects. Reduced report of a World Health Organization and March of Dimes Foundation meeting. *Rev. Med. Chile* **2007**, *135*, 806–813.
3. Zheng, X.Y.; Song, X.M.; Chen, G.; Chen, J.P.; Ji, Y.; Wu, J.L.; Liu, J.F.; Zhang, L.; Fan, X.H. Epidemiology of birth defects in high-prevalence areas of China. *Zhonghua Liu Xing Bing Xue Za Zhi* **2007**, *28*, 5–9.
4. Wills, L. Treatment of "pernicious anaemia of pregnancy" and "tropical anaemia" with special reference to yeast extract as a curative agent. 1931. *Natl. Med. J. India* **2013**, *26*, 117–122.
5. Czeizel, A.E.; Dudas, I. Prevention of the first occurrence of neural-tube defects by periconceptional vitamin supplementation. *N. Engl. J. Med.* **1992**, *327*, 1832–1835.
6. Ionescu-Ittu, R.; Marelli, A.J.; Mackie, A.S.; Pilote, L. Prevalence of severe congenital heart disease after folic acid fortification of grain products: Time trend analysis in Quebec, Canada. *BMJ* **2009**, *338*.
7. Tolarova, M.; Harris, J. Reduced recurrence of orofacial clefts after periconceptional supplementation with high-dose folic acid and multivitamins. *Teratology* **1995**, *51*, 71–78.
8. Martinez-Frias, M.L.; Perez, B.; Desviat, L.R.; Castro, M.; Leal, F.; Rodriguez, L.; Mansilla, E.; Martinez-Fernandez, M.L.; Bermejo, E.; Rodriguez-Pinilla, E.; *et al.* Maternal polymorphisms 677C-T and 1298A-C of MTHFR, and 66A-G MTRR genes: Is there any relationship between polymorphisms of the folate pathway, maternal homocysteine levels, and the risk for having a child with Down syndrome? *Am. J. Med. Genet. A* **2006**, *140*, 987–997.
9. Hibbard, B.M.; Hibbard, E.D.; Hwa, T.S.; Tan, P. Abruptio placentae and defective folate metabolism in Singapore women. *Int. J. Obstet. Gynaecol. Br. Commonw.* **1969**, *76*, 1003–1007.
10. Mignini, L.E.; Latthe, P.M.; Villar, J.; Kilby, M.D.; Carroli, G.; Khan, K.S. Mapping the theories of preeclampsia: The role of homocysteine. *Obstet. Gynecol.* **2005**, *105*, 411–425.

11. George, L.; Mills, J.L.; Johansson, A.L.; Nordmark, A.; Olander, B.; Granath, F.; Cnattingius, S. Plasma folate levels and risk of spontaneous abortion. *JAMA* **2002**, *288*, 1867–1873.

12. Lindblad, B.; Zaman, S.; Malik, A.; Martin, H.; Ekstrom, A.M.; Amu, S.; Holmgren, A.; Norman, M. Folate, vitamin B12, and homocysteine levels in South Asian women with growth-retarded fetuses. *Acta Obstet. Gynecol. Scand.* **2005**, *84*, 1055–1061.

13. Gao, R.; Ding, Y.; Liu, X.; Chen, X.; Wang, Y.; Long, C.; Li, S.; Guo, L.; He, J. Effect of folate deficiency on promoter methylation and gene expression of Esr1, Cdh1 and Pgr, and its influence on endometrial receptivity and embryo implantation. *Hum. Reprod.* **2012**, *27*, 2756–2765.

14. Winterhager, E.; Gellhaus, A.; Blois, S.M.; Hill, L.A.; Barr, K.J.; Kidder, G.M. Decidual angiogenesis and placental orientation are altered in mice heterozygous for a dominant loss-of-function Gja1 (connexin43) mutation. *Biol. Reprod.* **2013**, *89*, 111.

15. Kim, M.; Park, H.J.; Seol, J.W.; Jang, J.Y.; Cho, Y.S.; Kim, K.R.; Choi, Y.; Lydon, J.P.; Demayo, F.J.; Shibuya, M.; *et al.* VEGF-A regulated by progesterone governs uterine angiogenesis and vascular remodelling during pregnancy. *EMBO Mol. Med.* **2013**, *5*, 1415–1430.

16. Charnock-Jones, D.S.; Kaufmann, P.; Mayhew, T.M. Aspects of human fetoplacental vasculogenesis and angiogenesis. I. Molecular regulation. *Placenta* **2004**, *25*, 103–113.

17. Senger, D.R.; Ledbetter, S.R.; Claffey, K.P.; Papadopoulos-Sergiou, A.; Peruzzi, C.A.; Detmar, M. Stimulation of endothelial cell migration by vascular permeability factor/vascular endothelial growth factor through cooperative mechanisms involving the alphavbeta3 integrin, osteopontin, and thrombin. *Am. J. Pathol.* **1996**, *149*, 293–305.

18. Zhao, S.; Yuan, H.; Xie, C.; Xiao, D. Determination of folic acid by capillary electrophoresis with chemiluminescence detection. *J. Chromatogr. A* **2006**, *1107*, 290–293.

19. Livak, K.J.; Schmittgen, T.D. Analysis of relative gene expression data using real-time quantitative PCR and the $2^{-\Delta\Delta C_T}$ Method. *Methods* **2001**, *25*, 402–408.

20. Liao, X.G.; Li, Y.L.; Gao, R.F.; Geng, Y.Q.; Chen, X.M.; Liu, X.Q.; Ding, Y.B.; Mu, X.Y.; Wang, Y.X.; He, J.L. Folate deficiency decreases apoptosis of endometrium decidual cells in pregnant mice via the mitochondrial pathway. *Nutrients* **2015**, *7*, 1916–1932.

21. Chandana, E.P.; Maeda, Y.; Ueda, A.; Kiyonari, H.; Oshima, N.; Yamamoto, M.; Kondo, S.; Oh, J.; Takahashi, R.; Yoshida, Y.; *et al.* Involvement of the Reck tumor suppressor protein in maternal and embryonic vascular remodeling in mice. *BMC Dev. Biol.* **2010**, *10*, 84.

22. Burri, P.H.; Hlushchuk, R.; Djonov, V. Intussusceptive angiogenesis, its emergence, its characteristics, and its significance. *Dev. Dyn.* **2004**, *231*, 474–488.

23. Hyder, S.M.; Stancel, G.M. Regulation of angiogenic growth factors in the female reproductive tract by estrogens and progestins. *Mol. Endocrinol.* **1999**, *13*, 806–811.

24. Willmott, M.; Bartosik, D.B.; Romanoff, E.B. The effect of folic acid on superovulation in the immature rat. *J. Endocrinol.* **1968**, *41*, 439–445.

25. Mohanty, D.; Das, K.C. Effect of folate deficiency on the reproductive organs of female rhesus monkeys: A cytomorphological and cytokinetic study. *J. Nutr.* **1982**, *112*, 1565–1576.

26. Mooij, P.N.; Wouters, M.G.; Thomas, C.M.; Doesburg, W.H.; Eskes, T.K. Disturbed reproductive performance in extreme folic acid deficient golden hamsters. *Eur. J. Obstet. Gynecol. Reprod. Biol.* **1992**, *43*, 71–75.

27. Xiao, S.; Hansen, D.K.; Horsley, E.T.; Tang, Y.S.; Khan, R.A.; Stabler, S.P.; Jayaram, H.N.; Antony, A.C. Maternal folate deficiency results in selective upregulation of folate receptors and heterogeneous nuclear ribonucleoprotein-E1 associated with multiple subtle aberrations in fetal tissues. *Birth Defects Res. A Clin. Mol. Teratol.* **2005**, *73*, 6–28.

28. Abrahamsohn, P.A.; Zorn, T.M. Implantation and decidualization in rodents. *J. Exp. Zool.* **1993**, *266*, 603–628.

29. Folkman, J.; Klagsbrun, M. Angiogenic factors. *Science* **1987**, *235*, 442–447.

30. Reynolds, L.P.; Killilea, S.D.; Redmer, D.A. Angiogenesis in the female reproductive system. *FASEB J.* **1992**, *6*, 886–892.

31. Plaisier, M.; Rodrigues, S.; Willems, F.; Koolwijk, P.; van Hinsbergh, V.W.; Helmerhorst, F.M. Different degrees of vascularization and their relationship to the expression of vascular endothelial growth factor, placental growth factor, angiopoietins, and their receptors in first-trimester decidual tissues. *Fertil. Steril.* **2007**, *88*, 176–187.

32. Cooper, J.C.; Sharkey, A.M.; McLaren, J.; Charnock-Jones, D.S.; Smith, S.K. Localization of vascular endothelial growth factor and its receptor, flt, in human placenta and decidua by immunohistochemistry. *J. Reprod. Fertil.* **1995**, *105*, 205–213.

33. Douglas, N.C.; Tang, H.; Gomez, R.; Pytowski, B.; Hicklin, D.J.; Sauer, C.M.; Kitajewski, J.; Sauer, M.V.; Zimmermann, R.C. Vascular endothelial growth factor receptor 2 (VEGFR-2) functions to promote uterine decidual angiogenesis during early pregnancy in the mouse. *Endocrinology* **2009**, *150*, 3845–3854.

34. Torry, D.S.; Wang, H.S.; Wang, T.H.; Caudle, M.R.; Torry, R.J. Preeclampsia is associated with reduced serum levels of placenta growth factor. *Am. J. Obstet. Gyneco.l* **1998**, *179*, 1539–1544.

35. Khaliq, A.; Li, X.F.; Shams, M.; Sisi, P.; Acevedo, C.A.; Whittle, M.J.; Weich, H.; Ahmed, A. Localisation of placenta growth factor (PlGF) in human term placenta. *Growth Factors* **1996**, *13*, 243–250.

36. Torry, D.S.; Ahn, H.; Barnes, E.L.; Torry, R.J. Placenta growth factor: Potential role in pregnancy. *Am. J. Reprod. Immunol.* **1999**, *41*, 79–85.

37. Carmeliet, P.; Moons, L.; Luttun, A.; Vincenti, V.; Compernolle, V.; De Mol, M.; Wu, Y.; Bono, F.; Devy, L.; Beck, H.; *et al.* Synergism between vascular endothelial growth factor and placental growth factor contributes to angiogenesis and plasma extravasation in pathological conditions. *Nat. Med.* **2001**, *7*, 575–583.

38. Luttun, A.; Tjwa, M.; Moons, L.; Wu, Y.; Angelillo-Scherrer, A.; Liao, F.; Nagy, J.A.; Hooper, A.; Priller, J.; De Klerck, B.; *et al.* Revascularization of ischemic tissues by PlGF treatment, and inhibition of tumor angiogenesis, arthritis and atherosclerosis by anti-Flt1. *Nat. Med.* **2002**, *8*, 831–840.

39. Edirimanne, V.E.; Woo, C.W.; Siow, Y.L.; Pierce, G.N.; Xie, J.Y.; O, K. Homocysteine stimulates NADPH oxidase-mediated superoxide production leading to endothelial dysfunction in rats. *Can. J. Physiol. Pharmacol.* **2007**, *85*, 1236–1247.

40. Outinen, P.A.; Sood, S.K.; Pfeifer, S.I.; Pamidi, S.; Podor, T.J.; Li, J.; Weitz, J.I.; Austin, R.C. Homocysteine-induced endoplasmic reticulum stress and growth arrest leads to specific changes in gene expression in human vascular endothelial cells. *Blood* **1999**, *94*, 959–967.

41. Jacques, P.F.; Bostom, A.G.; Wilson, P.W.; Rich, S.; Rosenberg, I.H.; Selhub, J. Determinants of plasma total homocysteine concentration in the Framingham Offspring cohort. *Am. J. Clin. Nutr.* **2001**, *73*, 613–621.

42. Miller, J.W.; Nadeau, M.R.; Smith, J.; Smith, D.; Selhub, J. Folate-deficiency-induced homocysteinaemia in rats: Disruption of S-adenosylmethionine's co-ordinate regulation of homocysteine metabolism. *Biochem. J.* **1994**, *298*, 415–419.

43. Lentz, S.R.; Sadler, J.E. Inhibition of thrombomodulin surface expression and protein C activation by the thrombogenic agent homocysteine. *J. Clin. Invest.* **1991**, *88*, 1906–1914.

44. Malhotra, J.D.; Kaufman, R.J. The endoplasmic reticulum and the unfolded protein response. *Semin. Cell Dev. Biol.* **2007**, *18*, 716–731.

45. Zhang, C.; Cai, Y.; Adachi, M.T.; Oshiro, S.; Aso, T.; Kaufman, R.J.; Kitajima, S. Homocysteine induces programmed cell death in human vascular endothelial cells through activation of the unfolded protein response. *J. Biol. Chem.* **2001**, *276*, 35867–35874.

46. Oosterbaan, A.M.; Steegers, E.A.; Ursem, N.T. The effects of homocysteine and folic acid on angiogenesis and VEGF expression during chicken vascular development. *Microvasc. Res.* **2012**, *83*, 98–104.

47. Yan, T.T.; Li, Q.; Zhang, X.H.; Wu, W.K.; Sun, J.; Li, L.; Zhang, Q.; Tan, H.M. Homocysteine impaired endothelial function through compromised vascular endothelial growth factor/Akt/endothelial nitric oxide synthase signalling. *Clin. Exp. Pharmacol. Physiol.* **2010**, *37*, 1071–1077.

48. Wang, H.; Dey, S.K. Roadmap to embryo implantation: Clues from mouse models. *Nat. Rev. Genet.* **2006**, *7*, 185–199.

49. Bagchi, I.C.; Li, Q.; Cheon, Y.P. Role of steroid hormone-regulated genes in implantation. *Ann. N. Y. Acad. Sci.* **2001**, *943*, 68–76.

50. Ramathal, C.Y.; Bagchi, I.C.; Taylor, R.N.; Bagchi, M.K. Endometrial decidualization of mice and men. *Semin. Reprod. Med.* **2010**, *28*, 17–26.

51. Critchley, H.O.; Saunders, P.T. Hormone receptor dynamics in a receptive human endometrium. *Reprod. Sci.* **2009**, *16*, 191–199.

52. Shweiki, D.; Itin, A.; Neufeld, G.; Gitay-Goren, H.; Keshet, E. Patterns of expression of vascular endothelial growth factor (VEGF) and VEGF receptors in mice suggest a role in hormonally regulated angiogenesis. *J. Clin. Invest.* **1993**, *91*, 2235–2243.

53. Wetendorf, M.; DeMayo, F.J. The progesterone receptor regulates implantation, decidualization, and glandular development via a complex paracrine signaling network. *Mol. Cell. Endocrinol.* **2012**, *357*, 108–118.

54. Zhao, Y.; Park, S.; Bagchi, M.K.; Taylor, R.N.; Katzenellenbogen, B.S. The coregulator, repressor of estrogen receptor activity (REA), is a crucial regulator of the timing and magnitude of uterine decidualization. *Endocrinology* **2013**, *154*, 1349–1360.

55. Zhao, Y.; Chen, X.; Liu, X.; Ding, Y.; Gao, R.; Qiu, Y.; Wang, Y.; He, J. Exposure of mice to benzo(a)pyrene impairs endometrial receptivity and reduces the number of implantation sites during early pregnancy. *Food Chem. Toxicol.* **2014**, *69*, 244–251.

56. Kumar, T.R.; Wang, Y.; Lu, N.; Matzuk, M.M. Follicle stimulating hormone is required for ovarian follicle maturation but not male fertility. *Nat. Genet.* **1997**, *15*, 201–204.

57. Niswender, G.D.; Juengel, J.L.; Silva, P.J.; Rollyson, M.K.; McIntush, E.W. Mechanisms controlling the function and life span of the corpus luteum. *Physiol. Rev.* **2000**, *80*, 1–29.

58. Petroff, M.G.; Petroff, B.K.; Pate, J.L. Mechanisms of cytokine-induced death of cultured bovine luteal cells. *Reproduction* **2001**, *121*, 753–760.

59. Mahesh, V.B.; Brann, D.W.; Hendry, L.B. Diverse modes of action of progesterone and its metabolites. *J. Steroid Biochem. Mol. Biol.* **1996**, *56*, 209–219.

60. Golub, M.S.; Kaufman, F.L.; Campbell, M.A.; Li, L.H.; Donald, J.M. "Natural" progesterone: Information on fetal effects. *Birth Defects Res. B Dev. Reprod. Toxicol.* **2006**, *77*, 455–470.

61. Da Silva, R.P.; Kelly, K.B.; Al Rajabi, A.; Jacobs, R.L. Novel insights on interactions between folate and lipid metabolism. *Biofactors* **2014**, *40*, 277–283.

62. Obeid, R.; Herrmann, W. Homocysteine and lipids: S-adenosyl methionine as a key intermediate. *FEBS Lett.* **2009**, *583*, 1215–1225.

Section 2:

New Studies of Vitamin D and Its Role in Fetal Development

Regulation of Calcitriol Biosynthesis and Activity: Focus on Gestational Vitamin D Deficiency and Adverse Pregnancy Outcomes

Andrea Olmos-Ortiz, Euclides Avila, Marta Durand-Carbajal and Lorenza Díaz

Abstract: Vitamin D has garnered a great deal of attention in recent years due to a global prevalence of vitamin D deficiency associated with an increased risk of a variety of human diseases. Specifically, hypovitaminosis D in pregnant women is highly common and has important implications for the mother and lifelong health of the child, since it has been linked to maternal and child infections, small-for-gestational age, preterm delivery, preeclampsia, gestational diabetes, as well as imprinting on the infant for life chronic diseases. Therefore, factors that regulate vitamin D metabolism are of main importance, especially during pregnancy. The hormonal form and most active metabolite of vitamin D is calcitriol. This hormone mediates its biological effects through a specific nuclear receptor, which is found in many tissues including the placenta. Calcitriol synthesis and degradation depend on the expression and activity of CYP27B1 and CYP24A1 cytochromes, respectively, for which regulation is tissue specific. Among the factors that modify these cytochromes expression and/or activity are calcitriol itself, parathyroid hormone, fibroblast growth factor 23, cytokines, calcium and phosphate. This review provides a current overview on the regulation of vitamin D metabolism, focusing on vitamin D deficiency during gestation and its impact on pregnancy outcomes.

Reprinted from *Nutrients*. Cite as: Olmos-Ortiz, A.; Avila, E.; Durand-Carbajal, M.; Díaz, L. Regulation of Calcitriol Biosynthesis and Activity: Focus on Gestational Vitamin D Deficiency and Adverse Pregnancy Outcomes. *Nutrients* **2015**, *7*, 443–480.

1. Vitamin D Synthesis and Metabolism

UVB radiation from sunlight initiates vitamin D (VD) biosynthesis in the skin by bioconverting 7-dehydrocholesterol to previtamin D_3, which is thermally isomerized to VD_3. VD may also be obtained from the diet to a lesser extent. The nutritional forms of VD include both VD_3 (cholecalciferol) from animal origin and VD_2 (ergocalciferol) from fungi and plant origin. Once formed in the skin or absorbed in the intestine, VD is released into the circulation and transported by the VD-binding protein (DBP) to the liver, where it is converted by the VD-25-hydroxylase (CYP2R1) into 25-hydroxyvitamin D (calcidiol, 25OHD). Calcidiol is the major vitamin D metabolite present in the circulation and the best indicator of VD nutritional status. Nevertheless, this metabolite is not the active form of VD, and therefore needs further activation by a second hydroxylation step catalyzed by the enzyme 25OHD-1-α-hydroxylase (CYP27B1) in order to generate 1,25-$(OH)_2D_3$ (calcitriol), which is the hormonal form and most active VD metabolite. CYP27B1 is primarily expressed in the kidney but also may be found in different tissues including the placenta. The bioavailability of calcitriol is tightly regulated to restrict the biological actions of this hormone in target cells while maintaining calcium and phosphate homeostasis, and the enzyme in charge of degrading calcitriol to water-soluble and less active metabolites is the 1,25-$(OH)_2D_3$-24-hydroxylase (CYP24A1), which in turn is highly upregulated by calcitriol itself, as a negative feedback mechanism [1,2].

Importantly, in order for CYP27B1 to fulfill its duty of producing calcitriol, there must be enough substrate available. This requirement is readily accomplished by the endocytic receptors megalin/cubilin and the adaptor protein disabled-2 (Dab2) present in the kidney, where 25OHD in complex with DBP is filtered through the glomerulus and reabsorbed in the proximal tubules by the cooperative action of these proteins [3–5]. Inside the cell, DBP is degraded and 25OHD is released and hydroxylated by CYP27B1. This specialized mechanism allowing renal uptake and activation of 25OHD is paramount for calcitriol production, as demonstrated by Nykjaer A. *et al.* [3] in rats infused with [3]H-25OHD/DBP and where megalin activity was blocked. In these animals, no conversion products (*i.e.*, ^{3}H-calcitriol) were recovered from serum samples. In contrast, in animals with intact and active megalin that were also infused, ^{3}H-calcitriol was readily detected in their plasma samples. Similarly, the importance of cubilin in the 25OHD reabsorption process is evident in human patients carrying inactivating mutations in cubilin gene (Imerslund–Gräsbeck disease), which exhibit abnormal urinary excretion of 25OHD and DBP [4].

2. Calcitriol Biological Effects

Calcitriol actions are mediated through the vitamin D receptor (VDR), a high-affinity ligand-activated transcription factor. Once bound to its ligand, the VDR heterodimerizes with the retinoid X receptor (RXR). This complex recognizes vitamin D response elements (VDRE) in the promoter regions of VD target genes and recruits co-activators or co-repressors in order to induce or repress gene transcription [6]. In addition, non-genomic calcitriol-dependent biological effects can also take place in cells, involving second messengers generated by membrane-initiated signaling pathways [7,8]. Indeed, the classic VDR and the membrane-associated rapid response steroid-binding protein (MARRS) found in the cell membrane may bind calcitriol and initiate the activation of numerous pathways involving protein kinase C (PKC) [9], mitogen-activated protein kinase (MAPK) [10], protein kinase A (PKA) [11,12], phosphatidyl inositol phosphate [13] and Ca^{2+} and chloride channels [8,14]. Very important processes are mediated through these rapid signaling cascades, such as insulin secretion and transcaltachia [15–17]. In general, the known VDRE-containing genes can be grouped in very diverse biological networks including bone and mineral metabolism (*i.e.*, osteopontin [18]); cell life and death (comprising proliferation, differentiation, migration and apoptosis, *i.e.*, p21 [19]), metabolism and cardiovascular health (*i.e.*, cystathionine β-synthase [20], renin [21] and VEGF [22]), immune function (*i.e.*, cathelicidin hCTD, LL-37 [23,24]) and detoxification (*i.e.*, CYP3A4, CYP24A1 [25]).

3. Regulation of the VD-Metabolizing Enzymes

Renal CYP27B1, which is responsible for the most part of circulating calcitriol, is mainly regulated by parathyroid hormone (PTH) -as a signal of calcium status-, fibroblast growth factor 23 (FGF23) -as a signal of serum phosphate levels- and calcitriol itself -as a negative feedback regulatory loop- [26]. When serum calcium levels are low, PTH is secreted by the parathyroid gland in order to stimulate renal CYP27B1 by a cyclic AMP (cAMP)-dependent mechanism [27]. PTH also causes CYP24A1 mRNA degradation in the kidney [28]. Calcitriol production is then boosted, thereby increasing blood calcium levels by promoting absorption of dietary calcium from the gastrointestinal tract, increasing renal tubular calcium reabsorption and stimulating the release of calcium from bone. As feedback effects, the synthesis and secretion of PTH are then inhibited by calcitriol and FGF23, the latter being produced in the bone [29]. FGF23 also potently inhibits CYP27B1 in response to elevated phosphate levels [30]. Finally, calcitriol inhibits its own production by different mechanisms comprising PTH inhibition, direct transcriptional repression of the CYP27B1 gene, and FGF23 and CYP24A1 induction [31]. Other factors that stimulate renal CYP27B1 activity and/or expression are insulin-like growth factor type I (IGF-I) and calcitonin [32–34].

4. Extra-Renal Regulation of Vitamin D-Hydroxylases

Extra-renal CYP27B1 is regulated in different ways than those observed in the kidney, in a tissue-specific manner. For instance, macrophage and monocyte CYP27B1 is not stimulated by PTH but rather by cytokines such as interferon-γ (INF-γ) and tumor necrosis factor-α (TNF-α) [35–38]. In addition, CYPB7B1 in immune cells is not readily negatively regulated by calcitriol. Likewise, the negative regulatory loop exerted by CYP24A1 is not very effective; therefore, 25OHD availability is the limiting factor for calcitriol synthesis in these cells [38]. In a similar manner as in immune cells, in keratinocytes, TNF-α and INF-γ potently induce CYP27B1 whereas calcitriol does not directly inhibit this gene [39–41]. Nevertheless, CYP24A1 is induced by calcitriol and efficiently degrades bioactive calcitriol, thus regulating calcitriol availability in the epidermis [39]. The transcriptional induction of CYP24A1 by calcitriol is

179

feasible considering the existence of multiple VDREs within its promoter. However, other regulatory mechanisms can also play a role in CYP24A1 regulation, such as alternative splicing, epigenetic gene silencing and metabolism of its mRNA [42–45].

In a comparable fashion as immune cells and keratinocytes, proinflammatory cytokines induce CYP27B1 gene expression in the human placenta [46]. Interestingly, in this tissue, CYP24A1 expression is also stimulated by these factors, suggesting that both synthesis and catabolism of placental calcitriol are locally affected by inflammatory cytokines [46]. Nevertheless, we have shown that TNF-α increased significantly the expression of CYP24A1 over CYP27B1, whereas IFN-γ preferentially stimulated CYP27B1. These observations, together with those showing that cultured trophoblasts secrete significantly more TNF-α than INF-γ, suggest that in the placenta, increased TNF-α secretion may limit calcitriol bioavailability [46]. The latter agrees with *in vivo* evidence showing low serum calcitriol and low placental CYP27B1 expression and calcitriol production in preeclampsia (PE), a pregnancy-associated condition characterized by an exacerbated pro-inflammatory profile.

In contrast to immune and epidermal cells, calcitriol in the placenta is able to transcriptionally inhibit CYP27B1 expression, which is mediated by both the VDR and a cAMP-dependent mechanism [12]. In this tissue, CYP24A1 gene expression is also potently induced by calcitriol [12]. However, it is also recognized that the CYP24A1 gene is methylated in the human placenta, suggesting that epigenetic decoupling of VD feedback catabolism may play an important role in maximizing calcitriol bioavailability at the feto-maternal interface [43]. Nevertheless, as discussed previously by Rosen *et al.* [47], this assumption is not supported by functional studies, since there is unequivocal evidence for human placental synthesis of 24,25-dihydroxyvitamin D_3, the main metabolic product of CYP24A1 [48]. Moreover, in this seminal article by Rubin and colleagues, under physiologic concentrations of 25OHD, placental trophoblasts preferentially synthesize 24,25-dihydroxyvitamin D_3 over calcitriol [48], which may explain why fetal levels of 24-hydroxylated VD metabolites are 40-fold higher than calcitriol [47,49,50]. These studies strongly suggested that placental CYP24A1 expression and activity, together with substrate availability are important limiting factors for calcitriol synthesis in the feto-maternal interface. Other hormonal factors affecting placental VD-metabolism are IGF-I and the natural occurring calciotropic hormones calcitonin and PTH [12,51]. IGF-I stimulates biotransformation of 25OHD into calcitriol [51], while both calcitonin and PTH regulate the placental VD-hydroxylases in the same manner as calcitriol and cAMP, inducing CYP24A1 while repressing CYP27B1 gene expression, thereby favoring VD catabolism [12].

5. Physiological Changes of 25OHD, Calcitriol, DBP and VDR during Pregnancy

During pregnancy, significant changes in maternal serum calcitriol, DBP and placental VDR take place and interact to acquire extra calcium for adequate fetal bone mineralization (for a recent review see Brannon PM and Picciano MF [52]). Indeed, the fetus may accumulate up to 30 g of calcium at term, and to satisfy this demand, VD metabolism is boosted in order to increase calcium intestinal absorption [53]. Collectively, these changes include increased maternal serum calcitriol, DBP, placental VDR and renal and placental CYP27B1 activity, without changes in serum 25OHD or calcium levels. In fact, maternal ionized calcium does not increase despite higher circulating calcitriol [54–57]; instead, serum calcium remains normal as calcium is transferred to the fetus. This equilibrium could be attributed to the concomitant normal rise in calciuria [55–59], precluding the risk of hypercalcemia. Fetal serum calcium levels are higher than those observed in the mother, a situation that requires specific mechanisms for calcium transport against a concentration gradient. In this regard, the active transplacental passage of calcium to the fetus is mediated by placental expression of calcium binding proteins such as calbindin-D9k and 28k [60–62]. Interestingly, placental VDR has shown to be a positive predictor of fetal femur length and is positively correlated with maternal-to-fetal transfer of calcium [63], suggesting that fetal skeletal growth could be affected by VDR-dependent mechanisms; and therefore, the relative VDR placental abundance would be a preponderant feature for fetal bone health.

Maternal 25OHD serum levels remain constant across pregnancy [56,57,59,64], suggesting that the increment observed in serum calcitriol levels is independent of changes in its precursor synthesis. Maternal 25OHD crosses the placental barrier and represents the main pool of VD in the fetus. In fact, serum fetal (cord blood) 25OHD levels are on average 25% reduced compared to maternal serum and correlate well with mother 25OHD levels [65,66]; therefore, VD deficiency in the mother could be vertically transmitted to the fetus.

During pregnancy, serum calcitriol rises from the first trimester, doubling its concentration compared to non-gravid women by the end of the third trimester and returning to normal values after delivery [54,56,58,59,64,67]. This physiological rise in calcitriol levels observed during pregnancy could be related to increased synthesis rather than decreased clearance [68]. Increased synthesis of calcitriol is linked to higher CYP27B1 activity in maternal kidney, placental trophoblasts and decidua [69–71].

The mechanisms underlying improved CYP27B1 activity during pregnancy remain elusive, partly because its known regulatory factors stay unchanged during this period, such as PTH [54–56,59], which may be even lower with respect to non-gravid women [58,64]. Also, a murine PTH null model supports that PTH does not contribute to increased calcitriol levels during pregnancy [72]. It has been hypothesized [64,73] that a potential regulatory factor for CYP27B1 could be the PTH analog PTH-related peptide (PTH-rP), which is synthesized by fetal parathyroids and placenta [74] and increases throughout pregnancy. PTH-rP could reach the maternal circulation and, after binding to PTH type 1 receptor (PTHR1), it may induce gene expression of CYP27B1 in the kidney and catalyze calcitriol synthesis for endocrine actions. However, this mechanism could not completely explain the higher activity of CYP27B1 in placenta because, as previously described, this tissue has its own mechanisms governing VD metabolism. In fact, PTH downregulates placental CYP27B1 gene expression [12].

The placental contribution to maternal calcitriol levels was demonstrated in 1978 by Weisman and colleagues in a nephrectomized pregnant rat model. In that study, the authors showed that anephric rats can synthesize calcitriol and 24,25-dihydroxyvitamin D_3 from 25OHD and that the fetoplacental unit is the most likely site of production of such metabolites [75]. Later, the *in vitro* synthesis of 24,25-dihydroxyvitamin D_3 and calcitriol by the human placenta was demonstrated [69]. Interestingly, in a model of chronic renal failure by Blum and colleagues [76], nephrectomized rats had lower calcitriol levels in comparison with normal rats, but during pregnancy the nephrectomized group reached similar levels to those observed in pregnant controls, despite kidney absence, which emphasized the important contribution of the placenta [76]. In 2000, studies in cultured human placental syncytiotrophoblasts showed that the synthesis of calcitriol from its endogenous precursor was driven by an enzymatic 1α-hydroxylation mechanism, since these cells expressed a CYP27B1 gene transcription product with a nucleotide sequence identical to that of transcripts previously characterized in the human kidney [70]. Later, the CYP27B1 protein localization was demonstrated in human placental decidual and trophoblastic cells [77].

In relation to VDR, it has been shown that its gene and protein expression is higher in placental and decidual tissue during the first and second trimesters in comparison with term placentas [78,79], in a similar manner as CYP27B1, with highest levels of expression occurring in first trimester decidua [78], thus suggesting a more preponderant role for calcitriol during the first part of pregnancy. It is likely that this is related to the importance of maintaining an anti-inflammatory setting for the acceptance of the fetal allograft. This is discussed further in Section 6.

Regarding DBP, two longitudinal studies indicate that this protein increases 25% to 56% during pregnancy [59,67], but the mechanisms leading to this increment are still unknown. It has been hypothesized that the DBP rise may be due to increased calcitriol concentration in gestation. In support of this assumption, serum DBP levels in pregnant women correlated with serum calcitriol levels [80].

The rise in DBP during pregnancy is intriguing and should be taken into consideration for the analysis of VD homeodynamics and physiological impact during this period. Actually, a great debate has been taking place regarding which form of 25OHD is the more suitable for activation, the "free" or the DBP-bound form. In this regard, the "free hormone" hypothesis sustains that the free steroid, by diffusing freely through the cell membrane, is the one available for activation and thereafter capable of performing biological effects, while the hormone bound to its carrier protein is considered to be sequestered and therefore, not bioavailable. However, this hypothesis has been confronted in the last years, given the important transporting and interacting mechanisms existing between the megalin/cubilin complex and DBP/25OHD, together with the observed disparity between the expected amounts of free hormone available for passive diffusion and the levels required to efficiently occupy intracellular target receptors. For an excellent review see: Chun *et al.* [81]. Interestingly, Chun and colleagues have recently proposed a viable hypothesis considering a role for DBP in tissue discrimination of $25OHD_2$ and $25OHD_3$. Given that $25OHD_2$ binds to DBP with lower affinity than $25OHD_3$, the kidney would preferentially use the latter metabolite, while cells in the immune system might profit of a greater pool of $25OHD_2$ for antimicrobial peptide induction [81].

It is noteworthy mentioning that megalin/cubilin-mediated 25OHD/DBP endocytosis may also take place in the placenta, since these receptors are expressed in this tissue [82–84] and placental calcitriol production has been proved [69,75], suggesting that circulating 25OHD is accessible to placental CYP27B1 by active transport. However, trophoblastic production of calcitriol may also be explained by the steroid freely diffusing through the cell membrane, and consequently both free and bound-25OHD might represent a bioavailable material for placental CYP27B1. Therefore, even if the uptake of 25OHD by proximal tubule cells evidently depends on the internalization of DBP, the functional significance of the placental megalin/cubilin endocitic complex expression and functionality remains far from clear.

Interestingly, mice with genetic ablation of the DBP gene only presented classic VD-associated problems when maintained under a low VD diet, supporting a role for DBP in maintaining stable serum stores of VD metabolites while modulating the rates of its bioavailability, activation, and end-organ responsiveness [85].

6. Calcitriol Effects during Pregnancy

One of the main activities attributed to calcitriol during pregnancy is to increase calcium absorption and to upregulate placental calcium transport. However, since VDR and CYP27B1 are also expressed in reproductive feminine tissues like the uterus, ovary, endometrium, fallopian epithelial cells and placenta [86–88], other potential paracrine and autocrine actions of calcitriol cannot be discarded. In this regard, during gestation, VD-dependent regulation of the immune function is paramount, since an adequate balance of the cytokine profile is necessary for pregnancy success. Specifically, calcitriol plays a dual role aimed at improving the innate immune response while restraining exacerbated inflammation. Calcitriol achieves this by inhibiting pro-inflammatory cytokines such as TNF-α, IFN-γ and interleukin-6 (IL-6), while at the same time induces the potent antimicrobial peptide hCTD in the fetoplacental unit [89–92]. In this tissue, calcitriol also stimulates other antimicrobial peptides known as β-defensins (HBDs), in particular HBD2 and HBD3 [93].

Calcitriol biological effects in the placenta are also related to hormonogenesis and overall placental physiology. In particular, calcitriol induces endometrial decidualization and estradiol and progesterone synthesis, but also regulates the expression of human chorionic gonadotropin and placental lactogen expression [94–97]. Table 1 lists currently known targets regulated by calcitriol in human placenta.

Considering these important effects of calcitriol on human pregnancy, it is not surprising that VD inadequacy may contribute to many gestation-associated disorders. Herein, we revise some common adverse pregnancy outcomes associated with maternal VD deficiency.

7. Vitamin D Deficiency and Adverse Pregnancy Outcomes

As previously mentioned, circulating 25OHD represents the best indicator of VD status. This metabolite was eligible instead of calcitriol for two principal reasons [98]: (1) 25OHD is present in a higher concentration than calcitriol (ng/mL $vs.$ pg/mL); and (2) in a deficient 25OHD scenario, PTH is stimulated and consequently induces renal CYP27B1 expression and, therefore, calcitriol synthesis. Consequently, this could derive in a relative and transient "normality" in calcitriol levels, given its short half-life (few hours for calcitriol instead of 2–3 weeks for 25OHD [99,100]).

The spectrum of VD status has been established considering the known risk for adverse consequences [101]. 25OHD values lesser than 25 nmol/L are related to rickets and osteomalacia and therefore are labeled as "severe deficiency". 25OHD values lesser than 50 nmol/L may sustain long-term adverse health consequences and are classified as "deficiency." The 75 nmol/L cut-off is the point above which there is no upper stimulation of PTH [102] and was thereafter designated as "sufficient." However, Heaney pointed out that 25OHD concentrations < 80 nmol/L are associated with reduced calcium absorption and osteoporosis risk [103]; therefore, values lesser than 75 nmol/L are considered as "insufficient." The conversion factor between 25OHD nmol/L and ng/mL is 2.5 (Table 2).

Table 1. Targets modulated by calcitriol in the human placenta (+ = Stimulation; − = Inhibition).

Target	Biological Network	Regulation	Bioeffect	Cell Type	Reference
Placental lactogen	Cell life and death	+	Growth control	Trophoblast	[97]
TNF-α	Immune function	−	Restraining inflammation	Trophoblast	[91,92]
		−	Immunosuppression	Decidual cells	[89]
IL-6	Immune function	−	Restraining inflammation	Trophoblast	[91,92]
		−	Immunosuppression	Decidual cells	[89]
CSF2 (colony stimulating factor 2)	Immune function	−	Immunosuppression	Decidual cells	[89]
hCTD	Immune function	+	Restraining infection	Trophoblast	[90]
				Decidual cells	[89]
CYP24A1	Bone and mineral metabolism	+	Calcitriol catabolism	Trophoblast	[12]
				Decidual cells	[104]
CYP27B1	Bone and mineral metabolism	−	Calcitriol synthesis	Trophoblast	[12]
IL-10 (Interleukin 10)	Immune function	−	Reducing risk of infection	Trophoblast	[105]
KCNH1 (Potassium voltage-gated channel)	Cell life and death		Unknown	Trophoblast	[106]
Calbindin-D 28 kDa	Bone and mineral metabolism	+	Calcium transfer	Trophoblast	[61,62]
Calbindin-D 9 kDa	Bone and mineral metabolism	+	Calcium transfer	Trophoblast	[61]
hCG (human chorionic gonadotrophin)	Cell life and death	+, −	Maintenance of pregnancy	Trophoblast	[96]
3β-HSD (3β-hydroxysteroid dehydrogenase) *	Cell life and death	+	Progesterone synthesis	Trophoblast	[95]
CYP19 (aromatase) *	Cell life and death	+	Estradiol synthesis	Trophoblast	[95]
Prolactin	Cell life and death	+	Establishment of pregnancy	Decidual cells	[107]
VDR	Bone and mineral metabolism	+	Allowing calcitriol actions	Trophoblast	[62]
Platelet-activating factor acetylhydrolase	Cell life and death	−	Inactivation of platelet-activating factor	Decidual macrophages	[108]
HOXA10 (Homeobox A10)	Cell life and death	+	Embryo implantation	Decidual cells	[109]
Osteopontin	Bone and mineral metabolism	+	Embryo implantation	Decidual cells	[104]
HBD2	Immune function	+	Restraining infection	Trophoblast	[93]
HBD3	Immune function	+	Restraining infection	Trophoblast	[93]

* Only observed at the enzyme activity level.

185

Table 2. Cut-offs in vitamin D status according to the Endocrine Society [110].

Vitamin D Status	25OHD (nmol/L)	25OHD (ng/mL)
Severe deficiency	<25	<10
Deficiency	<50	<20
Insufficiency	<75	<30
Sufficiency	75–110	30–44
Toxicity	>250	>100

Table 2 shows the criteria for VD status as proposed by the Endocrine Society. We believe this criteria is more applicable to this review since it provides guidance for clinicians caring for patients, as compared to the reference proposed by the Institute of Medicine, more likely intended for normal healthy populations only to ensure skeletal health [111].

Observational studies have described an association between insufficiency or deficiency in 25OHD levels and adverse pregnancy and neonatal outcomes including PE, gestational diabetes, bacterial vaginosis, recurrent abortion, premature rupture of membranes (PROM), preterm delivery, cesarean section, intrauterine growth restriction and also impaired fertility treatment.

The VD literature is growing rapidly and there are some recent and detailed reviews and meta-analyses about adverse pregnancy outcomes and VD [52,112–119]. The purpose of this section is therefore to show a broad overview of VD status and its relationship with epidemiological and observational data in adverse pregnancy outcomes.

7.1. VD and Preeclampsia (PE)

PE is a hypertensive disease associated to gestation. It is clinically diagnosed by new-onset hypertension (140/90 mmHg) and proteinuria (300 mg/24 h or protein dipstick 1+ or greater) after the 20th gestational week [120,121]. The major cause related to this disease is abnormal placentation secondary to insufficient throphoblastic invasion that disrupts the endocrine, immunologic and angiogenic environment, resulting in the clinical manifestation of PE [122,123]. Interestingly, a multicenter study with 2030 pregnant women of an American cohort from 1959 to 1966 showed that higher maternal circulating 25OHD levels were associated with a significantly lower risk of placental vascular pathology (hemorrhage, infarcts, microinfarcts, decidual atheromas or thrombosis of cord vessels) in pregnant women carrying male fetuses [124]. From this perspective, VD could be a protective factor for the correct development of placental vasculature.

There is a general consensus in the literature about preeclamptic women having lower 25OHD and calcitriol serum levels compared to normotensive normoevolutive pregnant women [125–129]. Indeed, VD deficiency is more common among preeclamptic women [130–135]. This could partially be explained by significantly lower CYP27B1 placental expression and therefore, lower calcitriol biosynthesis in preeclamptic *versus* normal placentas [136].

The relationship between VD, especially 25OHD serum levels, and the risk of PE development has been extensively analyzed in the medical literature. Herein, we resume the studies that positively correlate VD deficiency and PE risk (Table 3).

Table 3. Observational studies on 25OHD serum levels and the risk for PE development.

Reference	Sample Size (PE Cases *vs.* Controls)	Weeks of Gestation for Blood Sampling	25OHD Cut off	Risk for PE Development (OR (95% CI))
[130]	100 PE and 100 controls	>24	<75 nmol/L	3.26 (1.12–9.54)
			<37.5 nmol/L	4.23 (1.4–12.8)
[131]	33 PE, 79 eclamptic and 76 control	≥ 20 weeks, prior to magnesium sulfate therapy	<5 nmol/L	3.9 (1.18–12.87) for PE
				5.14 (1.98–13.37) for eclampsia
[132]	32 PE and 665 controls	24–26	<50 nmol/L	3.24 (1.37–7.69)
[133]	51 severe PE and 204 controls	15–20	<50 nmol/L	3.63 (1.52–8.65)
[134]	55 PE and 219 controls	22	<37.5 nmol/L	5.0 (1.7–14.1)

PE = Preeclampsia; OR = odds ratio; CI = confidence interval.

Interestingly, Robinson and colleagues [129] found that a 10 ng/mL increase in 25OHD levels yields a 63% decrease in the risk of severe PE, strongly suggesting that pregnant women should have VD sufficiency in order to lower the risk for PE development. In support of this postulation, recently, Bodnar and coworkers [137] studied a large cohort with 717 PE women and 2,986 control women, concluding that maternal VD deficiency is a clear risk factor for severe PE development. Specifically, they found that maternal 25OHD levels ≥ 50 nmol/L reduce in 40% the risk of severe PE development in comparison to women with 25OHD < 30 nmol/L. Another study reports that both 25OHD and soluble VEGF receptor type 1/placental growth factor (sFlt-1/PlGF) ratio at 15–20 weeks of gestation were significant predictors of severe PE [138]. Similarly, a Norwegian study [139] revealed that increased VD intake (15–20 µg/day) decreases about 25% the risk for PE development, and four independent meta-analyses showed a significant association between PE and 25OHD insufficiency or deficiency compared with control groups [112,119,140,141].

Despite all these reports, other authors inform they did not find any relation between maternal 25OHD levels and risk of PE development [142,143].

In summary, this data supports that maintaining VD sufficiency is a relatively simple measure (by cholecalciferol supplementation or reasonable skin sun exposure) for preventing one of the major causes in mother and baby morbidity-mortality, namely, preeclampsia.

7.2. VD and Bacterial Vaginosis

Bacterial vaginosis (BV) is a common infectious disease in reproductive-aged women. It is caused by the replacement of normal vaginal flora (especially Lactobacillus) for mixed anaerobic bacteria [144]. Its importance during pregnancy resides in the association of BV with adverse gynecologic and obstetric outcomes such as PROM, which can cause spontaneous or induced preterm delivery [145].

Interestingly, the National Health and Nutrition Examination Survey (NHANES) 2001–2004 reported that black women suffer two-fold more BV cases in comparison to white women (51.6% *vs.* 23.2%, respectively) [146]. This proportion could be explained by the fact that high melanin levels in darkly pigmented skin blocks ultraviolet radiation reducing cutaneous VD photosynthesis and consequently, decreasing the well-known antimicrobial activity of endogenous calcitriol [147,148]. Observational studies support this hypothesis. A prospective cohort study [149] developed at Pittsburgh University followed 469 pregnant women from <16th gestational week to term. It was observed that mothers with 25OHD serum levels <20 nmol/L had a 65% increased risk of developing BV compared to 25OHD sufficient women (>80 nmol/L), and similarly, in a subsample of the Nashville Birth Cohort [150], 25OHD serum levels were lower in women who developed BV during pregnancy. In a secondary analysis of data from the NHANES 2001–2004, Hensel and coworkers [151] described that VD insufficiency or deficiency had a statistically significant association with BV only among pregnant women (adjusted OR 2.87, 95% CI 1.13–7.28). Interestingly, a meta-analysis comprising 16 independent studies showed that women with bacterial or viral infections presented 2.1 increased risk (95% CI: 1.6–2.7) of PE development [152], suggesting a probable common risk factor which could be VD deficiency.

Besides BV, calcitriol can prevent other kinds of infections during pregnancy. In human bladder biopsies and established bladder cell lines, 25OHD treatment induced hCTD gene expression, which diminished uropathogenic *E. coli* infection, suggesting that adequate 25OHD serum levels could help prevent urinary tract infections [153].

In addition, a case-control study [154] reports that pregnant women with 25OHD insufficiency at 14–16 gestational week had 2.1-fold increased risk in developing severe to moderate periodontal disease (95% CI: 0.99–4.5).

The physiological mechanisms underlying these observations are possibly related to immune responses regulated by calcitriol. In fact, as previously mentioned, calcitriol can induce innate immune responses by activating hCTD in placenta, macrophages and dendritic cells [90,155]. The antimicrobial hCTD is an active peptide with broad spectrum antimicrobial activity (anti-Gram-positive and Gram-negative bacteria, mycobacterias, spirochetas and yeasts). Its mechanism of action includes bacterial membrane disruption and activation of toll-like receptors and macrophage and neutrophil chemotaxis [156]. Recently, it was also found that calcitriol can induce hCTD expression, multivesicular endosomes and phagolysosome biogenesis in macrophages, leading to microbial killing through autophagy [157–159]. Other important antimicrobial peptides induced by calcitriol in the placenta are HBD2 and HBD3, which also play a shielding role upon infections. Conjointly, these endogenous antibiotics provide an efficient mechanism of front-line defense since they have the capacity to kill a wide variety of microorganisms throughout the female reproductive tract [160]. Interestingly, it has been shown that IL-10, a physiological suppressor of maternal active immunity, downregulates placental antimicrobial peptides expression, which may be permissive for microbial invasion, since the placenta represents a mechanical and immunological barrier essential to restrict infection progress. However, calcitriol is able to antagonize IL-10 suppressive effects upon placental innate defenses by downregulating IL-10 expression, while at the same time restraining exacerbated inflammation and subsequently helping pregnancy to continue in quiescence [93,105]. These data indicate that adequate VD levels are crucial to enhance immunity.

By reducing infections, calcitriol may exert protective effects upon PROM. However, another mechanism might be involved in PROM prevention: calcitriol, either alone or combined with lipopolysaccharide endotoxin, decreases oxitocin and connexin 43 expression in myometrial smooth muscle cells, both proteins are associated with uterine contractions [161]. These results suggest that calcitriol can modulate uterine quiescence even under bacterial infection and therefore can prevent the abnormal uterine contractions that favor PROM and preterm delivery. In this sense, 25OHD could exert a protective role in preterm birth but this still remains unclear, since in a multicenter American cohort with twin-gestation women [162], it was observed that women with sufficiency in 25OHD (>75 nmol/L) had a 60% lower risk of preterm labor in comparison to those <75 nmol/L (OR 0.4, 95% CI 0.2–0.8). However, in a case-control study with women at high risk for prior preterm birth, VD status at 16–22 gestational weeks was not associated with recurrent preterm birth [163].

7.3. Vitamin D and Gestational Diabetes

Gestational diabetes mellitus (GDM) is defined as carbohydrate intolerance resulting in hyperglycemia of variable severity with new-onset or first recognition during pregnancy [164,165]. GDM, one of the most common complications of pregnancy, is related to adverse outcomes that increase morbidity and mortality in mothers and neonates, including hypertension, PE, urinary tract infection, caesarean delivery, fetal macrosomia, neonatal hypoglycemia and high long-term risk for metabolic syndrome or diabetes mellitus type 2 (DM2) development [165–167].

The classic risk factors known for GDM include maternal overweight status or obesity, prior history of GDM, family history of DM2, antecedent of macrosomic infant, and increased maternal age [165]. However, since 1980 [168], there is a constantly growing body of evidence that supports a connection between VD and insulin or glucose metabolism.

Some observational studies reported lower 25OHD levels in pregnant women with GDM in comparison with normal pregnant women [169–176]. In Table 4, studies that evaluated serum 25OHD levels and the risk for GDM are shown.

Table 4. Observational studies on 25OHD serum levels and risk for GDM development.

Reference	Sample Size (GDM Cases *vs.* Controls)	Weeks of Gestation for Blood Sampling	25OHD Cut off	Risk for GDM Development (OR (95% CI))
[169]	20 GDM and 40 controls	At delivery	<50 nmol/L	30.78 (4.65–203.90)
[177]	68 GDM and 1,246 controls	26–28	<25 nmol/L	3.6 (1.7–7.8)
[171]	116 GDM and 219 controls	15–18	<73.5 nmol/L	2.21 (1.19–4.13)
[178]	200 GDM and 200 controls	26–28	<25 nmol/L	1.80 (1.209–2.678)
[172]	54 GDM and 111 controls	24–28	<37.5 nmol/L	2.66 (1.26–5.6)
			<50 nmol/L	2.02 (0.88–4.6)
[173]	57 GDM and 114 controls	16	<50 nmol/L	3.74 (1.47–9.50)
[170]	81 GDM and 226 controls	Between 2nd and 3rd trimester	<50 nmol/L	1.92 (0.89–4.17)

GDM = Gestational diabetes mellitus; OR = odds ratio; CI = confidence interval.

In a meta-analysis made by Poel and coworkers [179], the mean odds ratio calculated for GDM from 7 independent observational studies about 25OHD deficiency was 1.61 (95% CI 1.19–2.17). Similarly, a review on VD status and GDM risk concluded that maternal VD deficiency and insufficiency are associated with markers of altered glucose homeostasis [180].

Other studies correlated serum 25OHD levels with a significant inverse association with glucose metabolic response in women with GDM: higher serum 25OHD was found to be associated with at least one of the following parameters: lower fasting glucose, lower 2 h glucose (*post* oral glucose tolerance test), lower glycosylated hemoglobin, lower serum insulin, lower insulin resistance or lower homeostasis model of assessment of insulin resistance HOMA-IR [170,171,174,175, 178,181–184].

In the future, the VD and lifestyle intervention (DALI) protocol could provide interesting information about VD supplementation and GDM risk. DALI is a multicenter European protocol in which the risk of GDM is being evaluated in 880 pregnant women divided into eight intervention groups considering physical activity, healthy eating habits and VD_3 supplementation (1600 IU/day or placebo). Unfortunately, the results from this study are still unpublished [185]. To our knowledge, there is only one published double-blind randomized controlled clinical trial which supplemented VD_3 on pregnant women with GDM [186]. In this study, pregnant women received two oral doses of 50,000 IU (baseline and day 21) or placebo capsules after 24 weeks of gestation. Women treated with VD_3 had a significant increase in 25OHD serum levels and a significant decrease in fasting glucose, insulin serum and HOMA-IR, which supports positive glucose metabolic effects on mothers by VD_3 supplementation. Similarly, Mozzafari and coworkers [187] administered a single intramuscular VD_3 dose (300,000 IU) post-partum in 45 women with GDM. After three months of intervention, treated women presented significantly higher 25OHD levels and lower HOMA-IR than women with GDM in the control group.

Contradictorily to this background, there are some studies which concluded that there are no significant differences between VD status in women with GDM or controls [182,188,189], or conclude that VD deficiency is not a risk factor for GDM [190,191].

There is little consensus about the physiological mechanisms governing calcitriol and glucose metabolism connections. The classic mechanism known is that calcitriol can regulate intracellular calcium flux on β-pancreatic cells and therefore can modulate depolarization-stimulated insulin release [17]. However, there are recent evidences that include other VD-dependent mechanisms: (a) diminished inflammatory state in obesity and enhanced expression of genes involved in glucose and lipid metabolism like peroxisome proliferator-activated receptor gamma (PPARγ) or its coactivator (PGC1α) in peripheral blood mononuclear cells [192]; (b) weight reduction and muscle insulin receptor substrate 1 (IRS-1) upregulation [193]; (c) upregulation of adipocyte glucose transporter 4 (GLUT4) protein and its translocation to the cell surface [194]; and d) returning to normal liver activity of glucose metabolic enzymes hexokinase, fructose 1,6-bisphosphatase and glucose 6-phosphatase [195]. In GDM, these VD-modulated beneficial mechanisms could be altered, at least in part, because placentas from GDM mothers have higher CYP24A1 protein and gene expression which can derivate in lower calcitriol bioavailability [169].

7.4. Vitamin D and Low Birth Weight or Small for Gestational Age

Newborns small for gestational age (SGA) are defined as those with a birth weight for gestational age below to the 10th percentile in standard growth curves (<5th and 3rd percentiles are also used), whereas low birth weight is defined as newborn weight lower than 2500 g independently of gestational age [196,197]. These complications are associated with substantially higher rates of perinatal morbidity and mortality, including cerebral palsy, neonatal polycythemia, hyperbilirubinemia, and hypoglycemia [197].

The associations between serum maternal 25OHD levels and birth weight of SGA newborns have not been extensively studied. Epidemiological analyses support that black infants had lower birth weight than white infants, which suggests a possible role of VD [198]. However, there are still controversial opinions about lower VD levels failing to modulate fetal growth or if external parameters as maternal obesity, lower socioeconomic status or poor nutrition contribute to lower 25OHD levels and also to SGA and low birth weight development [199]. Herein, we present the major findings in this area. Few studies did not find a significant relation between birth weight for SGA proportion and 25OHD levels [190,200–202]; however, many observational studies did. A multicenter cohort study indicated that maternal 25OHD levels > 37.5 nmol/L are associated with higher birth weight infants in comparison to newborns from women with lesser than 37.5 nmol/L [203]. Another study indicates that pregnant women who delivered SGA infants had lower serum 25OHD levels at 11–13 gestational weeks [204]. Also, umbilical cord serum calcitriol concentrations were lower in SGA than in adequate weight for gestational age infants [205]. In this study, maternal 25OHD levels were also lower in the SGA group but did not reach statistical significance. Similarly, in a birth cohort study, women with 25OHD levels between 8.5 and 48 nmol/L were more likely to give birth to SGA offspring (OR 1.57, 95% CI 1.03–2.39) [206].

Dietary analysis of total VD_3 intake was a significant predictor of infant birth weight adjusted for gestation [207], whereas milk or VD intake during pregnancy were significant independent predictors of birth weight [208]. However, it seems that placental weight is not related to 25OHD levels [203].

In a case-control study, Bodnar and colleagues [209] also observed that pregnant women with 25OHD deficiency (<37.5 nmol/L) had an increased significant risk of SGA development in offspring. Interestingly, this effect was more evident in white women (OR 7.5, 95% CI 1.8–31.9) in comparison to black women (OR 1.5, 95% CI 0.6–3.5). Unexpectedly, the women with 25OHD insufficiency (37.5–75 nmol/L) presented a lower risk of SGA than women with 25OHD sufficiency (>75 nmol/L) in both black and white women. The authors discuss that the potential mechanisms which can explain this U-shaped SGA risk remain uncertain, but the risk of other diseases such as allergic responses or atopic disorders present a similar pattern.

We only found one interventional study about VD and birth weight. In a partially randomized assay on pregnant women, the intervention with one single oral dose of 1500 µg VD$_3$ (equal to 60,000 IU) or two doses of 3000 µg each (equal to 120,000 IU) in the 2nd and 3rd trimesters resulted in higher birth weight and length in comparison to newborns of mothers treated with usual care [210].

Interestingly, interventional studies with calcium and VD$_3$ performed in pregnant adolescents showed that both nutrients positively influenced fetal bone growth *in utero*, and that even if both factors were needed for fetal bone health, one could partially compensate for the other [211]. This study suggests that special attention should be paid to pregnant adolescents in order to fulfill adequate VD and calcium requirements, since not only fetal but also maternal bone health may be at risk. This is supported by other studies showing that lactating adolescents lose more bone mineral density when suffering from VD deficiency or low calcium intake [212].

Interestingly, Morley and colleagues suggested that studies on maternal VD status and birth weight should consider neonatal VDR polymorphism, since differences in this feature could help explain why findings from different populations regarding maternal VD status and neonate birth weight have been inconsistent [213].

8. Vitamin D Expenditure and Homeodynamics: Considerations for VD Supplementation

8.1. Endogenous and Exogenous Factors Affecting the VD Status Equation

Considering the high risk of adverse events during pregnancy associated to VD deficiency, it is also important to analyze additional factors that may significantly modify the bioavailability of VD and its metabolites in our body. Indeed, the VD endocrine system is not in constant equilibrium; instead, it is under dynamic regulation and interaction with different factors. For example, the half-life of 25OHD is strongly influenced by DBP concentration, since 25OHD binds to DBP with high affinity [81,214]. Moreover, 25OHD is also affected by DBP genotype [214]. Indeed, the genetic variations that occur in DBP modify its binding affinity for VD metabolites, and the lesser affinity, a shorter half-life is expected. Similarly, genetic variations in CYP27B1, CYP24A1, CYP2R1 and the VDR differentially impact on VD metabolism and biological effects. Single nucleotide polymorphisms have been reported for each of these proteins and may be found as population-specific variants that result in modification of the final VD status. For reviews on this issue please see [215–217]. Considering this, and as previously suggested [215], it is feasible that optimal concentrations of 25OHD required to reduce disease outcomes may vary according to genotype. Other endogenous elements that may predict serum 25OHD half-life are factors known to affect 25OHD metabolism, such as PTH, plasma phosphate and albumin-adjusted calcium [218].

Besides the endogenous factors previously described, exogenous aspects affecting 25OHD plasma concentration include dietary intake, type of clothing and sunshine protection [219], lifestyle and geophysical conditions, this last one interpreted as UVB exposure. In this regard, a study performed with pregnant women in Germany showed that during the winter months, 98% of the maternal blood samples and 94% of the cord blood samples had 25OHD levels < 50 nmol/L, while in the summer months, only 49% of the women and 35% of the cord blood samples were vitamin D deficient [220]. Interestingly, in the same study, the authors found that a significant risk factor for maternal VD deficiency was physical inactivity (adjusted OR 2.67, 95% CI 1.06–6.69, $p = 0.032$), which might be related to less sun exposure. However, a sedentary lifestyle may also be associated with obesity, which has been found to be linked to VD deficiency. Indeed, obese subjects normally have lower basal 25OHD serum concentrations than lean individuals [221], which is possibly explained by the fact that VD is readily stored in adipose tissue due to its fat-soluble nature. In this manner, VD may be sequestered in the greater body pool of fat present in obese individuals, which is supported by previous studies showing that after equal whole-body irradiation or VD supplementation, the increase in serum VD was more than 50% lower in obese than in non-obese subjects [221]. While this occurs in body fat, the muscle cells protect 25OHD from degradation by binding it to actin fibers, in a megalin-dependent process [222]. This may explain why 25OHD concentrations are usually positively associated to muscle-related parameters such as lean body mass and exercise [223].

Unfortunately, during pregnancy, the toll of VD deficiency in obese mothers affects also their child's VD status and health [224,225]. Many studies have shown an array of adverse health outcomes in the offspring of obese women; for example, lower maternal VD status may be linked to programmed differences in offspring fat mass [224,226]. Among the more important adverse effects of maternal VD deficiency upon their offspring, impaired fetal growth and bone development, altered growth and bone mass later in childhood, neonatal hypocalcemia or tetany and respiratory tract infections have been reported [227].

8.2. Dose Regimens and Vitamin D Supplementation in Pregnant Women

Despite the health advantages associated with a sufficient VD status during pregnancy, as described previously, at this time general consensus supporting a guideline for VD supplementation in pregnant population has not yet been reached. In the literature, a broad spectrum for dosage and periodicity in cholecalciferol supplementation schemes has been reported: 2000 IU, 4000 IU, 14,000 IU, 60,000 IU, 120,000 IU or 200,000 IU administered daily, weekly, monthly or in a single mega-dose. Herein, we resume the more recent randomized clinical trials on VD supplementation in pregnancy. Table 5 includes doses and frequency for supplementation together with the outcome as percentage of women who achieved VD sufficiency at the end of intervention and those who developed hypercalcemia.

Based on these data, it seems that 4000 IU given daily results in the highest proportion of pregnant women reaching VD sufficiency without developing hypercalcemia. An exception to this observation is the study by Hossain *et al.* [228], in which only 15% women reached sufficiency under this regimen. Regarding this, we should mention that the group of Pakistani women included in the Hossain study were severely VD deficient (<25 nmol/L) and were an ethnic group in which particular genetic variants might be affecting VD metabolism, which remains to be further studied. Moreover, the cases of hypercalcemia were comparable in both control and supplemented groups, while hypercalcemia persisted despite VD deficiency, suggesting independence of the pharmacological intervention. On the other hand, it should be noted that in the study by Wagner *et al.* [229], the percentage of women considered to attain sufficiency might be underestimated, since their cut-off value was 25OHD serum levels > 100 nmol/L. As in the case of 4000 IU given daily, the weekly regimen of 50,000 IU seems to be also a good therapeutic strategy, since 100% women reached sufficiency without hypercalcemia. However, more studies are needed to confirm these findings.

In contrast, monthly and unique dose regimens do not seem to adequately fulfill VD sufficiency. It is noteworthy that under the single-dose regimen, some authors included in their analyses serum levels below 75 nmol/L (identified with * and ** in Table 5), which under the Endocrine Society parameters is still considered deficiency. Indeed, in the study by Sahu *et al.* [230], which considered a cut-off of 75 nmol/L, only 34.2% of women reached sufficiency with the highest dose, which is very low. Similarly, in the study by Yu *et al.* [231], the observed proportion of 93% in the supplemented group might be misleading, since this number includes women with serum 25OHD levels > 25 nmol/L.

The recent evidence discussed in Section 8.1 may help us to understand the differences in VD expenditure and homeodynamics in order to reach a general consensus on VD supplementation in a tailored manner. We believe, that at this moment, the ideal scheme for VD supplementation will depend on particular endogenous and exogenous factors, on the available formulations of VD (*i.e.*, in Mexico only tablets with 400 IU are available), and on the personal VD metabolism, which should be monitored periodically by serum 25OHD analyses. By taking all these considerations into account, and under medical counseling and supervision, every woman may modulate their VD levels for acquiring sufficiency and avoiding possible toxicity that could lead to hypercalcemia.

Table 5. Cholecalciferol supplementation and VD status in randomized clinical trials in healthy pregnant women.

Reference	Sample Size	Period of Supplementation	Cholecalciferol Supplemented (IU)	% Women with Serum 25OHD > 75 nmol/L at Delivery (No Asterisk)	Hypercalcemia
		Unique Dose			
[210]	97	2nd trimester Two doses at 2nd and 3rd trimester	60,000 120,000	27% ** 62.5% **	No evaluated
[230]	84	No supplementation 5th month Two doses at 5th and 7th month	- 60,000 120,000	7% 5.7% 34.2%	No evaluated
[231]	180	No supplementation 27 week	- 200,000	60% * 93% *	No indicated
		Daily			
[232]	228	27 weeks to term	0 1000 2000	50% 89% 91%	No
[228]	175	Less than 20 weeks to term	0 4000	1% 15%	3 cases 9 cases
[233]	162 deficient women	12–16 weeks to term	400 2000 4000	9.5% 24.4% 65.1%	No
[229]	257	12–16 weeks to term	2000 4000	37.4% *** 46.2% ***	No
[234]	350	12–16 weeks to term	400 2000 4000	50% 70.8% 82%	No
[231]	180	27 weeks to term	800	86% *	No indicated

Table 5. *Cont.*

Reference	Sample Size	Period of Supplementation	Cholecalciferol Supplemented (IU)	% Women with Serum 25OHD >75 nmol/L at Delivery (No Asterisk)	Hypercalcemia
Weekly					
[235]	109 deficient women	26–28 weeks to term (8 weeks)	400 50,000	3.70% 100%	No
[236]	28	26–28 weeks to term	Basement 70,000 + 35,000 weekly 14,000 weekly	90% 56%	No
Monthly					
[237]	51 deficient women	From 2nd month to term	50,000 100,000	35% **** 59% ****	No evaluated

* 25OHD serum > 25 nmol/L; ** 25OHD serum > 50 nmol/L; *** 25OHD serum > 100 nmol/L; **** in cord blood.

197

9. Methods of Serum VD Measurement

Since four decades ago, numerous analytical methods have been developed for 25OHD measurement, including competitive protein binding assay, enzyme-linked immunoassay (ELISA), radioimmunoassay (RIA), chemiluminescence assay, gas chromatography-mass spectrometry (GC-MS), high performance liquid chromatography (HPLC) and, more recently, liquid chromatography coupled with mass spectrometry (LC-MS) or tandem mass spectrometry (LC-MS/MS). A good review of accuracy, sensibility and technical description of these methods was made by Hollis [238].

LC-MS/MS is the most promising technique for VD analysis since it is a highly specific, reliable, reproducible and robust method and is considered the new gold standard for 25OHD quantification [239,240]. Despite its major field of application being research, LC-MS/MS technology is also currently being applied in clinical laboratories [241]. In addition, LC-MS/MS offers the possibility for quantifying other metabolites of VD in serum samples, such as $25OHD_2$, $25OHD_3$, 3-epi-$25OHD_2$, 3-epi-$25OHD_3$, 24R,25 dihydroxyvitamin D_3 [242,243] and $25OHD_3$ 3-sulfate [244]. Other metabolites as VD_2, VD_3, $1\alpha,25(OH)_2D_2$ and $1\alpha,25(OH)_2D_3$ may also be detected and discriminated.

One limitation of this technique is the interference with 3-epi $25(OH)D_3$ that can lead to 25OHD overestimation. This could be a problem especially in pediatric samples which are known to have significant amounts of this epimer. Recently, van den Ouweland and colleagues developed a LC-MS/MS method which eliminates this limitation [245].

Interestingly, new technology developed to be used in our daily life will allow us to measure 25OHD easily at home. The proposed system is a gold-nanoparticle-immunoassay developed at Cornell University, adapted to a device that couples to smartphones allowing them to calculate in a small drop of blood 25OHD serum concentrations with 10 nM sensitivity [246].

In the aftermath of what is discussed in Sections 5 and 8.1, it seems that 25OHD should not be exclusively considered for the assessment of VD, but rather, the equation for VD status may also consider DBP levels. Powe and coworkers [247] recently suggested that free 25OHD (25OHD minus DBP) is a better indicator for VD status since free 25OHD offers a strong correlation with PTH than total 25OHD. However, this article has been criticized by other authors [248]. Indeed, as previously discussed, Weintraub [248] pointed out that the 25OHD/DBP complex is necessary for the endocytosis by megalin/cubilin in the kidney, so 25OHD bound to DBP may be the real substrate mediating final calcitriol biosynthesis. Nevertheless, this would only apply to those cells expressing megalin/cubilin, and definitive further studies are needed in order to clarify the participation of other mechanisms of 25OHD storage and internalization into the cell.

10. Final Considerations

Maintaining adequate VD serum concentrations within the recommended levels is mandatory during pregnancy, since it is involved in many important biological processes, including fetal programming and development. Indeed, the benefits of maintaining adequate VD serum levels are not circumscribed to the mother, but also to the offspring. It is noteworthy mentioning that epidemiological studies have shown controversial results about the benefits of prescribing VD supplements to prevent adverse pregnancy outcomes associated with maternal deficiency. We believe that the controversy may be explained because the biological phenomena can be affected not only by serum concentrations, but also by many factors, such as racial, climatological, or genetic reasons; nutritional status; lifestyle; physical activity; or health status during pregnancy. On the other hand, the few studies that do not corroborate benefits lack sustained clinical evidence of real risks due to VD supplementation. Conversely, systematic reviews and meta-analyses demonstrate a strong association between VD adequate levels and health benefits. Regarding this controversy, recently, two debated articles concluded that the proposed adverse health outcomes related to VD deficiency might be, in fact, the result of reverse causation, understanding by this that low VD levels are a consequence of ill health rather than a cause, and that the evidence does not really support VD supplementation for prevention of disease [249–251]. In response to these articles, Gillie, with straightforward arguments, demonstrated that the aforementioned articles had made a type 2 statistical error, and that VD deficiency, especially at critical times such as pregnancy and early childhood, could derive in serious health harm [252]. An example of the arguments exposed by Gillie is rickets, a disease characterized by bone deformation in children caused by VD deficiency. This illness may be corrected by adequate VD supplementation during childhood, but the alterations in bones cannot be reversed by this intervention once adulthood is reached. Another example discussed by Gillie is diabetes type 1, which occurs in children and is thought to be caused by VD deficiency in the womb, causing irreversible changes to biochemistry, immune status or organ structure.

A final consideration is the fact that VD supplementation is useful to prevent adverse pregnancy outcomes, but it might not always be necessary, especially when lifestyle recommendations are good enough to prevent them. In order to take the adequate decision about VD supplementation, every clinical individual situation must be analyzed and placed in the correct balance of risk and benefit before prescribing VD supplementation. However, when controversies about clinical decisions are involved, scientists must avoid creating medical barriers about the use of preventive strategies in medicine.

11. Conclusions

Although the importance of VD in the regulation of calcium homeostasis in pregnant women is well established, there is now increasing evidence that calcitriol is also important for the prevention of several adverse scenarios that could potentially threaten pregnancy such as infection and preeclampsia. Even though more interventional and basic studies are needed in order to understand the role of VD in pregnancy health and disease, through the information resumed herein it is clear that many of the beneficial effects of calcitriol during gestation involve its immunomodulatory properties as well as its capacity to regulate hormonogenesis. Despite the protective role of VD in pregnancy outcomes and that several epidemiological studies have documented highly prevalent gestational hypovitaminosis D around the world, routine VD screening is still not mandatory and not enough interventional studies have been undertaken to achieve a consensus for VD supplementation in pregnant women, highlighting the need for further studies and establishment of screening guidelines during pregnancy. Given that the human placenta expresses CYP27B1, which catalyzes the local synthesis of calcitriol, the supplementation with VD during pregnancy might be an accessible and safe way to reduce the incidence of some adverse events associated with mother and baby morbidity-mortality, such as PE, GDM, PROM and infections; while, at the same time, both the mother and the child will profit from the physiological benefits of calcitriol. Notably, adequate sun exposure, a VD-rich diet and physical activity should always be considered as the first recommendation, while supplementation with cholecalciferol may be advised for persistent VD deficient women.

Acknowledgments: This work was supported by the Consejo Nacional de Ciencia y Tecnología (CONACyT), México grant number 153862 to LD. AOO is a PhD. student from Posgrado en Ciencias Biológicas at Universidad Nacional Autónoma de México (UNAM) and is receiving a scholarship from CONACyT (231018).

Author Contributions: All of the authors contributed in the writing and proof-reading of this review article.

Conflicts of Interest: The authors declare no conflict of interest.

References

1. Bikle, D. Highlights from the 16th vitamin D workshop, San Francisco, CA, June 11–14, 2013. *J. Steroid Biochem. Mol. Biol.* **2014**, *144*, 1–4.
2. Wacker, M.; Holick, M.F. Sunlight and vitamin D: A global perspective for health. *Derm. Endocrinol.* **2013**, *5*, 51–108.
3. Nykjaer, A.; Dragun, D.; Walther, D.; Vorum, H.; Jacobsen, C.; Herz, J.; Melsen, F.; Christensen, E.I.; Willnow, T.E. An endocytic pathway essential for renal uptake and activation of the steroid 25-(OH) vitamin D3. *Cell* **1999**, *96*, 507–515.

4. Nykjaer, A.; Fyfe, J.C.; Kozyraki, R.; Leheste, J.R.; Jacobsen, C.; Nielsen, M.S.; Verroust, P.J.; Aminoff, M.; de la Chapelle, A.; Moestrup, S.K.; *et al.* Cubilin dysfunction causes abnormal metabolism of the steroid hormone 25(OH) vitamin D(3). *Proc. Natl. Acad. Sci. USA* **2001**, *98*, 13895–13900.

5. Morris, S.M.; Tallquist, M.D.; Rock, C.O.; Cooper, J.A. Dual roles for the dab2 adaptor protein in embryonic development and kidney transport. *EMBO J.* **2002**, *21*, 1555–1564.

6. Dusso, A.S.; Brown, A.J.; Slatopolsky, E. Vitamin D. *Am. J. Physiol. Ren. Physiol.* **2005**, *289*, 8–28.

7. Costa, J.L.; Eijk, P.P.; van de Wiel, M.A.; ten Berge, D.; Schmitt, F.; Narvaez, C.J.; Welsh, J.; Ylstra, B. Anti-proliferative action of vitamin D in MCF7 is still active after siRNA-VDR knock-down. *BMC Genomics* **2009**, *10*, 499.

8. Haussler, M.R.; Jurutka, P.W.; Mizwicki, M.; Norman, A.W. Vitamin D receptor (VDR)-mediated actions of 1alpha,25(OH)(2)vitamin D(3): Genomic and non-genomic mechanisms. *Best Pract. Res. Clin. Endocrinol. Metab.* **2011**, *25*, 543–559.

9. Sylvia, V.L.; Schwartz, Z.; Ellis, E.B.; Helm, S.H.; Gomez, R.; Dean, D.D.; Boyan, B.D. Nongenomic regulation of protein kinase C isoforms by the vitamin D metabolites 1 alpha,25-(OH)2D3 and 24R,25-(OH)2D3. *J. Cell. Physiol.* **1996**, *167*, 380–393.

10. Beno, D.W.; Brady, L.M.; Bissonnette, M.; Davis, B.H. Protein kinase C and mitogen-activated protein kinase are required for 1,25-dihydroxyvitamin D3-stimulated EGR induction. *J. Biol. Chem.* **1995**, *270*, 3642–3647.

11. Berg, J.P.; Haug, E. Vitamin D: A hormonal regulator of the cAMP signaling pathway. *Crit. Rev. Biochem. Mol. Biol.* **1999**, *34*, 315–323.

12. Avila, E.; Diaz, L.; Barrera, D.; Halhali, A.; Mendez, I.; Gonzalez, L.; Zuegel, U.; Steinmeyer, A.; Larrea, F. Regulation of vitamin D hydroxylases gene expression by 1,25-dihydroxyvitamin D3 and cyclic AMP in cultured human syncytiotrophoblasts. *J. Steroid Biochem. Mol. Biol.* **2007**, *103*, 90–96.

13. Morelli, S.; de Boland, A.R.; Boland, R.L. Generation of inositol phosphates, diacylglycerol and calcium fluxes in myoblasts treated with 1,25-dihydroxyvitamin D3. *Biochem. J.* **1993**, *289*, 675–679.

14. Zanello, L.P.; Norman, A.W. 1 alpha,25(OH)2 vitamin D3-mediated stimulation of outward anionic currents in osteoblast-like ROS 17/2.8 cells. *Biochem. Biophys. Res. Commun.* **1996**, *225*, 551–556.

15. Nemere, I.; Dormanen, M.C.; Hammond, M.W.; Okamura, W.H.; Norman, A.W. Identification of a specific binding protein for 1 alpha,25-dihydroxyvitamin D3 in basal-lateral membranes of chick intestinal epithelium and relationship to transcaltachia. *J. Biol. Chem.* **1994**, *269*, 23750–23756.

16. Quesada, J.M.; Martin-Malo, A.; Santiago, J.; Hervas, F.; Martinez, M.E.; Castillo, D.; Barrio, V.; Aljama, P. Effect of calcitriol on insulin secretion in uraemia. *Nephrol. Dial. Transplant.* **1990**, *5*, 1013–1017.

17. Sergeev, I.N.; Rhoten, W.B. 1,25-dihydroxyvitamin D3 evokes oscillations of intracellular calcium in a pancreatic beta-cell line. *Endocrinology* **1995**, *136*, 2852–2861.

18. Noda, M.; Vogel, R.L.; Craig, A.M.; Prahl, J.; DeLuca, H.F.; Denhardt, D.T. Identification of a DNA sequence responsible for binding of the 1,25-dihydroxyvitamin D3 receptor and 1,25-dihydroxyvitamin D3 enhancement of mouse secreted phosphoprotein 1 (spp-1 or osteopontin) gene expression. *Proc. Natl. Acad. Sci. USA* **1990**, *87*, 9995–9999.

19. Liu, M.; Lee, M.H.; Cohen, M.; Bommakanti, M.; Freedman, L.P. Transcriptional activation of the Cdk inhibitor p21 by vitamin D3 leads to the induced differentiation of the myelomonocytic cell line U937. *Genes Dev.* **1996**, *10*, 142–153.

20. Kriebitzsch, C.; Verlinden, L.; Eelen, G.; van Schoor, N.M.; Swart, K.; Lips, P.; Meyer, M.B.; Pike, J.W.; Boonen, S.; Carlberg, C.; *et al.* 1,25-dihydroxyvitamin D3 influences cellular homocysteine levels in murine preosteoblastic MC3T3-E1 cells by direct regulation of cystathionine beta-synthase. *J. Bone Miner. Res.* **2011**, *26*, 2991–3000.

21. Yuan, W.; Pan, W.; Kong, J.; Zheng, W.; Szeto, F.L.; Wong, K.E.; Cohen, R.; Klopot, A.; Zhang, Z.; Li, Y.C. 1,25-dihydroxyvitamin D3 suppresses renin gene transcription by blocking the activity of the cyclic AMP response element in the renin gene promoter. *J. Biol. Chem.* **2007**, *282*, 29821–29830.

22. Garcia-Quiroz, J.; Rivas-Suarez, M.; Garcia-Becerra, R.; Barrera, D.; Martinez-Reza, I.; Ordaz-Rosado, D.; Santos, N.; Villanueva, O.; Santos-Cuevas, C.L.; Avila, E.; *et al.* Calcitriol reduces thrombospondin-1 and increases vascular endothelial growth factor in breast cancer cells: Implications for tumor angiogenesis. *J. Steroid Biochem. Mol. Biol.* **2014**, *144*, 215–222.

23. Liu, P.T.; Stenger, S.; Tang, D.H.; Modlin, R.L. Cutting edge: Vitamin D-mediated human antimicrobial activity against mycobacterium tuberculosis is dependent on the induction of cathelicidin. *J. Immunol.* **2007**, *179*, 2060–2063.

24. Wang, T.T.; Nestel, F.P.; Bourdeau, V.; Nagai, Y.; Wang, Q.; Liao, J.; Tavera-Mendoza, L.; Lin, R.; Hanrahan, J.W.; Mader, S.; *et al.* Cutting edge: 1,25-dihydroxyvitamin D3 is a direct inducer of antimicrobial peptide gene expression. *J. Immunol.* **2004**, *173*, 2909–2912.

25. Thompson, P.D.; Jurutka, P.W.; Whitfield, G.K.; Myskowski, S.M.; Eichhorst, K.R.; Dominguez, C.E.; Haussler, C.A.; Haussler, M.R. Liganded VDR induces CYP3A4 in small intestinal and colon cancer cells via DR3 and ER6 vitamin D responsive elements. *Biochem. Biophys. Res. Commun.* **2002**, *299*, 730–738.

26. Henry, H.L. Regulation of vitamin D metabolism. *Best Pract. Res. Clin. Endocrinol. Metab.* **2011**, *25*, 531–541.

27. Rost, C.R.; Bikle, D.D.; Kaplan, R.A. In vitro stimulation of 25-hydroxycholecalciferol 1 alpha-hydroxylation by parathyroid hormone in chick kidney slices: Evidence for a role for adenosine 3',5'-monophosphate. *Endocrinology* **1981**, *108*, 1002–1006.

28. Zierold, C.; Mings, J.A.; DeLuca, H.F. Parathyroid hormone regulates 25-hydroxyvitamin D(3)-24-hydroxylase mRNA by altering its stability. *Proc. Natl. Acad. Sci. USA* **2001**, *98*, 13572–13576.

29. Shimada, T.; Kakitani, M.; Yamazaki, Y.; Hasegawa, H.; Takeuchi, Y.; Fujita, T.; Fukumoto, S.; Tomizuka, K.; Yamashita, T. Targeted ablation of FGF23 demonstrates an essential physiological role of FGF23 in phosphate and vitamin D metabolism. *J. Clin. Invest.* **2004**, *113*, 561–568.

30. Shimada, T.; Hasegawa, H.; Yamazaki, Y.; Muto, T.; Hino, R.; Takeuchi, Y.; Fujita, T.; Nakahara, K.; Fukumoto, S.; Yamashita, T. FGF-23 is a potent regulator of vitamin D metabolism and phosphate homeostasis. *J. Bone Miner. Res.* **2004**, *19*, 429–435.

31. Bikle, D.D. Vitamin D metabolism, mechanism of action, and clinical applications. *Chem. Biol.* **2014**, *21*, 319–329.

32. Nesbitt, T.; Drezner, M.K. Insulin-like growth factor-I regulation of renal 25-hydroxyvitamin D-1-hydroxylase activity. *Endocrinology* **1993**, *132*, 133–138.

33. Menaa, C.; Vrtovsnik, F.; Friedlander, G.; Corvol, M.; Garabedian, M. Insulin-like growth factor I, a unique calcium-dependent stimulator of 1,25-dihydroxyvitamin D3 production. Studies in cultured mouse kidney cells. *J. Biol. Chem.* **1995**, *270*, 25461–25467.

34. Kawashima, H.; Torikai, S.; Kurokawa, K. Calcitonin selectively stimulates 25-hydroxyvitamin D3-1 alpha-hydroxylase in proximal straight tubule of rat kidney. *Nature* **1981**, *291*, 327–329.

35. Overbergh, L.; Stoffels, K.; Valckx, D.; Giulietti, A.; Bouillon, R.; Mathieu, C. Regulation of 25-hydroxyvitamin D-1alpha-hydroxylase by IFNgamma in human monocytic THP1 cells. *J. Steroid Biochem. Mol. Biol.* **2004**, *89–90*, 453–455.

36. Gyetko, M.R.; Hsu, C.H.; Wilkinson, C.C.; Patel, S.; Young, E. Monocyte 1 alpha-hydroxylase regulation: Induction by inflammatory cytokines and suppression by dexamethasone and uremia toxin. *J. Leukoc. Biol.* **1993**, *54*, 17–22.

37. Pryke, A.M.; Duggan, C.; White, C.P.; Posen, S.; Mason, R.S. Tumor necrosis factor-alpha induces vitamin D-1-hydroxylase activity in normal human alveolar macrophages. *J. Cell. Physiol.* **1990**, *142*, 652–656.

38. Adams, J.S.; Gacad, M.A. Characterization of 1 alpha-hydroxylation of vitamin D3 sterols by cultured alveolar macrophages from patients with sarcoidosis. *J. Exp. Med.* **1985**, *161*, 755–765.

39. Xie, Z.; Munson, S.J.; Huang, N.; Portale, A.A.; Miller, W.L.; Bikle, D.D. The mechanism of 1,25-dihydroxyvitamin D(3) autoregulation in keratinocytes. *J. Biol. Chem.* **2002**, *277*, 36987–36990.

40. Bikle, D.D.; Pillai, S.; Gee, E.; Hincenbergs, M. Tumor necrosis factor-alpha regulation of 1,25-dihydroxyvitamin D production by human keratinocytes. *Endocrinology* **1991**, *129*, 33–38.

41. Bikle, D.D.; Pillai, S.; Gee, E.; Hincenbergs, M. Regulation of 1,25-dihydroxyvitamin D production in human keratinocytes by interferon-gamma. *Endocrinology* **1989**, *124*, 655–660.

42. Ren, S.; Nguyen, L.; Wu, S.; Encinas, C.; Adams, J.S.; Hewison, M. Alternative splicing of vitamin D-24-hydroxylase: A novel mechanism for the regulation of extrarenal 1,25-dihydroxyvitamin D synthesis. *J. Biol. Chem.* **2005**, *280*, 20604–20611.

43. Novakovic, B.; Sibson, M.; Ng, H.K.; Manuelpillai, U.; Rakyan, V.; Down, T.; Beck, S.; Fournier, T.; Evain-Brion, D.; Dimitriadis, E.; *et al.* Placenta-specific methylation of the vitamin D 24-hydroxylase gene: Implications for feedback autoregulation of active vitamin D levels at the fetomaternal interface. *J. Biol. Chem.* **2009**, *284*, 14838–14848.

44. Chung, I.; Karpf, A.R.; Muindi, J.R.; Conroy, J.M.; Nowak, N.J.; Johnson, C.S.; Trump, D.L. Epigenetic silencing of CYP24 in tumor-derived endothelial cells contributes to selective growth inhibition by calcitriol. *J. Biol. Chem.* **2007**, *282*, 8704–8714.

45. Matilainen, J.M.; Malinen, M.; Turunen, M.M.; Carlberg, C.; Vaisanen, S. The number of vitamin D receptor binding sites defines the different vitamin D responsiveness of the CYP24 gene in malignant and normal mammary cells. *J. Biol. Chem.* **2010**, *285*, 24174–24183.

46. Noyola-Martinez, N.; Diaz, L.; Zaga-Clavellina, V.; Avila, E.; Halhali, A.; Larrea, F.; Barrera, D. Regulation of CYP27B1 and CYP24A1 gene expression by recombinant pro-inflammatory cytokines in cultured human trophoblasts. *J. Steroid Biochem. Mol. Biol.* **2014**, *144*, 106–109.

47. Rosen, C.J.; Adams, J.S.; Bikle, D.D.; Black, D.M.; Demay, M.B.; Manson, J.E.; Murad, M.H.; Kovacs, C.S. The nonskeletal effects of vitamin D: An endocrine society scientific statement. *Endocr. Rev.* **2012**, *33*, 456–492.

48. Rubin, L.P.; Yeung, B.; Vouros, P.; Vilner, L.M.; Reddy, G.S. Evidence for human placental synthesis of 24,25-dihydroxyvitamin D3 and 23,25-dihydroxyvitamin D3. *Pediatr. Res.* **1993**, *34*, 98–104.

49. Higashi, T.; Mitamura, K.; Ohmi, H.; Yamada, N.; Shimada, K.; Tanaka, K.; Honjo, H. Levels of 24,25-dihydroxyvitamin D3, 25-hydroxyvitamin D3 and 25-hydroxyvitamin D3 3-sulphate in human plasma. *Ann. Clin. Biochem.* **1999**, *36*, 43–47.

50. Lester, G.E.; Gray, T.K.; Lorenc, R.S. Evidence for maternal and fetal differences in vitamin D metabolism. *Proc. Soc. Exp. Biol. Med.* **1978**, *159*, 303–307.

51. Halhali, A.; Diaz, L.; Sanchez, I.; Garabedian, M.; Bourges, H.; Larrea, F. Effects of IGF-I on 1,25-dihydroxyvitamin D(3) synthesis by human placenta in culture. *Mol. Hum. Reprod.* **1999**, *5*, 771–776.

52. Brannon, P.M.; Picciano, M.F. Vitamin D in pregnancy and lactation in humans. *Ann. Rev. Nutr.* **2011**, *31*, 89–115.

53. Kumar, R.; Cohen, W.R.; Silva, P.; Epstein, F.H. Elevated 1,25-dihydroxyvitamin D plasma levels in normal human pregnancy and lactation. *J. Clin. Invest.* **1979**, *63*, 342–344.

54. Seki, K.; Makimura, N.; Mitsui, C.; Hirata, J.; Nagata, I. Calcium-regulating hormones and osteocalcin levels during pregnancy: A longitudinal study. *Am. J. Obstet. Gynecol.* **1991**, *164*, 1248–1252.

55. Dahlman, T.; Sjoberg, H.E.; Bucht, E. Calcium homeostasis in normal pregnancy and puerperium. A longitudinal study. *Acta Obstet. Gynecol. Scand.* **1994**, *73*, 393–398.

56. Cross, N.A.; Hillman, L.S.; Allen, S.H.; Krause, G.F.; Vieira, N.E. Calcium homeostasis and bone metabolism during pregnancy, lactation, and postweaning: A longitudinal study. *Am. J. Clin. Nutr.* **1995**, *61*, 514–523.

57. Kovacs, C.S. Calcium and bone metabolism disorders during pregnancy and lactation. *Endocrinol. Metab. Clin. North Am.* **2011**, *40*, 795–826.

58. Moller, U.K.; Streym, S.; Mosekilde, L.; Heickendorff, L.; Flyvbjerg, A.; Frystyk, J.; Jensen, L.T.; Rejnmark, L. Changes in calcitropic hormones, bone markers and insulin-like growth factor I (IGF-I) during pregnancy and postpartum: A controlled cohort study. *Osteoporos. Int.* **2013**, *24*, 1307–1320.

59. Ritchie, L.D.; Fung, E.B.; Halloran, B.P.; Turnlund, J.R.; Van Loan, M.D.; Cann, C.E.; King, J.C. A longitudinal study of calcium homeostasis during human pregnancy and lactation and after resumption of menses. *Am. J. Clin. Nutr.* **1998**, *67*, 693–701.

60. Tuan, R.S.; Moore, C.J.; Brittingham, J.W.; Kirwin, J.J.; Akins, R.E.; Wong, M. In vitro study of placental trophoblast calcium uptake using JEG-3 human choriocarcinoma cells. *J. Cell Sci.* **1991**, *98*, 333–342.

61. Halhali, A.; Figueras, A.G.; Diaz, L.; Avila, E.; Barrera, D.; Hernandez, G.; Larrea, F. Effects of calcitriol on calbindins gene expression and lipid peroxidation in human placenta. *J. Steroid Biochem. Mol. Biol.* **2010**, *121*, 448–451.

62. Belkacemi, L.; Zuegel, U.; Steinmeyer, A.; Dion, J.P.; Lafond, J. Calbindin-D28k (CaBP28k) identification and regulation by 1,25-dihydroxyvitamin D3 in human choriocarcinoma cell line JEG-3. *Mol. Cell. Endocrinol.* **2005**, *236*, 31–41.

63. Young, B.E.; Cooper, E.M.; McIntyre, A.W.; Kent, T.; Witter, F.; Harris, Z.L.; O'Brien, K.O. Placental vitamin D receptor (VDR) expression is related to neonatal vitamin D status, placental calcium transfer, and fetal bone length in pregnant adolescents. *FASEB J.* **2014**, *28*, 2029–2037.

64. Ardawi, M.S.; Nasrat, H.A.; HS, B.A.A. Calcium-regulating hormones and parathyroid hormone-related peptide in normal human pregnancy and postpartum: A longitudinal study. *Eur. J. Endocrinol.* **1997**, *137*, 402–409.

65. Ron, M.; Menczel, J.; Schwartz, L.; Palti, Z.; Kidroni, G. Vitamin D3 metabolites in amniotic fluid in relation with maternal and fetal sera in term pregnancies. *J. Perinat. Med.* **1987**, *15*, 282–290.

66. Gupta, M.M.; Kuppuswamy, G.; Subramanian, A.R. Transplacental transfer of 25-hydroxy-cholecalciferol. *Postgrad. Med. J.* **1982**, *58*, 408–410.

67. Wilson, S.G.; Retallack, R.W.; Kent, J.C.; Worth, G.K.; Gutteridge, D.H. Serum free 1,25-dihydroxyvitamin D and the free 1,25-dihydroxyvitamin D index during a longitudinal study of human pregnancy and lactation. *Clin. Endocrinol. (Oxf.)* **1990**, *32*, 613–622.

68. Paulson, S.K.; Ford, K.K.; Langman, C.B. Pregnancy does not alter the metabolic clearance of 1,25-dihydroxyvitamin D in rats. *Am. J. Physiol.* **1990**, *258*, E158–E162.

69. Weisman, Y.; Harell, A.; Edelstein, S.; David, M.; Spirer, Z.; Golander, A. 1 alpha, 25-dihydroxyvitamin D3 and 24,25-dihydroxyvitamin D3 *in vitro* synthesis by human decidua and placenta. *Nature* **1979**, *281*, 317–319.

70. Diaz, L.; Sanchez, I.; Avila, E.; Halhali, A.; Vilchis, F.; Larrea, F. Identification of a 25-hydroxyvitamin D3 1alpha-hydroxylase gene transcription product in cultures of human syncytiotrophoblast cells. *J. Clin. Endocrinol. Metab.* **2000**, *85*, 2543–2549.

71. Whitsett, J.A.; Ho, M.; Tsang, R.C.; Norman, E.J.; Adams, K.G. Synthesis of 1,25-dihydroxyvitamin D3 by human placenta *in vitro*. *J. Clin. Endocrinol. Metab.* **1981**, *53*, 484–488.

72. Kirby, B.J.; Ma, Y.; Martin, H.M.; Buckle Favaro, K.L.; Karaplis, A.C.; Kovacs, C.S. Upregulation of calcitriol during pregnancy and skeletal recovery after lactation do not require parathyroid hormone. *J. Bone Miner. Res.* **2013**, *28*, 1987–2000.

73. Sanz-Salvador, L.; Garcia-Perez, M.A.; Tarin, J.J.; Cano, A. Endocrinology in pregnancy: Bone metabolic changes during pregnancy: A period of vulnerability to osteoporosis and fracture. *Eur. J. Endocrinol.* **2015**, *172*, 53–65.

74. Simmonds, C.S.; Kovacs, C.S. Role of parathyroid hormone (PTH) and PTH-related protein (PTHrP) in regulating mineral homeostasis during fetal development. *Crit. Rev. Eukaryot. Gene Expr.* **2010**, *20*, 235–273.

75. Weisman, Y.; Vargas, A.; Duckett, G.; Reiter, E.; Root, A.W. Synthesis of 1,25-dihydroxyvitamin D in the nephrectomized pregnant rat. *Endocrinology* **1978**, *103*, 1992–1996.

76. Blum, M.; Weisman, Y.; Turgeman, S.; Cabili, S.; Wollman, Y.; Peer, G.; Stern, N.; Silverberg, D.; Schwartz, D.; Iaina, A. Pregnancy decreases immunoreactive parathyroid hormone level in rats with chronic renal failure. *Clin. Sci. (Lond.)* **1999**, *96*, 427–430.

77. Zehnder, D.; Bland, R.; Williams, M.C.; McNinch, R.W.; Howie, A.J.; Stewart, P.M.; Hewison, M. Extrarenal expression of 25-hydroxyvitamin D(3)-1 alpha-hydroxylase. *J. Clin. Endocrinol. Metab.* **2001**, *86*, 888–894.

78. Zehnder, D.; Evans, K.N.; Kilby, M.D.; Bulmer, J.N.; Innes, B.A.; Stewart, P.M.; Hewison, M. The ontogeny of 25-hydroxyvitamin D(3) 1alpha-hydroxylase expression in human placenta and decidua. *Am. J. Pathol.* **2002**, *161*, 105–114.

79. Evans, K.N.; Bulmer, J.N.; Kilby, M.D.; Hewison, M. Vitamin D and placental-decidual function. *J. Soc. Gynecol. Investig.* **2004**, *11*, 263–271.

80. Bikle, D.D.; Gee, E.; Halloran, B.; Haddad, J.G. Free 1,25-dihydroxyvitamin D levels in serum from normal subjects, pregnant subjects, and subjects with liver disease. *J. Clin. Invest.* **1984**, *74*, 1966–1971.

81. Chun, R.F.; Peercy, B.E.; Orwoll, E.S.; Nielson, C.M.; Adams, J.S.; Hewison, M. Vitamin D and DBP: The free hormone hypothesis revisited. *J. Steroid Biochem. Mol. Biol.* **2014**, *144*, 132–137.

82. Burke, K.A.; Jauniaux, E.; Burton, G.J.; Cindrova-Davies, T. Expression and immunolocalisation of the endocytic receptors megalin and cubilin in the human yolk sac and placenta across gestation. *Placenta* **2013**, *34*, 1105–1109.

83. Akour, A.A.; Gerk, P.; Kennedy, M.J. Megalin expression in human term and preterm placental villous tissues: Effect of gestational age and sample processing and storage time. *J. Pharmacol. Toxicol. Methods* **2014**.

84. Christensen, E.I.; Birn, H. Megalin and cubilin: Multifunctional endocytic receptors. *Nat. Rev. Mol. Cell Biol.* **2002**, *3*, 256–266.

85. Safadi, F.F.; Thornton, P.; Magiera, H.; Hollis, B.W.; Gentile, M.; Haddad, J.G.; Liebhaber, S.A.; Cooke, N.E. Osteopathy and resistance to vitamin D toxicity in mice null for vitamin D binding protein. *J. Clin. Invest.* **1999**, *103*, 239–251.

86. Johnson, J.A.; Grande, J.P.; Roche, P.C.; Kumar, R. Immunohistochemical detection and distribution of the 1,25-dihydroxyvitamin D3 receptor in rat reproductive tissues. *Histochem. Cell Biol.* **1996**, *105*, 7–15.

87. Shahbazi, M.; Jeddi-Tehrani, M.; Zareie, M.; Salek-Moghaddam, A.; Akhondi, M.M.; Bahmanpoor, M.; Sadeghi, M.R.; Zarnani, A.H. Expression profiling of vitamin D receptor in placenta, decidua and ovary of pregnant mice. *Placenta* **2011**, *32*, 657–664.

88. Zarnani, A.H.; Shahbazi, M.; Salek-Moghaddam, A.; Zareie, M.; Tavakoli, M.; Ghasemi, J.; Rezania, S.; Moravej, A.; Torkabadi, E.; Rabbani, H.; *et al.* Vitamin D3 receptor is expressed in the endometrium of cycling mice throughout the estrous cycle. *Fertil. Steril.* **2010**, *93*, 2738–2743.

89. Evans, K.N.; Nguyen, L.; Chan, J.; Innes, B.A.; Bulmer, J.N.; Kilby, M.D.; Hewison, M. Effects of 25-hydroxyvitamin D3 and 1,25-dihydroxyvitamin D3 on cytokine production by human decidual cells. *Biol. Reprod.* **2006**, *75*, 816–822.

90. Liu, N.; Kaplan, A.T.; Low, J.; Nguyen, L.; Liu, G.Y.; Equils, O.; Hewison, M. Vitamin D induces innate antibacterial responses in human trophoblasts via an intracrine pathway. *Biol. Reprod.* **2009**, *80*, 398–406.

91. Diaz, L.; Noyola-Martinez, N.; Barrera, D.; Hernandez, G.; Avila, E.; Halhali, A.; Larrea, F. Calcitriol inhibits TNF-alpha-induced inflammatory cytokines in human trophoblasts. *J. Reprod. Immunol.* **2009**, *81*, 17–24.

92. Noyola-Martinez, N.; Diaz, L.; Avila, E.; Halhali, A.; Larrea, F.; Barrera, D. Calcitriol downregulates TNF-alpha and IL-6 expression in cultured placental cells from preeclamptic women. *Cytokine* **2013**, *61*, 245–250.

93. Olmos-Ortiz, A.; Noyola-Martinez, N.; Barrera, D.; Zaga-Clavellina, V.; Avila, E.; Halhali, A.; Biruete, B.; Larrea, F.; Diaz, L. IL-10 inhibits while calcitriol reestablishes placental antimicrobial peptides gene expression. *J. Steroid Biochem. Mol. Biol.* **2014**.

94. Halhali, A.; Acker, G.M.; Garabedian, M. 1,25-dihydroxyvitamin D3 induces *in vivo* the decidualization of rat endometrial cells. *J. Reprod. Fertil.* **1991**, *91*, 59–64.

95. Barrera, D.; Avila, E.; Hernandez, G.; Halhali, A.; Biruete, B.; Larrea, F.; Diaz, L. Estradiol and progesterone synthesis in human placenta is stimulated by calcitriol. *J. Steroid Biochem. Mol. Biol.* **2007**, *103*, 529–532.

96. Barrera, D.; Avila, E.; Hernandez, G.; Mendez, I.; Gonzalez, L.; Halhali, A.; Larrea, F.; Morales, A.; Diaz, L. Calcitriol affects hCG gene transcription in cultured human syncytiotrophoblasts. *Reprod. Biol. Endocrinol.* **2008**, *6*, 3.

97. Stephanou, A.; Ross, R.; Handwerger, S. Regulation of human placental lactogen expression by 1,25-dihydroxyvitamin D3. *Endocrinology* **1994**, *135*, 2651–2656.

98. Binkley, N.; Ramamurthy, R.; Krueger, D. Low vitamin D status: Definition, prevalence, consequences, and correction. *Endocrinol. Metab. Clin. North Am.* **2010**, *39*, 287–301.

99. Levine, B.S.; Song, M. Pharmacokinetics and efficacy of pulse oral *versus* intravenous calcitriol in hemodialysis patients. *J. Am. Soc. Nephrol.* **1996**, *7*, 488–496.

100. Batchelor, A.J.; Watson, G.; Compston, J.E. Changes in plasma half-life and clearance of 3h-25-hydroxyvitamin D3 in patients with intestinal malabsorption. *Gut* **1982**, *23*, 1068–1071.

101. Dawson-Hughes, B.; Heaney, R.P.; Holick, M.F.; Lips, P.; Meunier, P.J.; Vieth, R. Estimates of optimal vitamin D status. *Osteoporos. Int.* **2005**, *16*, 713–716.

102. Pepe, J.; Romagnoli, E.; Nofroni, I.; Pacitti, M.T.; de Geronimo, S.; Letizia, C.; Tonnarini, G.; Scarpiello, A.; D'Erasmo, E.; Minisola, S. Vitamin D status as the major factor determining the circulating levels of parathyroid hormone: A study in normal subjects. *Osteoporos. Int.* **2005**, *16*, 805–812.

103. Heaney, R.P. Functional indices of vitamin D status and ramifications of vitamin D deficiency. *Am. J. Clin. Nutr.* **2004**, *80*, 1706–1709.

104. Vigano, P.; Lattuada, D.; Mangioni, S.; Ermellino, L.; Vignali, M.; Caporizzo, E.; Panina-Bordignon, P.; Besozzi, M.; di Blasio, A.M. Cycling and early pregnant endometrium as a site of regulated expression of the vitamin D system. *J. Mol. Endocrinol.* **2006**, *36*, 415–424.

105. Barrera, D.; Noyola-Martinez, N.; Avila, E.; Halhali, A.; Larrea, F.; Diaz, L. Calcitriol inhibits interleukin-10 expression in cultured human trophoblasts under normal and inflammatory conditions. *Cytokine* **2012**, *57*, 316–321.

106. Avila, E.; Garcia-Becerra, R.; Rodriguez-Rasgado, J.A.; Diaz, L.; Ordaz-Rosado, D.; Zugel, U.; Steinmeyer, A.; Barrera, D.; Halhali, A.; Larrea, F.; *et al.* Calcitriol down-regulates human ether a go-go 1 potassium channel expression in cervical cancer cells. *Anticancer Res.* **2010**, *30*, 2667–2672.

107. Delvin, E.E.; Gagnon, L.; Arabian, A.; Gibb, W. Influence of calcitriol on prolactin and prostaglandin production by human decidua. *Mol. Cell Endocrinol.* **1990**, *71*, 177–183.

108. Narahara, H.; Miyakawa, I.; Johnston, J.M. The inhibitory effect of 1,25-dihydroxyvitamin D3 on the secretion of platelet-activating factor acetylhydrolase by human decidual macrophages. *J. Clin. Endocrinol. Metab.* **1995**, *80*, 3121–3126.

109. Daftary, G.S.; Taylor, H.S. Endocrine regulation of HOX genes. *Endocr. Rev.* **2006**, *27*, 331–355.

110. Holick, M.F.; Binkley, N.C.; Bischoff-Ferrari, H.A.; Gordon, C.M.; Hanley, D.A.; Heaney, R.P.; Murad, M.H.; Weaver, C.M. Evaluation, treatment, and prevention of vitamin D deficiency: An Endocrine Society clinical practice guideline. *J. Clin. Endocrinol. Metab.* **2011**, *96*, 1911–1930.

111. Ross, A.C.; Manson, J.E.; Abrams, S.A.; Aloia, J.F.; Brannon, P.M.; Clinton, S.K.; Durazo-Arvizu, R.A.; Gallagher, J.C.; Gallo, R.L.; Jones, G.; *et al.* The 2011 Report on dietary reference intakes for calcium and vitamin D from the Institute of Medicine: What clinicians need to know. *J. Clin. Endocrinol. Metab.* **2011**, *96*, 53–58.

112. Aghajafari, F.; Nagulesapillai, T.; Ronksley, P.E.; Tough, S.C.; O'Beirne, M.; Rabi, D.M. Association between maternal serum 25-hydroxyvitamin D level and pregnancy and neonatal outcomes: Systematic review and meta-analysis of observational studies. *BMJ* **2013**, *346*, 1169.

113. Barrett, H.; McElduff, A. Vitamin D and pregnancy: An old problem revisited. *Best Pract. Res. Clin. Endocrinol. Metab.* **2010**, *24*, 527–529.

114. Bodnar, L.M.; Simhan, H.N. Vitamin D may be a link to black-white disparities in adverse birth outcomes. *Obstet. Gynecol. Surv.* **2010**, *65*, 273–284.

115. Christesen, H.T.; Falkenberg, T.; Lamont, R.F.; Jorgensen, J.S. The impact of vitamin D on pregnancy: A systematic review. *Acta Obstet. Gynecol. Scandinav.* **2012**, *91*, 1357–1367.

116. Nassar, N.; Halligan, G.H.; Roberts, C.L.; Morris, J.M.; Ashton, A.W. Systematic review of first-trimester vitamin D normative levels and outcomes of pregnancy. *Am. J. Obstet. Gynecol.* **2011**, *205*, 208.e201–208.e207.

117. Thorne-Lyman, A.; Fawzia, W.W. Vitamin D during pregnancy and maternal, neonatal and infant health outcomes: A systematic review and meta-analysis. *Paediatr. Perinat. Epidemiol.* **2012**, *26*, 75–90.

118. Urrutia, R.P.; Thorp, J.M. Vitamin D in pregnancy: Current concepts. *Curr. Opin. Obstet. Gynecol.* **2012**, *24*, 57–64.

119. Wei, S.Q.; Qi, H.P.; Luo, Z.C.; Fraser, W.D. Maternal vitamin D status and adverse pregnancy outcomes: A systematic review and meta-analysis. *J Matern. Fetal Neonatal Med.* **2013**, *26*, 889–899.

120. Report of the National high blood pressure Education Program Working Group on high blood pressure in pregnancy. *Am. J. Obstet. Gynecol.* **2000**, *183*, 1–22.

121. ACOG practice bulletin. Diagnosis and management of preeclampsia and eclampsia. Number 33, january 2002. American College of Obstetricians and Gynecologists. *Int. J. Gynaecol. Obstet.* **2002**, *77*, 67–75.

122. Baumwell, S.; Karumanchi, S.A. Pre-eclampsia: Clinical manifestations and molecular mechanisms. *Nephron Clin. Pract.* **2007**, *106*, c72–c81.

123. Palei, A.C.; Spradley, F.T.; Warrington, J.P.; George, E.M.; Granger, J.P. Pathophysiology of hypertension in pre-eclampsia: A lesson in integrative physiology. *Acta Physiol.* **2013**, *208*, 224–233.

124. Gernand, A.D.; Bodnar, L.M.; Klebanoff, M.A.; Parks, W.T.; Simhan, H.N. Maternal serum 25-hydroxyvitamin D and placental vascular pathology in a multicenter US cohort. *Am. J. Clin. Nutr.* **2013**, *98*, 383–388.

125. Halhali, A.; Bourges, H.; Carrillo, A.; Garabedian, M. Lower circulating insulin-like growth factor I and 1,25-dihydroxyvitamin D levels in preeclampsia. *Rev. Invest. Clin.* **1995**, *47*, 259–266.

126. Halhali, A.; Diaz, L.; Avila, E.; Ariza, A.C.; Garabedian, M.; Larrea, F. Decreased fractional urinary calcium excretion and serum 1,25-dihydroxyvitamin D and IGF-I levels in preeclampsia. *J. Steroid Biochem. Mol. Biol.* **2007**, *103*, 803–806.

127. Halhali, A.; Tovar, A.R.; Torres, N.; Bourges, H.; Garabedian, M.; Larrea, F. Preeclampsia is associated with low circulating levels of insulin-like growth factor I and 1,25-dihydroxyvitamin D in maternal and umbilical cord compartments. *J. Clin. Endocrinol. Metab.* **2000**, *85*, 1828–1833.

128. Diaz, E.; Halhali, A.; Luna, C.; Diaz, L.; Avila, E.; Larrea, F. Newborn birth weight correlates with placental zinc, umbilical insulin-like growth factor I, and leptin levels in preeclampsia. *Arch. Med. Res.* **2002**, *33*, 40–47.

129. Robinson, C.J.; Alanis, M.C.; Wagner, C.L.; Hollis, B.W.; Johnson, D.D. Plasma 25-hydroxyvitamin D levels in early-onset severe preeclampsia. *Am. J. Obstet. Gynecol.* **2010**, *203*, 366.e361–366.e366.

130. Xu, L.; Lee, M.; Jeyabalan, A.; Roberts, J.M. The relationship of hypovitaminosis D and IL-6 in preeclampsia. *Am. J. Obstet. Gynecol.* **2014**, *210*, 149.e141–149.e147.

131. Ullah, M.I.; Koch, C.A.; Tamanna, S.; Rouf, S.; Shamsuddin, L. Vitamin D deficiency and the risk of preeclampsia and eclampsia in Bangladesh. *Horm. Metab. Res.* **2013**, *45*, 682–687.

132. Wei, S.Q.; Audibert, F.; Luo, Z.C.; Nuyt, A.M.; Masse, B.; Julien, P.; Fraser, W.D. Maternal plasma 25-hydroxyvitamin D levels, angiogenic factors, and preeclampsia. *Am. J. Obstet. Gynecol.* **2013**, *208*, 390.e391–390.e396.

133. Baker, A.M.; Haeri, S.; Camargo, C.A., Jr.; Espinola, J.A.; Stuebe, A.M. A nested case-control study of midgestation vitamin D deficiency and risk of severe preeclampsia. *J. Clin. Endocrinol. Metab.* **2010**, *95*, 5105–5109.

134. Bodnar, L.M.; Catov, J.M.; Simhan, H.N.; Holick, M.F.; Powers, R.W.; Roberts, J.M. Maternal vitamin D deficiency increases the risk of preeclampsia. *J. Clin. Endocrinol. Metab.* **2007**, *92*, 3517–3522.

135. Abedi, P.; Mohaghegh, Z.; Afshary, P.; Latifi, M. The relationship of serum vitamin D with pre-eclampsia in the iranian women. *Matern. Child. Nutr.* **2014**, *10*, 206–212.

136. Diaz, L.; Arranz, C.; Avila, E.; Halhali, A.; Vilchis, F.; Larrea, F. Expression and activity of 25-hydroxyvitamin D-1 alpha-hydroxylase are restricted in cultures of human syncytiotrophoblast cells from preeclamptic pregnancies. *J. Clin. Endocrinol. Metab.* **2002**, *87*, 3876–3882.

137. Bodnar, L.M.; Simhan, H.N.; Catov, J.M.; Roberts, J.M.; Platt, R.W.; Diesel, J.C.; Klebanoff, M.A. Maternal vitamin D status and the risk of mild and severe preeclampsia. *Epidemiology* **2014**, *25*, 207–214.

138. Woodham, P.C.; Brittain, J.E.; Baker, A.M.; Leann Long, D.; Haeri, S.; Camargo, C.A.J.; Boggess, K.A.; Stuebe, A.M. Midgestation maternal serum 25-hydroxyvitamin D level and soluble fms-like tyrosine kinase 1/placental growth factor ratio as predictors of severe preeclampsia. *Hypertension* **2011**, *58*, 1120–1125.

139. Haugen, M.; Brantsæter, A.L.; Trogstad, L.; Alexander, J.; Roth, C.; Magnus, P.; Meltzera, H.M. Vitamin D supplementation and reduced risk of preeclampsia in nulliparous women. *Epidemiology* **2009**, *20*, 720–726.

140. Hyppönen, E.; Cavadino, A.; Williams, D.; Fraser, A.; Vereczkey, A.; Fraser, W.D.; Bánhidy, F.; Lawlor, D.; Czeizel, A.E. Vitamin D and pre-eclampsia: Original data, systematic review and meta-analysis. *Ann. Nutr. Metab.* **2013**, *63*, 331–340.

141. Tabesh, M.; Salehi-Abargouei, A.; Esmaillzadeh, A. Maternal vitamin D status and risk of pre-eclampsia: A systematic review and meta-analysis. *J. Clin. Endocrinol. Metab.* **2013**, *98*, 3165–3173.

142. Shand, A.W.; Nassar, N.; von Dadelszen, P.; Innis, S.M.; Green, T.J. Maternal vitamin D status in pregnancy and adverse pregnancy outcomes in a group at high risk for pre-eclampsia. *BJOG* **2010**, *117*, 1593–1598.

143. Powe, C.E.; Seely, E.W.; Rana, S.; Bhan, I.; Ecker, J.; Karumanchi, S.A.; Thadhani, R. First trimester vitamin D, vitamin D binding protein, and subsequent preeclampsia. *Hypertension* **2010**, *56*, 758–763.

144. Mashburn, J. Vaginal infections update. *J. Midwifery Womens Health* **2012**, *57*, 629–634.

145. Denney, J.M.; Culhane, J.F. Bacterial vaginosis: A problematic infection from both a perinatal and neonatal perspective. *Semin. Fetal Neonatal Med.* **2009**, *14*, 200–203.

146. Allsworth, J.E.; Peipert, J.F. Prevalence of bacterial vaginosis: 2001–2004 National Health and Nutrition Examination Survey data. *Obstet. Gynecol.* **2007**, *109*, 114–120.

147. Prietl, B.; Treiber, G.; Pieber, T.R.; Amrein, K. Vitamin D and immune function. *Nutrients* **2013**, *5*, 2502–2521.

148. Hewison, M. Vitamin D and immune function: An overview. *Proc. Nutr. Soc.* **2012**, *71*, 50–61.

149. Bodnar, L.M.; Krohn, M.A.; Simhan, H.N. Maternal vitamin D deficiency is associated with bacterial vaginosis in the first trimester of pregnancy. *J. Nutr.* **2009**, *139*, 1157–1161.

150. Dunlop, A.L.; Taylor, R.N.; Tangpricha, V.; Fortunato, S.; Menon, R. Maternal vitamin D, folate, and polyunsaturated fatty acid status and bacterial vaginosis during pregnancy. *Infect. Dis. Obstet. Gynecol.* **2011**, *2011*, 216217.

151. Hensel, K.J.; Randis, T.M.; Gelber, S.E.; Ratner, A.J. Pregnancy-specific association of vitamin D deficiency and bacterial vaginosis. *Am. J. Obstet. Gynecol.* **2011**, *204*, 41–49.

152. Rustveld, L.O.; Kelsey, S.F.; Sharma, R. Association between maternal infections and preeclampsia: A systematic review of epidemiologic studies. *Matern. Child. Health J.* **2008**, *12*, 223–242.

153. Hertting, O.; Holm, A.; Luthje, P.; Brauner, H.; Dyrdak, R.; Jonasson, A.F.; Wiklund, P.; Chromek, M.; Brauner, A. Vitamin D induction of the human antimicrobial peptide cathelicidin in the urinary bladder. *PLoS One* **2010**, *5*, 15580.

154. Boggess, K.A.; Espinola, J.A.; Moss, K.; Beck, J.; Offenbacher, S.; Camargo, C.A. Vitamin D status and periodontal disease among pregnant women. *J. Periodontol.* **2011**, *82*, 195–200.

155. Lowry, M.B.; Guo, C.; Borregaard, N.; Gombart, A.F. Regulation of the human cathelicidin antimicrobial peptide gene by 1alpha,25-dihydroxyvitamin D in primary immune cells. *J. Steroid Biochem. Mol. Biol.* **2014**, *143*, 183–191.

156. Mendez-Samperio, P. The human cathelicidin hCAP18/LL-37: A multifunctional peptide involved in mycobacterial infections. *Peptides* **2010**, *31*, 1791–1798.

157. Campbell, G.R.; Spector, S.A. Autophagy induction by vitamin D inhibits both mycobacterium tuberculosis and human immunodeficiency virus type 1. *Autophagy* **2012**, *8*, 1523–1525.

158. Campbell, G.R.; Spector, S.A. Vitamin D inhibits human immunodeficiency virus type 1 and mycobacterium tuberculosis infection in macrophages through the induction of autophagy. *PLoS Pathog.* **2012**, *8*, 1002689.

159. Wan, M.; van der Does, A.M.; Tang, X.; Lindbom, L.; Agerberth, B.; Haeggstrom, J.Z. Antimicrobial peptide LL-37 promotes bacterial phagocytosis by human macrophages. *J. Leukoc. Biol.* **2014**, *95*, 971–981.

160. Frew, L.; Stock, S.J. Antimicrobial peptides and pregnancy. *Reproduction* **2011**, *141*, 725–735.

161. Thota, C.; Farmer, T.; Garfield, R.E.; Menon, R.; Al-Hendy, A. Vitamin D elicits anti-inflammatory response, inhibits contractile-associated proteins, and modulates Toll-like receptors in human myometrial cells. *Reprod. Sci.* **2013**, *20*, 463–475.

162. Bodnar, L.M.; Rouse, D.J.; Momirova, V.; Peaceman, A.M.; Sciscione, A.; Spong, C.Y.; Varner, M.W.; Malone, F.D.; Iams, J.D.; Mercer, B.M.; *et al.* Maternal 25-hydroxyvitamin D and preterm birth in twin gestations. *Obstet. Gynecol.* **2013**, *122*, 91–98.

163. Thorp, J.M.; Camargo, C.A.; McGee, P.L.; Harper, M.; Klebanoff, M.A.; Sorokin, Y.; Varner, M.W.; Wapner, R.J.; Caritis, S.N.; Iams, J.D.; *et al.* Vitamin D status and recurrent preterm birth: A nested case-control study in high-risk women. *BJOG* **2012**, *119*, 1617–1623.

164. American Diabetes Association. Gestational diabetes mellitus. *Diabetes Care* **2003**, *26* (Suppl. 1), 103–105.

165. American Diabetes Association. Standards of medical care in diabetes–2012. *Diabetes Care* **2012**, *35* (Suppl. 1), 11–63.

166. Wang, Z.; Kanguru, L.; Hussein, J.; Fitzmaurice, A.; Ritchie, K. Incidence of adverse outcomes associated with gestational diabetes mellitus in low- and middle-income countries. *Int. J. Gynaecol. Obstet.* **2013**, *121*, 14–19.

167. Wendland, E.M.; Torloni, M.R.; Falavigna, M.; Trujillo, J.; Dode, M.A.; Campos, M.A.; Duncan, B.B.; Schmidt, M.I. Gestational diabetes and pregnancy outcomes—A systematic review of the world health organization (WHO) and the International Association of Diabetes in Pregnancy Study Groups (IADPSG) diagnostic criteria. *BMC Pregnancy Childbirth* **2012**, *12*, 23.

168. Norman, A.W.; Frankel, J.B.; Heldt, A.M.; Grodsky, G.M. Vitamin D deficiency inhibits pancreatic secretion of insulin. *Science* **1980**, *209*, 823–825.

169. Cho, G.J.; Hong, S.C.; Oh, M.J.; Kim, H.J. Vitamin D deficiency in gestational diabetes mellitus and the role of the placenta. *Am. J. Obstet. Gynecol.* **2013**, *209*, 560 e561–560 e568.

170. Clifton-Bligh, R.J.; McElduff, P.; McElduff, A. Maternal vitamin D deficiency, ethnicity and gestational diabetes. *Diabetes Med.* **2008**, *25*, 678–684.

171. Parlea, L.; Bromberg, I.L.; Feig, D.S.; Vieth, R.; Merman, E.; Lipscombe, L.L. Association between serum 25-hydroxyvitamin D in early pregnancy and risk of gestational diabetes mellitus. *Diabetes Med.* **2012**, *29*, 25–32.

172. Soheilykhah, S.; Mojibian, M.; Rashidi, M.; Rahimi-Saghand, S.; Jafari, F. Maternal vitamin D status in gestational diabetes mellitus. *Nutr. Clin. Pract.* **2010**, *25*, 524–527.

173. Zhang, C.; Qiu, C.; Hu, F.B.; David, R.M.; van Dam, R.M.; Bralley, A.; Williams, M.A. Maternal plasma 25-hydroxyvitamin D concentrations and the risk for gestational diabetes mellitus. *PLoS One* **2008**, *3*, 3753.

174. Zuhur, S.S.; Erol, R.S.; Kuzu, I.; Altuntas, Y. The relationship between low maternal serum 25-hydroxyvitamin D levels and gestational diabetes mellitus according to the severity of 25-hydroxyvitamin D deficiency. *Clinics (Sao Paulo)* **2013**, *68*, 658–664.

175. Maghbooli, Z.; Hossein-Nezhad, A.; Karimi, F.; Shafaei, A.R.; Larijani, B. Correlation between vitamin D3 deficiency and insulin resistance in pregnancy. *Diabetes Metab. Res. Rev.* **2008**, *24*, 27–32.

176. Napartivaumnuay, N.; Niramitmahapanya, S.; Deerochanawong, C.; Suthornthepavarakul, T.; Sarinnapakorn, V.; Jaruyawongs, P. Maternal 25 hydroxyvitamin D level and its correlation in thai gestational diabetes patients. *J. Med. Assoc. Thail.* **2013**, *96* (Suppl. 3), 69–76.

177. Burris, H.H.; Rifas-Shiman, S.L.; Kleinman, K.; Litonjua, A.A.; Huh, S.Y.; Rich-Edwards, J.W.; Camargo, C.A., Jr.; Gillman, M.W. Vitamin D deficiency in pregnancy and gestational diabetes mellitus. *Am. J. Obstet. Gynecol.* **2012**, *207*, 182.e181–182.e188.

178. Wang, O.; Nie, M.; Hu, Y.Y.; Zhang, K.; Li, W.; Ping, F.; Liu, J.T.; Chen, L.M.; Xing, X.P. Association between vitamin D insufficiency and the risk for gestational diabetes mellitus in pregnant chinese women. *Biomed. Environ. Sci.* **2012**, *25*, 399–406.

179. Poel, Y.H.; Hummel, P.; Lips, P.; Stam, F.; van der Ploeg, T.; Simsek, S. Vitamin D and gestational diabetes: A systematic review and meta-analysis. *Eur. J. Intern. Med.* **2012**, *23*, 465–469.

180. Senti, J.; Thiele, D.K.; Anderson, C.M. Maternal vitamin D status as a critical determinant in gestational diabetes. *J. Obstet. Gynecol. Neonatal. Nurs.* **2012**, *41*, 328–338.

181. Lau, S.L.; Gunton, J.E.; Athayde, N.P.; Byth, K.; Cheung, N.W. Serum 25-hydroxyvitamin D and glycated haemoglobin levels in women with gestational diabetes mellitus. *Med. J. Aust.* **2011**, *194*, 334–337.

182. Makgoba, M.; Nelson, S.M.; Savvidou, M.; Messow, C.M.; Nicolaides, K.; Sattar, N. First-trimester circulating 25-hydroxyvitamin D levels and development of gestational diabetes mellitus. *Diabetes Care* **2011**, *34*, 1091–1093.

183. McLeod, D.S.; Warner, J.V.; Henman, M.; Cowley, D.; Gibbons, K.; McIntyre, H.D. Associations of serum vitamin D concentrations with obstetric glucose metabolism in a subset of the Hyperglycemia and Adverse Pregnancy Outcome (HAPO) study cohort. *Diabetes Med.* **2012**, *29*, 199–204.

184. Walsh, J.M.; McGowan, C.A.; Kilbane, M.; McKenna, M.J.; McAuliffe, F.M. The relationship between maternal and fetal vitamin D, insulin resistance, and fetal growth. *Reprod. Sci.* **2013**, *20*, 536–541.

185. Jelsma, J.G.; van Poppel, M.N.; Galjaard, S.; Desoye, G.; Corcoy, R.; Devlieger, R.; van Assche, A.; Timmerman, D.; Jans, G.; Harreiter, J.; *et al.* Dali: Vitamin D and lifestyle intervention for gestational diabetes mellitus (GDM) prevention: An european multicentre, randomised trial-study protocol. *BMC Pregnancy Childbirth* **2013**, *13*, 142.

186. Asemi, Z.; Hashemi, T.; Karamali, M.; Samimi, M.; Esmaillzadeh, A. Effects of vitamin D supplementation on glucose metabolism, lipid concentrations, inflammation, and oxidative stress in gestational diabetes: A double-blind randomized controlled clinical trial. *Am. J. Clin. Nutr.* **2013**, *98*, 1425–1432.

187. Mozaffari-Khosravi, H.; Hosseinzadeh-Shamsi-Anar, M.; Salami, M.A.; Hadinedoushan, H.; Mozayan, M.R. Effects of a single post-partum injection of a high dose of vitamin D on glucose tolerance and insulin resistance in mothers with first-time gestational diabetes mellitus. *Diabetes Med.* **2012**, *29*, 36–42.

188. Baker, A.M.; Haeri, S.; Camargo, C.A., Jr.; Stuebe, A.M.; Boggess, K.A. First-trimester maternal vitamin D status and risk for gestational diabetes (GDM) a nested case-control study. *Diabetes Metab. Res. Rev.* **2012**, *28*, 164–168.

189. Savvidou, M.D.; Akolekar, R.; Samaha, R.B.; Masconi, A.P.; Nicolaides, K.H. Maternal serum 25-hydroxyvitamin D levels at 11(+0) -13(+6) weeks in pregnant women with diabetes mellitus and in those with macrosomic neonates. *BJOG* **2011**, *118*, 951–955.

190. Farrant, H.J.; Krishnaveni, G.V.; Hill, J.C.; Boucher, B.J.; Fisher, D.J.; Noonan, K.; Osmond, C.; Veena, S.R.; Fall, C.H. Vitamin D insufficiency is common in indian mothers but is not associated with gestational diabetes or variation in newborn size. *Eur. J. Clin. Nutr.* **2009**, *63*, 646–652.

191. Tomedi, L.E.; Simhan, H.N.; Bodnar, L.M. Early-pregnancy maternal vitamin D status and maternal hyperglycaemia. *Diabetes Med.* **2013**, *30*, 1033–1039.

192. Mirzaei, K.; Hossein-Nezhad, A.; Keshavarz, S.A.; Eshaghi, S.M.; Koohdani, F.; Saboor-Yaraghi, A.A.; Hosseini, S.; Tootee, A.; Djalali, M. Insulin resistance via modification of PGC1alpha function identifying a possible preventive role of vitamin D analogues in chronic inflammatory state of obesity. A double blind clinical trial study. *Minerva Med.* **2014**, *105*, 63–78.

193. Alkharfy, K.M.; Al-Daghri, N.M.; Yakout, S.M.; Hussain, T.; Mohammed, A.K.; Krishnaswamy, S. Influence of vitamin D treatment on transcriptional regulation of insulin-sensitive genes. *Metab. Syndr. Relat. Disord.* **2013**, *11*, 283–288.

194. Manna, P.; Jain, S.K. Vitamin D up-regulates glucose transporter 4 (GLUT4) translocation and glucose utilization mediated by cystathionine-gamma-lyase (CSE) activation and H2Ss formation in 3T3L1 adipocytes. *J. Biol. Chem.* **2012**, *287*, 42324–42332.

195. Meerza, D.; Naseem, I.; Ahmed, J. Effect of 1, 25(OH)(2) vitamin D(3) on glucose homeostasis and DNA damage in type 2 diabetic mice. *J. Diabetes Complicat.* **2012**, *26*, 363–368.

196. Zhang, J.; Merialdi, M.; Platt, L.D.; Kramer, M.S. Defining normal and abnormal fetal growth: Promises and challenges. *Am. J. Obstet. Gynecol.* **2010**, *202*, 522–528.

197. Mayer, C.; Joseph, K.S. Fetal growth: A review of terms, concepts and issues relevant to obstetrics. *Ultrasound Obstet. Gynecol.* **2013**, *41*, 136–145.

198. Burris, H.H.; Mitchell, A.A.; Werler, M.M. Periconceptional multivitamin use and infant birth weight disparities. *Ann. Epidemiol.* **2010**, *20*, 233–240.

199. Kovacs, C.S. Maternal vitamin D deficiency: Fetal and neonatal implications. *Semin. Fetal Neonatal Med.* **2013**, *18*, 129–135.

200. Brunvand, L.; Quigstad, E.; Urdal, P.; Haug, E. Vitamin D deficiency and fetal growth. *Early Hum. Dev.* **1996**, *45*, 27–33.

201. Gale, C.R.; Robinson, S.M.; Harvey, N.C.; Javaid, M.K.; Jiang, B.; Martyn, C.N.; Godfrey, K.M.; Cooper, C. Maternal vitamin D status during pregnancy and child outcomes. *Eur. J. Clin. Nutr.* **2008**, *62*, 68–77.

202. Agarwal, R.; Virmani, D.; Jaipal, M.L.; Gupta, S.; Gupta, N.; Sankar, M.J.; Bhatia, S.; Agarwal, A.; Devgan, V.; Deorari, A.; *et al.* Vitamin D status of low birth weight infants in Delhi: A comparative study. *J. Trop. Pediatr.* **2012**, *58*, 446–450.

203. Gernand, A.D.; Simhan, H.N.; Klebanoff, M.A.; Bodnar, L.M. Maternal serum 25-hydroxyvitamin D and measures of newborn and placental weight in a U.S. multicenter cohort study. *J. Clin. Endocrinol. Metab.* **2013**, *98*, 398–404.

204. Ertl, R.; Yu, C.K.; Samaha, R.; Akolekar, R.; Nicolaides, K.H. Maternal serum vitamin D at 11–13 weeks in pregnancies delivering small for gestational age neonates. *Fetal Diagn. Ther.* **2012**, *31*, 103–108.

205. Namgung, R.; Tsang, R.C.; Specker, B.L.; Sierra, R.I.; Ho, M.L. Reduced serum osteocalcin and 1,25-dihydroxyvitamin D concentrations and low bone mineral content in small for gestational age infants: Evidence of decreased bone formation rates. *J. Pediatr.* **1993**, *122*, 269–275.

206. Van den Berg, G.; van Eijsden, M.; Vrijkotte, T.G.; Gemke, R.J. Suboptimal maternal vitamin D status and low education level as determinants of small-for-gestational-age birth weight. *Eur. J. Nutr.* **2013**, *52*, 273–279.

207. Scholl, T.O.; Chen, X. Vitamin D intake during pregnancy: Association with maternal characteristics and infant birth weight. *Early Hum. Dev.* **2009**, *85*, 231–234.

208. Mannion, C.A.; Gray-Donald, K.; Koski, K.G. Association of low intake of milk and vitamin D during pregnancy with decreased birth weight. *CMAJ* **2006**, *174*, 1273–1277.

209. Bodnar, L.M.; Catov, J.M.; Zmuda, J.M.; Cooper, M.E.; Parrott, M.S.; Roberts, J.M.; Marazita, M.L.; Simhan, H.N. Maternal serum 25-hydroxyvitamin D concentrations are associated with small-for-gestational age births in white women. *J. Nutr.* **2010**, *140*, 999–1006.

210. Kalra, P.; Das, V.; Agarwal, A.; Kumar, M.; Ramesh, V.; Bhatia, E.; Gupta, S.; Singh, S.; Saxena, P.; Bhatia, V. Effect of vitamin D supplementation during pregnancy on neonatal mineral homeostasis and anthropometry of the newborn and infant. *Br. J. Nutr.* **2012**, *108*, 1052–1058.

211. Young, B.E.; McNanley, T.J.; Cooper, E.M.; McIntyre, A.W.; Witter, F.; Harris, Z.L.; O'Brien, K.O. Maternal vitamin D status and calcium intake interact to affect fetal skeletal growth in utero in pregnant adolescents. *Am. J. Clin. Nutr.* **2012**, *95*, 1103–1112.

212. Diogenes, M.E.; Bezerra, F.F.; Rezende, E.P.; Taveira, M.F.; Pinhal, I.; Donangelo, C.M. Effect of calcium plus vitamin D supplementation during pregnancy in brazilian adolescent mothers: A randomized, placebo-controlled trial. *Am. J. Clin. Nutr.* **2013**, *98*, 82–91.

213. Morley, R.; Carlin, J.B.; Pasco, J.A.; Wark, J.D.; Ponsonby, A.L. Maternal 25-hydroxyvitamin D concentration and offspring birth size: Effect modification by infant VDR genotype. *Eur. J. Clin. Nutr.* **2009**, *63*, 802–804.

214. Jones, K.S.; Assar, S.; Harnpanich, D.; Bouillon, R.; Lambrechts, D.; Prentice, A.; Schoenmakers, I. 25(OH)D2 half-life is shorter than 25(OH)D3 half-life and is influenced by DBP concentration and genotype. *J. Clin. Endocrinol. Metab.* **2014**, *99*, 3373–3381.

215. McGrath, J.J.; Saha, S.; Burne, T.H.; Eyles, D.W. A systematic review of the association between common single nucleotide polymorphisms and 25-hydroxyvitamin D concentrations. *J. Steroid Biochem. Mol. Biol.* **2010**, *121*, 471–477.

216. Wang, T.J.; Zhang, F.; Richards, J.B.; Kestenbaum, B.; van Meurs, J.B.; Berry, D.; Kiel, D.P.; Streeten, E.A.; Ohlsson, C.; Koller, D.L.; *et al.* Common genetic determinants of vitamin D insufficiency: A genome-wide association study. *Lancet* **2010**, *376*, 180–188.

217. Barry, E.L.; Rees, J.R.; Peacock, J.L.; Mott, L.A.; Amos, C.I.; Bostick, R.M.; Figueiredo, J.C.; Ahnen, D.J.; Bresalier, R.S.; Burke, C.A.; *et al.* Genetic variants in CYP2R1, CYP24A1, and VDR modify the efficacy of vitamin D3 supplementation for increasing serum 25-hydroxyvitamin D levels in a randomized controlled trial. *J. Clin. Endocrinol. Metab.* **2014**, *99*, 2133–2137.

218. Jones, K.S.; Assar, S.; Vanderschueren, D.; Bouillon, R.; Prentice, A.; Schoenmakers, I. Predictors of 25(OH)D half-life and plasma 25(OH)D concentration in the Gambia and the UK. *Osteoporos. Int.* **2014**.

219. Karras, S.N.; Anagnostis, P.; Annweiler, C.; Naughton, D.P.; Petroczi, A.; Bili, E.; Harizopoulou, V.; Tarlatzis, B.C.; Persinaki, A.; Papadopoulou, F.; *et al.* Maternal vitamin D status during pregnancy: The mediterranean reality. *Eur. J. Clin. Nutr.* **2014**, *68*, 864–869.

220. Wuertz, C.; Gilbert, P.; Baier, W.; Kunz, C. Cross-sectional study of factors that influence the 25-hydroxyvitamin D status in pregnant women and in cord blood in Germany. *Br. J. Nutr.* **2013**, *110*, 1895–1902.

221. Wortsman, J.; Matsuoka, L.Y.; Chen, T.C.; Lu, Z.; Holick, M.F. Decreased bioavailability of vitamin D in obesity. *Am. J. Clin. Nutr.* **2000**, *72*, 690–693.

222. Abboud, M.; Puglisi, D.A.; Davies, B.N.; Rybchyn, M.; Whitehead, N.P.; Brock, K.E.; Cole, L.; Gordon-Thomson, C.; Fraser, D.R.; Mason, R.S. Evidence for a specific uptake and retention mechanism for 25-hydroxyvitamin D (25OHD) in skeletal muscle cells. *Endocrinology* **2013**, *154*, 3022–3030.

223. Abboud, M.; Gordon-Thomson, C.; Hoy, A.J.; Balaban, S.; Rybchyn, M.S.; Cole, L.; Su, Y.; Brennan-Speranza, T.C.; Fraser, D.R.; Mason, R.S. Uptake of 25-hydroxyvitamin D by muscle and fat cells. *J. Steroid Biochem. Mol. Biol.* **2014**, *144*, 232–236.

224. Josefson, J.L.; Feinglass, J.; Rademaker, A.W.; Metzger, B.E.; Zeiss, D.M.; Price, H.E.; Langman, C.B. Maternal obesity and vitamin D sufficiency are associated with cord blood vitamin D insufficiency. *J. Clin. Endocrinol. Metab.* **2013**, *98*, 114–119.

225. Bodnar, L.M.; Catov, J.M.; Roberts, J.M.; Simhan, H.N. Prepregnancy obesity predicts poor vitamin D status in mothers and their neonates. *J. Nutr.* **2007**, *137*, 2437–2442.

226. Crozier, S.R.; Harvey, N.C.; Inskip, H.M.; Godfrey, K.M.; Cooper, C.; Robinson, S.M. Maternal vitamin D status in pregnancy is associated with adiposity in the offspring: Findings from the Southampton Women's Survey. *Am. J. Clin. Nutr.* **2012**, *96*, 57–63.

227. Morales, E.; Romieu, I.; Guerra, S.; Ballester, F.; Rebagliato, M.; Vioque, J.; Tardon, A.; Rodriguez Delhi, C.; Arranz, L.; Torrent, M.; *et al.* Maternal vitamin D status in pregnancy and risk of lower respiratory tract infections, wheezing, and asthma in offspring. *Epidemiology* **2012**, *23*, 64–71.

228. Hossain, N.; Kanani, F.H.; Ramzan, S.; Kausar, R.; Ayaz, S.; Khanani, R.; Pal, L. Obstetric and neonatal outcomes of maternal vitamin D supplementation: Results of an open-label, randomized controlled trial of antenatal vitamin D supplementation in pakistani women. *J. Clin. Endocrinol. Metab.* **2014**, *99*, 2448–2455.

229. Wagner, C.L.; McNeil, R.; Hamilton, S.A.; Winkler, J.; Rodriguez Cook, C.; Warner, G.; Bivens, B.; Davis, D.J.; Smith, P.G.; Murphy, M.; *et al.* A randomized trial of vitamin D supplementation in 2 community health center networks in South Carolina. *Am. J. Obstet. Gynecol.* **2013**, *208*, 137.e1–137.e13.

230. Sahu, M.; Das, V.; Aggarwal, A.; Rawat, V.; Saxena, P.; Bhatia, V. Vitamin D replacement in pregnant women in rural north india: A pilot study. *Eur. J. Clin. Nutr.* **2009**, *63*, 1157–1159.

231. Yu, C.K.; Sykes, L.; Sethi, M.; Teoh, T.G.; Robinson, S. Vitamin D deficiency and supplementation during pregnancy. *Clin. Endocrinol. (Oxf.)* **2009**, *70*, 685–690.

232. Grant, C.C.; Stewart, A.W.; Scragg, R.; Milne, T.; Rowden, J.; Ekeroma, A.; Wall, C.; Mitchell, E.A.; Crengle, S.; Trenholme, A.; *et al.* Vitamin D during pregnancy and infancy and infant serum 25-hydroxyvitamin D concentration. *Pediatrics* **2014**, *133*, 143–153.

233. Dawodu, A.; Saadi, H.F.; Bekdache, G.; Javed, Y.; Altaye, M.; Hollis, B.W. Randomized controlled trial (RCT) of vitamin D supplementation in pregnancy in a population with endemic vitamin D deficiency. *J. Clin. Endocrinol. Metab.* **2013**, *98*, 2337–2346.

234. Hollis, B.W.; Johnson, D.; Hulsey, T.C.; Ebeling, M.; Wagner, C.L. Vitamin D supplementation during pregnancy: Double-blind, randomized clinical trial of safety and effectiveness. *J. Bone Min. Res.* **2011**, *26*, 2341–2357.

235. Hashemipour, S.; Lalooha, F.; Zahir Mirdamadi, S.; Ziaee, A.; Dabaghi Ghaleh, T. Effect of vitamin D administration in vitamin D-deficient pregnant women on maternal and neonatal serum calcium and vitamin d concentrations: A randomised clinical trial. *Br. J. Nutr.* **2013**, *110*, 1611–1616.

236. Roth, D.E.; al Mahmud, A.; Raqib, R.; Akhtar, E.; Black, R.E.; Baqui, A.H. Pharmacokinetics of high-dose weekly oral vitamin D3 supplementation during the third trimester of pregnancy in Dhaka, Bangladesh. *Nutrients* **2013**, *5*, 788–810.

237. Shakiba, M.; Iranmanesh, M.R. Vitamin D requirement in pregnancy to prevent deficiency in neonates: A randomised trial. *Singap. Med. J.* **2013**, *54*, 285–288.

238. Hollis, B.W. Assessment and interpretation of circulating 25-hydroxyvitamin D and 1,25-dihydroxyvitamin D in the clinical environment. *Endocrinol. Metab. Clin. North Am.* **2010**, *39*, 271–286.

239. Volmer, D.A.; Mendes, L.R.; Stokes, C.S. Analysis of vitamin D metabolic markers by mass spectrometry: Current techniques, limitations of the "gold standard" method, and anticipated future directions. *Mass Spectrom. Rev.* **2015**, *34*, 2–23.

240. Zhang, S.W.; Jian, W.; Sullivan, S.; Sankaran, B.; Edom, R.W.; Weng, N.; Sharkey, D. Development and validation of an LC-MS/MS based method for quantification of 25 hydroxyvitamin D2 and 25 hydroxyvitamin D3 in human serum and plasma. *J. Chromatogr. B Anal. Technol. Biomed. Life Sci.* **2014**, *961*, 62–70.

241. Adaway, J.E.; Keevil, B.G.; Owen, L.J. Liquid chromatography tandem mass spectrometry in the clinical laboratory. *Ann. Clin. Biochem.* **2015**, *52*, 18–38.

242. Baecher, S.; Leinenbach, A.; Wright, J.A.; Pongratz, S.; Kobold, U.; Thiele, R. Simultaneous quantification of four vitamin D metabolites in human serum using high performance liquid chromatography tandem mass spectrometry for vitamin D profiling. *Clin. Biochem.* **2012**, *45*, 1491–1496.

243. Shah, I.; Petroczi, A.; Naughton, D.P. Method for simultaneous analysis of eight analogues of vitamin D using liquid chromatography tandem mass spectrometry. *Chem. Cent. J.* **2012**, *6*, 112.

244. Higashi, T.; Goto, A.; Morohashi, M.; Ogawa, S.; Komatsu, K.; Sugiura, T.; Fukuoka, T.; Mitamura, K. Development and validation of a method for determination of plasma 25-hydroxyvitamin D3 3-sulfate using liquid chromatography/tandem mass spectrometry. *J. Chromatogr. B Anal. Technol. Biomed. Life Sci.* **2014**, *969*, 230–234.

245. Van den Ouweland, J.M.; Beijers, A.M.; van Daal, H. Overestimation of 25-hydroxyvitamin D3 by increased ionisation efficiency of 3-epi-25-hydroxyvitamin D3 in LC-MS/MS methods not separating both metabolites as determined by an LC-MS/MS method for separate quantification of 25-hydroxyvitamin D3, 3-epi-25-hydroxyvitamin D3 and 25-hydroxyvitamin D2 in human serum. *J. Chromatogr. B Anal. Technol. Biomed. Life Sci.* **2014**, *967*, 195–202.

246. Lee, S.; Oncescu, V.; Mancuso, M.; Mehta, S.; Erickson, D. A smartphone platform for the quantification of vitamin D levels. *Lab Chip* **2014**, *14*, 1437–1442.

247. Powe, C.E.; Evans, M.K.; Wenger, J.; Zonderman, A.B.; Berg, A.H.; Nalls, M.; Tamez, H.; Zhang, D.; Bhan, I.; Karumanchi, S.A.; *et al.* Vitamin D-binding protein and vitamin D status of black americans and white americans. *N. Engl. J. Med.* **2013**, *369*, 1991–2000.

248. Powe, C.E.; Karumanchi, S.A.; Thadhani, R. Vitamin D-binding protein and vitamin D in blacks and whites. *N. Engl. J. Med.* **2014**, *370*, 880–881.

249. Autier, P.; Boniol, M.; Pizot, C.; Mullie, P. Vitamin D status and ill health: A systematic review. *Lancet Diabet. Endocrinol.* **2014**, *2*, 76–89.

250. Bolland, M.J.; Grey, A.; Gamble, G.D.; Reid, I.R. The effect of vitamin D supplementation on skeletal, vascular, or cancer outcomes: A trial sequential meta-analysis. *Lancet Diabetes Endocrinol.* **2014**, *2*, 307–320.

251. Vitamin D: Chasing a myth? *Lancet Diabetes Endocrinol.* **2014**, *2*, 1.

252. Gillie, O. Controlled trials of vitamin D, causality and type 2 statistical error. *Public Health Nutr.* **2014**.

High Prevalence of Vitamin D Deficiency in Pregnant Korean Women: The First Trimester and the Winter Season as Risk Factors for Vitamin D Deficiency

Rihwa Choi, Seonwoo Kim, Heejin Yoo, Yoon Young Cho, Sun Wook Kim, Jae Hoon Chung, Soo-young Oh and Soo-Youn Lee

Abstract: We investigated the vitamin D status of Korean women during pregnancy and assessed the effects of vitamin D deficiency on two pregnancy outcomes; preterm births and the births of small for gestational age. We measured the serum 25-hydroxyvitamin D levels in 220 pregnant Korean women who were recruited prospectively and compared these levels with those of 500 healthy non-pregnant women. We analyzed vitamin D status according to patient demographics, season, and obstetrical characteristics; moreover, we also assessed pregnancy outcomes. The overall prevalence of vitamin D deficiency(<20 ng/mL) in pregnant women and healthy non-pregnant women was 77.3% and 79.2%; respectively; and the prevalence of severe vitamin D deficiency (<10 ng/mL) was 28.6% and 7.2%; respectively ($p < 0.05$). Vitamin D deficiency was more prevalent in the winter (100%) than in the summer (45.5%) in pregnant Korean women. A higher risk of vitamin D deficiency was observed in the first trimester than in the third trimester (adjusted OR 4.3; $p < 0.05$). No significant association was observed between vitamin D deficiency and any of the pregnancy outcomes examined. Further research focusing on the long-term consequences of vitamin D deficiency during pregnancy in Korean women is warranted.

Reprinted from *Nutrients*. Cite as: Choi, R.; Kim, S.; Yoo, H.; Cho, Y.Y.; Kim, S.W.; Chung, J.H.; Oh, S.-Y.; Lee, S.-Y. High Prevalence of Vitamin D Deficiency in Pregnant Korean Women: The First Trimester and the Winter Season as Risk Factors for Vitamin D Deficiency. *Nutrients* **2015**, *7*, 3427–3448.

1. Introduction

Vitamin D status is a well-known determinant of skeletal health and influences the risk of fracture, rickets, osteomalacia, and osteoporosis [1]. Humans obtain vitamin D from exposure to sunlight and diet, which are the two main determinants of vitamin D status in a population. Vitamin D3 is formed by exposure of the skin to sunlight and can also be obtained from the diet via animal products, whereas vitamin D2 is obtained from the diet via plant sources [1]. Vitamin D (hereafter used to refer to both D2 and D3) from the skin and diet is converted into the

219

circulating metabolite 25-hydroxyvitamin D—25(OH)D, including both 25(OH)D2 and 25(OH)D3—in the liver. This metabolite is often used as a biomarker to determine a patient's vitamin D status [2]. The 25(OH)D is metabolized in the kidneys into its active form, 1,25-dihydroxyvitamin D—1,25(OH)2D. The active form circulates in the blood at a significantly lower concentration (approximately 1/1000) compared with the concentration of 25(OH)D [1]. Circulating vitamin D, 25(OH)D, and 1,25(OH)2D are all bound to vitamin D-binding protein, a specific transporter protein. In target tissues, 1,25(OH)2D exerts its actions by associating with the VDR nuclear receptor (vitamin D receptor). Since the VDR is ubiquitously expressed in most cell types, including brain, prostate, breast, placenta, and immune, vitamin D has been hypothesized to have a number of functions outside the skeletal system [1].

Due to the importance of vitamin D, many concerns have been raised regarding the functional impacts of maternal vitamin D deficiency on multiple adverse health outcomes in mothers and their offspring. Moreover, low maternal levels of 25-hydroxyvitamin D have been suggested to be associated with a number of adverse obstetrical and neonatal outcomes [3,4]. Vitamin deficiency is a modifiable factor; therefore, it is important to determine the optimal vitamin D status during pregnancy. In the context of increasing clinical concern regarding the high prevalence of vitamin D deficiency worldwide, different prevalences of vitamin D deficiency have been reported in different geographic regions and latitudes. These prevalences have been determined by different diagnostic methods [5,6].

Multiple studies have shown that immunoassays may be limited by the cross-reactivity of antibodies and by non-equimolar recognition of the D2 and D3 forms of 25(OH)D, thereby overestimating the serum 25(OH)D concentration and the influence of vitamin D binding protein, which is known to circulate at higher concentrations in pregnant women [7,8]. Therefore, liquid chromatography-tandem mass spectrometry (LC-MS/MS) has been used as a reference method to accurately estimate patient vitamin D status [9,10].

However, a large population-based estimate of the vitamin D status of pregnant Korean women has not yet been performed. Therefore, this study aimed to investigate the vitamin D status of pregnant Korean women. This study also set out to investigate the determinants of vitamin D status during pregnancy and to assess the impact of vitamin D deficiency on pregnancy outcomes.

2. Methods

2.1. Ethics Statement

This study was conducted according to the guidelines laid down in the Declaration of Helsinki, and all procedures involving human subjects were approved by the Institutional Review Board of Samsung Medical Center (2011-12 & SMC

2011-12-041-001). All subjects provided written consent for their participation in this study.

2.2. Study Population

The target population of this study comprised pregnant women living in an urban area of South Korea (latitude 36°N) in any trimester of pregnancy. During the period of April 2012–September 2013, 282 pregnant women were prospectively recruited and followed. Among these women, 62 were excluded for one of the following reasons: Lack of information about basal characteristics such as prepregnancy body mass index (BMI), smoking, alcohol consumption, and occupation ($n = 5$), history of concurrent serious medical disease that could affect pregnancy outcomes ($n = 5$), history of intra-abdominal surgery ($n = 11$), history of surgery of the uterine cervix ($n = 24$) [11], and a lack of information regarding pregnancy outcomes due to follow-up loss ($n = 17$). As a result, 220 women were ultimately enrolled in the study. The vitamin D levels in these pregnant women were compared with those from healthy nonpregnant women of childbearing age ($n = 500$, 24–44 years) who visited a health-promotion center at Samsung Medical Center during the study period.

2.3. Data Collection

Blood samples were collected from the antecubital vein from pregnant women at the first prenatal consultation in any trimester of their pregnancy. Information about demographic characteristics, sociodemographic characteristics, smoking status, alcohol consumption during pregnancy and during the four weeks prior to the last menstrual period, diseases, medications, and obstetrical and gynecological history—i.e., parity (number of deliveries) and gravity (number of pregnancies)—was gathered by obstetrical nurses via questionnaires at the initial prenatal consultation. Some information was also obtained from electronic medical records. For all women included in the study, the prepregnant BMI was obtained from the self-reported weight and height recorded by the gynecologist during the prenatal consultation. BMIs were classified according to published cutoffs for Asian populations [12]. If the prepregnant body weight was not known, the first trimester BMI was used as a proxy for prepregnancy BMI for all women in their first, second, and third trimesters. Gestational age was determined according to the last menstrual period (LMP) and ultrasonography results. For the approximate 12% of all ultrasound gestational age estimates that differed by >10 days from LMP pregnancy dating, ultrasound dating was used. Neonatal outcomes were obtained from hospital medical records.

2.4. Definitions of Adverse Pregnancy Outcomes

A preterm birth was defined as a birth at less than 37 weeks of gestation. Neonates with birth weights below the 10th percentile for their gestational age as determined by birth weight percentile nomograms (National Data from Korean Health Insurance Review & Assessment Service 2009) were considered to be small for gestational age (SGA).

2.5. Laboratory Analyses

Approximately 500 μL serum was separated from 2 mL whole blood collected by venipuncture in a plain tube. Serum 25(OH)D2 and 25(OH)D3 concentrations were measured by LC-MS/MS with an Agilent 1200 LC 2D system connected to an Agilent 6460 Triple Quad MS (Agilent Technologies, Waldbronn, Germany). Vitamin D levels were detected in positive mode using the multiple reaction monitoring technique. The total 25(OH)D concentration was calculated as the sum of the serum 25(OH)D2 and 25(OH)D3 concentrations. The inter-assay and intra-assay coefficients of variation for this method were 5.5% and 7.1%, respectively. Based on published definitions of vitamin D status [1], we categorized 25(OH)D $\geq$30 ng/mL ($\geq$75 nmol/L) as sufficient and 25(OH)D 20–29.9 ng/mL(50–74.9 nmol/L) as suboptimal. Vitamin D deficiency was defined as 25(OH)D <20 ng/mL (<50 nmol/L) [13] and severe vitamin D deficiency was defined as 25(OH)D <10 ng/mL (<25 nmol/L) [14]. Since the optimal vitamin D concentration in pregnancy has been debated by groups such as the Institute of Medicine (IOM) and the Endocrine Society, no gold standard measurement method has been used to gather data regarding vitamin D status in large samples of Korean women, and little data are available regarding vitamin D status and adverse birth outcomes, the Endocrine Society's criteria for vitamin D status [1] were applied to assess the overall vitamin D status of pregnant women. The IOM's cutoff for vitamin D deficiency (<20 ng/mL) [13] was employed to analyze the association of vitamin D deficiency with adverse pregnancy and neonatal outcomes.

2.6. Statistical Analysis

Characteristics are presented as frequencies and percentages. Since age, prepregnancy BMI, and serum 25(OH)D levels were not normally distributed, nonparametric methods were used. The median was used as the measure of central tendency. Differences between trimesters, seasons of blood draw and of 25(OH)D measurements, and age groups were explored using the Kruskal-Wallis equality-of-populations rank test.

The odds of having a vitamin D deficiency (serum 25(OH)D < 20 ng/mL) *versus* a nondeficient vitamin D status were estimated through multivariable-adjusted logistic regression models. The following variables were entered as predictors in the model: Age, trimester, seasons of blood draw and of 25(OH)D measurements, education level, job, type of current pregnancy, concurrent pregnancy status, gravity, parity, previous or concurrent medical history (with the exception of intra-abdominal surgery), and gynecological disease history (with the exception of uterine cervix disease). The appropriateness of the sample size was validated by calculating the width of the confidence interval (CI). At the expected vitamin D deficiency rate of 80%, the 95% CI for vitamin D levels was calculated to be $\pm10\%$. The precisions of these two estimates were sufficient; thus, the size of this study was adequate for statistical analysis. A p value <0.05 was considered statistically significant. All p values were corrected by Bonferroni's method for multiple testing.

3. Results

3.1. General Characteristics

In total, 220 pregnant women in Korea participated in this study. The median age was 32.0 years old. Only 24 women (10.9%) had a prepregnancy BMI above 24 and no participant had a history of drinking alcohol during pregnancy. Only one participant had a history of smoking during pregnancy. More than three-quarters of all participants had more than 12 years of education, and over two-thirds had indoor jobs. The basal characteristics of the study population are summarized in Table 1.

3.2. Serum 25(OH)D Levels in Pregnant Korean Women

The median serum 25(OH)D concentration of all participants ($n = 220$) was 12.6 ng/mL. Serum 25(OH)D concentrations during the three trimesters are shown in Table 2 and Figure 1. According to pooled analysis, vitamin D concentrations differed significantly only between the first and third trimesters: 11.5 ng/mL during the first trimester *versus* 13.6 ng/mL during the third trimester ($p < 0.05$). Pooled analysis also revealed that the median serum 25(OH)D concentrations were 10.8 ng/mL in the spring, 20.5 ng/mL in the summer, 13.9 ng/mL in the fall, and 9.4 ng/mL in the winter. The serum 25(OH)D concentrations were significantly different between the spring and summer, the spring and fall, the summer and winter, and the fall and winter ($p < 0.05$). However, the serum 25(OH)D concentrations were not significantly different between the winter and spring or between the summer and fall ($p > 0.05$). Although no women in their third trimester of pregnancy were tested during the winter, peaks of 25(OH)D concentration were observed in the summer for all women who were tested in their first and third trimesters.

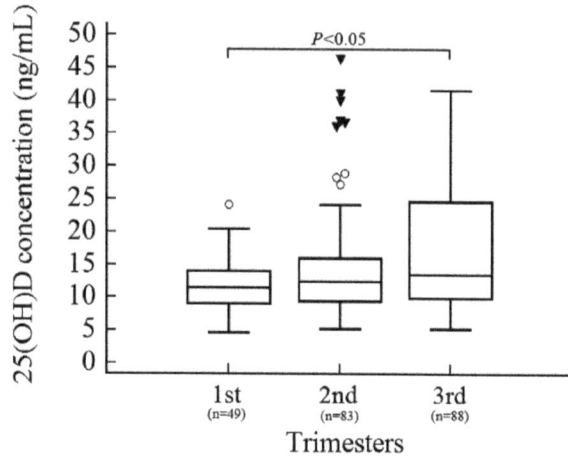

Figure 1. Serum 25-hydroxyvitamin D—25(OH)D—concentration according to trimester. Of particular note, the 25(OH)D concentration was significantly higher in the third trimester compared with the first trimester ($p < 0.05$).

3.3. Prevalences of Vitamin D Deficiency and Insufficiency in Pregnant Women

The percentages of vitamin D deficiency and insufficiency are shown in Table 2. A high prevalence of vitamin D deficiency was observed in pregnant women during all trimesters and also in healthy nonpregnant women. The overall prevalence of vitamin D deficiency—25(OH)D <20 ng/mL—in pregnant women was 77.3%; moreover, only 19 women (8.6%) had a serum 25(OH)D concentration >30 ng/mL, which is considered the optimal level. The median 25(OH)D concentration was higher in healthy nonpregnant women (15.4 ng/mL) compared with pregnant women (12.6 ng/mL). In contrast to pregnant women, among whom the prevalence of severe vitamin D deficiency was 28.6%, the prevalence of severe vitamin D deficiency among healthy nonpregnant women was 7.2%.

Table 1. Basic parameters of pregnant Korean women (n = 220).

Parameter	Total (n = 220) Median	Range	First Trimester (n = 49) Median	Range	Second Trimester (n = 83) Median	Range	Third Trimester (n = 88) Median	Range	p
Age, years	32.0	24.0–43.9	31.0	24.0–41.3	32.0	26.0–43.9	32.0	25.0–39.0	0.72
Prepregnant BMI (kg/m²)	20.2	16.0–28.5	20.3	16.0–26.3	20.8	16.3–28.5	19.8	16.0–27.5	0.21
Prepregnant BMI *	n	%	n	%	n	%	n	%	0.84
Underweight (BMI <18.0)	27	12.3	6	12.2	10	10.0	11	12.5	
Healthy normal (BMI 18.0–23.9)	169	76.8	38	77.6	63	75.9	68	77.3	
Overweight (BMI 24.0–26.9)	20	9.1	5	10.2	7	8.4	8	9.1	
Obese (BMI ≥ 27.0)	4	1.8	0	0.0	3	3.6	1	1.2	
Season †									0.10
Spring	98	44.5	20	40.8	35	42.2	43	48.9	
Summer	22	10.0	5	10.2	7	8.4	10	11.4	
Fall	87	39.5	18	39.7	34	40.9	35	39.8	
Winter	13	5.9	6	12.2	7	8.4	0	0.0	
Education level ‡									0.53
Low	12	5.5	3	6.1	6	7.2	3	3.4	
High	208	94.5	46	93.9	77	92.8	85	96.6	
Job									0.66
Any job	70	31.8	35	71.4	58	69.9	57	64.8	
Homemaker	150	68.2	14	28.6	25	30.1	31	35.2	
Type of current pregnancy									0.56
Spontaneous pregnancy	213	96.8	48	98.0	79	95.2	86	97.7	
Artificial pregnancy	7	3.2	1	2.0	4	4.8	2	2.3	
Single or multiple pregnancy									0.90
Singleton	217	98.6	48	98.0	82	98.8	87	98.9	
Twins	3	1.4	1	2.0	1	1.2	1	1.1	

Table 1. Cont.

Parameter	Total (n = 220) Median	Range	First Trimester (n = 49) Median	Range	Second Trimester (n = 83) Median	Range	Third Trimester (n = 88) Median	Range	p
Gravida									0.57
Primigravida	142	64.5	29	59.2	53	63.9	60	68.2	
Multigravida	78	35.5	20	40.8	30	36.1	28	31.8	
	n	%	n	%	n	%	n	%	
Parity									0.36
0 (nullipara)	136	61.8	27	55.1	50	60.2	59	67.0	
≥1	84	38.2	22	44.9	33	39.8	29	33.0	
Previous or concurrent medical history									0.30
Yes	68	30.9	17	34.7	29	34.9	22	25.0	
No	152	69.1	32	65.3	54	65.1	66	75.0	
Gynecological disease history									0.88
Yes	44	20.0	9	18.4	16	19.3	19	21.6	
No	176	80.0	40	81.6	67	80.7	69	78.4	

BMI: Body mass index; *: BMI classification for Asian populations was performed as described in [12]; †: Season of blood draw and of 25(OH)D measurements; ‡: Women who were educated ≤12 years were categorized as *low* and >12 years were categorized as *high*.

Table 2. The 25-hydroxyvitamin D—25(OH)D—concentrations in 220 pregnant Korean women across three trimesters and in 500 healthy nonpregnant women.

25(OH)D (ng/mL)	Healthy Nonpregnant Women * (n = 500)	All Pregnant Women (n = 220)	First Trimester (n = 49)	Second Trimester (n = 83)	Third Trimester (n = 88)
Median [†,‡]	15.4	12.6	11.5	12.5	13.6
IQR	12.7–19.7	9.7–17.3	9.1–14.0	9.5–16.0	9.9–24.7
95% CI	14.8–15.8	11.9–13.3	10.0–13.0	11.1–13.4	12.1–16.6
Range	5.8–40.4	4.7–46.3	4.7–24.2	5.3–46.3	5.3–41.6
% <10 ng/mL [†,§,¶,‖]	7.2	28.6	32.7	28.9	26.1
% <20 ng/mL [§]	79.2	77.3	91.8	80.7	65.9
% <30 ng/mL [†,§]	98.0	91.4	100.0	92.8	85.2

IQR: Interquartile range; *: Data were obtained from healthy nonpregnant women of childbearing age (24–44 years old) who visited a health-promotion center at Samsung Medical Center and volunteered to give blood during the study period; [†]: The serum 25(OH)D concentration, prevalence of vitamin D deficiency, and prevalence of women with suboptimal 25(OH)D levels (<30 ng/mL) were all significantly different between healthy nonpregnant women and pregnant women (p < 0.05); [‡]: The serum 25(OH)D concentration was significantly different between healthy nonpregnant women and pregnant women at each trimester (p < 0.05), except for pregnant women in their third trimester, after *post-hoc* analysis; §: The prevalences of severe vitamin D deficiency—25(OH)D <10 ng/mL, vitamin D deficiency—25(OH)D <20 ng/mL—and suboptimal 25(OH)D levels (<30 ng/mL) were significantly different among healthy nonpregnant women and pregnant women at each trimester; [¶]: A higher prevalence of severe vitamin D deficiency—25(OH)D <10 ng/mL—was observed in pregnant women than in healthy nonpregnant women; [‖]: The prevalences of severe vitamin D deficiency in the three trimesters were not significantly different among pregnant women (p > 0.05).

The percentage of vitamin D deficiency was higher in the first trimester (91.8%) than in the third trimester (65.9%) and was also higher in the winter (100.0%) than in the summer (45.5%) (p < 0.05). Interestingly, the prevalence of vitamin D deficiency decreased as pregnancy progressed: 91.8% during the first trimester, 80.7% during the second trimester, and 77.3% during the third trimester. All participants had vitamin D insufficiency in the first trimester. Pooled analyses of all blood samples revealed significant differences in the prevalences of vitamin D deficiency and the 25(OH)D concentrations across seasons. The prevalences of vitamin D deficiency were 84.7%, 45.5%, 73.7%, and 100% in the spring, summer, fall, and winter, respectively, with a significantly lower prevalence in the summer compared with the spring and fall (p < 0.05). The difference in the prevalence of vitamin D deficiency between the summer and the winter was not significant, probably because all women who were tested in the winter had a vitamin D deficiency and only 13 pregnant women were included during the winter. Thus, this statistical analysis was likely influenced by the small sample size (Figure 2). Additional analyses for potential interactions between season and trimester were performed for further statistical modeling. However, the effect of the first trimester occurring during winter was not significantly different than other season-trimester combinations (p = 0.4983). This finding could be due to the small sample size during winter (*i.e.*, no pregnant women in their third trimester were included in the winter in this study population). Thus, although an interaction term was included in an earlier iteration of the statistical model, it was not significant and thus, it was not included in the final model.

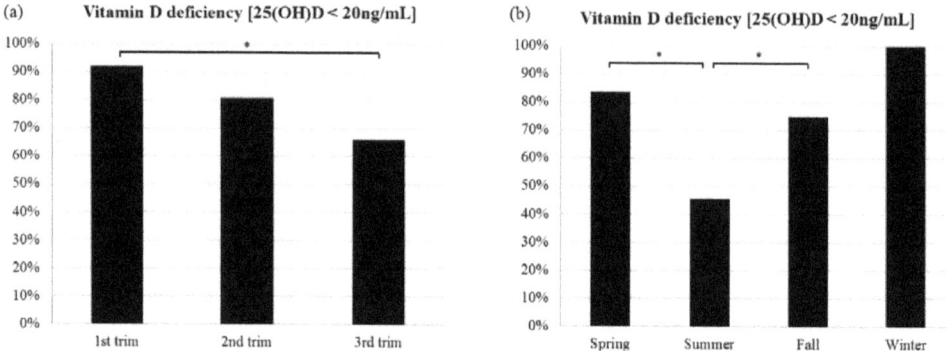

Figure 2. Prevalence of vitamin D deficiency (25(OH)D < 20 ng/mL) according to trimester and season. (**a**) Prevalence of vitamin D deficiency by trimester. The prevalence of vitamin D deficiency was significantly higher in the first trimester compared with the third trimester ($p < 0.05$); (**b**) Prevalence of vitamin D deficiency according to season of blood draw and 25(OH)D measurements. The prevalence of vitamin D deficiency was lower in the summer than in the spring or fall ($p < 0.05$); *: Statistically significant differences according to multivariable analysis ($p < 0.05$).

Table 3. Maternal characteristics and vitamin D status of 220 pregnant Korean women.

Vitamin D Cutoff	Total		Deficiency		Suboptimal		Optimal		*p*
			<20 ng/mL		20–29 ng/mL		30–100 ng/mL		
	n	%	*n*	%	*n*	%	*n*	%	
All women	220	100.0	170	77.3	31	14.1	19	8.6	>1
Prepregnant BMI *									
Underweight (BMI < 18.0)	27	12.3	21	77.8	5	18.5	1	3.7	
Healthy normal (BMI 18.0–23.9)	169	76.8	129	76.3	25	14.8	15	8.9	
Overweight (BMI 24.0–26.9)	20	9.1	17	85.0	1	5.0	2	10.0	
Obese (BMI ≥ 27.0)	4	1.9	3	75.0	0	0.0	1	25.0	
Age									0.53
<30 years	56	25.5	46	82.1	8	14.3	2	3.6	
30–35 years	119	54.1	86	72.3	19	16.0	14	11.8	
35–40 years	45	20.5	38	84.4	4	8.9	3	6.7	
Trimester									0.012
First trimester	49	22.3	45	91.8	4	8.2	0	0.0	
Second trimester	83	37.7	67	80.7	10	12.0	6	7.2	
Third trimester	88	40.0	58	65.9	17	19.3	13	14.8	
Season †									0.007
Spring	98	44.5	82	83.7	9	9.2	7	7.1	
Summer	22	10.0	10	45.5	8	36.4	4	18.2	
Fall	87	39.5	65	74.7	14	16.1	8	9.2	
Winter	13	5.9	13	100.0	0	0.0	0	0.0	
Education level									0.84
≤12 years	12	5.5	11	91.7	1	8.3	0	0.0	
>12 years	208	94.5	159	76.4	30	14.4	19	9.1	
Job									0.61
Any job	150	68.2	119	79.3	21	14.0	10	6.7	
Homemaker	70	31.8	51	72.9	10	14.3	9	12.9	

Table 3. Cont.

Vitamin D Cutoff	Total		Deficiency <20 ng/mL		Suboptimal 20–29 ng/mL		Optimal 30–100 ng/mL		p
	n	%	n	%	n	%	n	%	
Type of current pregnancy									0.13
Spontaneous	213	96.8	167	78.4	29	13.6	17	8.0	
Artificial insemination	7	3.2	3	42.9	2	28.6	2	28.6	
Single or multiple pregnancy									0.31
Singleton	217	98.6	169	77.9	30	13.8	18	8.3	
Twins	3	1.4	1	33.3	1	33.3	1	33.3	
Gravity									>1
Primigravida	142	64.5	107	75.4	21	14.8	14	9.9	
Multigravida	78	35.5	63	80.8	10	12.8	5	6.4	
Parity									0.96
0 (nullipara)	136	61.8	102	75.0	20	14.7	14	10.3	
≥1	84	38.2	68	81.0	11	13.1	5	6.0	
Previous or concurrent medical history									0.69
Yes	152	69.1	120	78.9	18	11.8	14	9.2	
No	68	30.9	50	73.5	13	19.1	5	7.4	
Gynecological disease history									0.18
Yes	176	80.0	131	74.4	29	16.5	16	9.1	
No	44	20.0	39	88.6	2	4.5	3	6.8	

*: BMI classification for Asian populations was performed as described in [12]. †: Season of blood draw and of 25(OH)D measurements.

Table 4. Risk of vitamin D deficiency during pregnancy in 220 Korean women.

Risk of Vitamin D Deficiency	Number of Subjects	VitD-Deficient Subjects (<20 ng/mL) n	%	Unadjusted Odds Ratio	95% CI Lower	95% CI Upper	p	Adjusted Odds Ratio	95% CI Lower	95% CI Upper	p
Age							0.16				0.27
<30 years	56	46	82.1	Reference				Reference			
30–35 years	119	86	72.3	0.567	0.229	1.403		0.523	0.186	1.475	
35–40 years	45	38	84.4	1.180	0.352	3.953		0.926	0.242	3.553	
Prepregnant BMI *							0.86				0.74
Underweight (BMI < 18.0)	27	21	77.8	1.085	0.330	3.567		0.628	0.168	2.345	
Healthy normal (BMI 18.0–23.9)	169	129	76.3	Reference				Reference			
Overweight (BMI 24.0–26.9)	20	17	85.0	1.757	0.369	8.3670		0.789	0.148	4.217	
Obese (BMI ≥ 27.0)	4	3	75.0	0.930	0.058	15.271		0.326	0.010	11.007	
Trimester							0.003				0.023
First trimester	49	45	91.8	5.819	1.629	20.792		4.274	1.205	15.159	
Second trimester	83	67	80.7	2.166	0.971	4.830		2.013	0.818	4.957	
Third trimester	88	58	65.9	Reference				Reference			
Season †							0.002				0.003
Spring	98	82	83.7	5.952	1.770	20.018		8.026	1.973	32.650	
Summer	22	10	45.5	Reference				Reference			
Fall	87	65	74.7	3.465	1.063	11.296		4.346	1.113	16.970	
Winter	13	13	100.0	32.157	0.777	1330.6	26.322	0.596	1161.7		
Education level							0.25				0.40
≤12 years	12	11	91.7	Reference				Reference			
>12 years	208	159	76.4	0.295	0.037	2.343		0.446	0.067	2.969	
Job							0.29				0.10
Any job	150	119	79.3	1.430	0.740	2.763		1.932	0.880	4.242	
Homemaker	70	51	72.9	Reference				Reference			

Table 4. *Cont.*

Risk of Vitamin D Deficiency	Number of Subjects	VitD-Deficient Subjects (<20 ng/mL)		Unadjusted Odds Ratio	95% CI		*p*	Adjusted Odds Ratio	95% CI		*p*
		n	%		Lower	Upper			Lower	Upper	
Type of current pregnancy							0.044				0.11
Spontaneous	213	167	78.4	Reference				Reference			
Artificial insemination	7	3	42.9	0.207	0.045	0.956		0.127	0.010	1.610	
Single or multiple pregnancy							0.11				0.78
Singleton	217	169	77.9	Reference				Reference			
Twins	3	1	33.3	0.142	0.013	1.601		0.559	0.009	35.596	
Gravity ‡							0.72				
Primigravida	142	107	75.4	Reference							
Multigravida	78	63	80.8	1.374	0.631	2.991					
Parity							0.62				0.27
0 (nullipara)	136	102	75.0	Reference				Reference			
≥1	84	68	81.0	1.417	0.659	3.0436		1.586	0.702	3.580	
Previous or concurrent medical history							0.38				0.36
Yes	152	120	78.9	0.741	0.381	1.4400		0.698	0.324	1.503	
No	68	50	73.5	Reference				Reference			
Gynecological disease history							0.05				0.027
Yes	176	131	74.4	2.679	0.995	7.2150		3.466	1.155	10.399	
No	44	39	88.6	Reference				Reference			

*: BMI classification for Asian populations was performed as described in [12]; †: Season of blood draw and of 25(OH)D measurements; ‡: The adjusted odds ratio for multivariate analysis was not calculated due to multicolinearity between gravity and parity.

232

3.4. Factors Associated with Vitamin D Deficiency during Pregnancy

Maternal characteristics, stratified by vitamin D status, are shown in Table 3. Age, education level, occupation, type of current pregnancy, number of concurrent pregnancies, gravity, parity, previous/concurrent medical history (with the exception of intra-abdominal surgery), and gynecological disease history (with the exception of uterine cervix disease) were not significantly different among the three groups of pregnant women as stratified by vitamin D status.

Factors associated with vitamin D deficiency over the course of pregnancy are shown in Table 4. Multiple logistic regression models for identifying independent predictors of vitamin D deficiency revealed that the winter season and the first trimester were independent predictors of vitamin D deficiency. The risk of vitamin D deficiency was significantly higher in the first *vs.* the third trimester (adjusted OR 4.2744; $p < 0.05$) and in the spring (adjusted OR 8.0258; $p < 0.05$). Artificial insemination pregnancies had a lower risk of vitamin D deficiency than spontaneous pregnancies according to univariate analysis, but this association was not seen in multivariate analysis. No significant associations were observed between any other factors and vitamin D deficiency.

3.5. Associations between Vitamin D Deficiency and Pregnancy Outcomes

The associations between adverse pregnancy outcomes and vitamin D deficiency (<20 ng/mL) during pregnancy were analyzed (Table 5). Among the 220 pregnant women, 54 (24.5%) had adverse pregnancy outcomes. Specifically, nine delivered preterm babies (4.1%) and 24 had babies small for their gestational age (10.9%). The prevalences of vitamin D deficiency were 77.8% (7/9) among the women who delivered preterm babies and 62.5% (15/24) among the women who had babies small for their gestational age.

Table 5. Associations between vitamin D deficiency, preterm babies, and SGA babies.

Outcomes	Preterm			SGA		
	Preterm (−)	Preterm (+)	p	SGA (−)	SGA (+)	p
Number of subjects	211	9		196	24	
Number with VitD deficiency *	163	7		155	15	
% with VitD deficiency *	77.3	77.8		79.1	62.5	
Unadjusted OR (95% CI)	Reference	1.030 (0.207–5.124)	0.97	Reference	0.441 (0.180–1.079)	0.07
Adjusted OR (95% CI)	Reference	0.699 (0.144–3.402)	0.66	Reference	0.448 (0.149–1.351)	0.15

SGA: Small for gestational age; OR: Odds ratio; *: 25(OH)D < 20 ng/mL.

No significant associations were observed between vitamin D deficiency and preterm delivery or SGA babies according to univariate or multivariate logistic regression analyses.

4. Discussion

The strengths of this study include its prospective study design, the fairly ethnically homogenous sample of adult Koreans, and the use of the gold standard LC-MS/MS method to measure 25(OH)D concentrations. Also, to the best of our knowledge, this is the first report of vitamin D status in Korean pregnant women, the first risk assessment for vitamin D deficiency during pregnancy, and the first investigation of the effect of vitamin D deficiency on pregnancy outcomes.

This study showed a high prevalence (77.3%) of vitamin D deficiency during pregnancy. Although many reports have reported high prevalences of vitamin D deficiency among pregnant women, most of these studies have focused on white and black pregnant women. Only a few studies have assessed vitamin D status in pregnant women living in Asia [15–19]. Sunlight exposure at different latitudes is likely to be an important factor that influences vitamin D status. The results of previous studies of vitamin D status among pregnant women in Asia at variable latitudes and in other regions near 36°N [3,4,20–24], which is similar to the latitude of the present study, are summarized in Table 6. The high prevalence of vitamin D deficiency observed in the present study is comparable with the findings of previous studies of Asian populations [15–19]. These studies tested vitamin D status at different gestational periods and used different cutoffs to define vitamin D deficiency. Moreover, most studies measured vitamin D levels by immunoassays rather than LC-MS/MS, thereby hindering direct comparisons of reported values of 25(OH)D concentrations. A recent study of 311 pregnant Chinese women in Guiyang, China reported a slightly higher prevalence of vitamin D deficiency (83.6%) with a slightly higher mean 25(OH)D concentration (14.69 ng/mL) [19]. This study used LC-MS/MS for measurement and sampled during the second and third trimesters. Additional studies using accurate measurement methods are needed to obtain more robust estimates of vitamin D status among Asian populations. In the present study, we found that the median 25(OH)D level among pregnant Korean women was significantly lower in the winter (9.4 ng/mL) than in the summer (20.5 ng/mL) or the fall (13.9 ng/mL) ($p < 0.05$). Consistent with this finding, the prevalence of vitamin D deficiency was much higher in the winter (100%) than in the summer (45.5%) ($p < 0.05$). Even in the summer, a vitamin D deficiency was still found in 45.5% of all women in our cohort. These results are comparable with those of previous studies in China, Greece, Iran, the Spanish Mediterranean seacoast, and California (USA) [15,19,22,23]. One previous study in Japan found no significant seasonal variation of vitamin D levels in pregnant women [16], although the highest concentration occurred in the fall. Moreover, a high prevalence of vitamin D deficiency was seen in all four seasons. Thus, it appears to be a general trend that the vitamin D levels in Asian populations are higher in the summer than in the winter.

Table 6. Serum 25(OH)D concentrations in pregnant women in Asian populations and in regions at latitudes near 36°N.

Ref.	Region	Lat. (°N) *	N of Preg	GA at Blood Sampling	25(OH)D Concentration Presented as	Reported Value	Units †	Converted to ng/mL ‡	% <20 ng/mL § (% <50 nmol/L)	Pregnancy and Birth Outcome	Significant Association (p < 0.05)	Method
Asia												
This study	South Korea	36	220	First, Second, Third trimesters	median (IQR)	12.6 (9.65–17.30)	ng/mL	12.6	77.3%	PROM, preterm delivery, SGA	No	LC-MS/MS
[16]	Tokai, Japan	35.3	93 ¶	30 weeks	mean ± SD	14.5 ± 5.0	ng/mL	14.5	89.5%	premature delivery	premature delivery	RIA
[17]	Beijing, China **	39.9	125	15–20 weeks	mean ± SD	28.4 ± 9.5	nmol/L	11.42	96.8%	NA		ELISA
[19]	Guiyang, China	NA *	311	Second and third trimesters	mean ± SD	14.69 ± 6.81	ng/mL	14.69	83.6%	NA		LC-MS/MS
[17]	Beijing, China	39.9	70	Prior to labor	mean ± SE	28.64 ± 1.41	nmol/L	11.47	90.2%	birth weight, birth length, HC	birth weight, birth length	ELISA
[15].	Nanjing, China	31	152	24–28 weeks	mean ± SD	10.9 ± 4.78	ng/mL	10.9	in winter 96.1% in summer 94.7%	NA		ELISA
[18]	Chengdu, China	30.7	77	Before labor	mean ± SD	35.95 ± 19.7	nmol/L	14.40	NA	NA		EIA
Studies at regions near 36°N												
[21]	Tehran, Iran **	NA *	552	Delivery	mean ± 2 SD	27.8 ± 21.71	nmol/L	11.1	NA	birth height, weight, HC, post. & ant. fontanel diameter, Apgar score	No	RIA
[20]	USA	NA *	928	First, second, third trimesters	mean (95% CI)	65 (61–68)	nmol/L	26.0	33.8%	NA		RIA
[23]	Almeria, Spain	36	502	11–14 weeks	median (IQR)	27.4 (20.9–32.8)	ng/mL	27.4	22.7%	NA		ECLIA
[3]	Almeria, Spain ‡‡	36	466	First, third trimesters	NA	NA	ng/mL	NA	23.4%	§§ PROM, preterm delivery, SGA, etc.	No	ECLIA

235

Table 6. Cont.

Ref.	Region	Lat. (°N)*	N of Preg	GA at Blood Sampling	25(OH)D Concentration					Pregnancy and Birth Outcome	Significant Association (p < 0.05)	Method
					Presented as	Reported Value	Units†	Converted to ng/mL‡	% <20 ng/mL§ (% <50 nmol/L)			
[22]	Athens, Greece	NA*	123	Delivery	median (IQR)	16.4 (11–21.1)	ng/mL	16.4	NA	NA		CLIA
[4]	Izmir, Turkey	38.25	300	≥37 weeks	mean ± SD	11.5 ± 5.4	ng/mL	11.5	90.3%	NA		CLIA
[24]	Ankara, Turkey**	40	79	Third trimester	mean ± SD	11.95 + 7.20	ng/mL	11.95	NA	birth height, weight, HC, post. & ant. fontanel diameter, MUAC, Apgar score	No	HPLC

Ref.: Reference; Lat.: Latitude; N of preg.: Number of enrolled pregnant women; GA: Gestational age; IQR: Interquartile range; PROM: Premature rupture of membranes; SGA: Small for gestational age; LC-MS/MS: Liquid chromatography-tandem mass spectrometry; EIA: Enzyme immunoassay; RIA: Radioimmunoassay; ELISA: Enzyme linked immunosorbent assay; ECLIA: Electrochemiluminescence assay; CLIA: Chemiluminescence immunoassay; early, first measurement (early stage of pregnancy); late, second measurement (late stage of pregnancy); NA: Not available; HC: Head circumference; MUAC: Mid-upper arm circumference; *: Latitude information was obtained from maps, but was not reported in the referenced articles themselves; †: Reported units for 25(OH)D concentration in the referenced articles; ‡: To convert the 25(OH)D values to nanomoles per liter, the values were multiplied by 2.496 (1 ng/mL is equivalent to 2.496 nmol/L). Only median or mean values were included in the table; §: A 25(OH)D concentration <20 ng/mL (<50 nmol/L) was defined as vitamin D deficiency; ¶: Including 14 cases with threatened premature delivery; **: Sampled only in winter; ‡‡: This study was the second phase of a study performed using a subset of participants recruited in a study by Perez-Lopez et al. [23]; §§: Obstetric and neonatal outcomes included labor initiation, route of delivery, PROM, hypertensive state, presence of gestational diabetes, intrauterine fetal demise, preterm birth, neonatal gender, Apgar score at birth, SGA, and congenital malformation.

In the present study, analysis of vitamin D status according to trimester revealed that being in the first trimester was a risk factor for vitamin D deficiency in pregnant Korean women. During pregnancy, the serum levels of 1,25(OH)D increase up to 2-fold starting at 10–12 weeks of gestation and reaching a maximum in the third trimester [25]. However, it is unclear whether 25(OH)D levels steadily increase throughout pregnancy [20]. The lower vitamin D concentration in the first trimester observed in the present study is comparable with previous studies in Thailand [26] and the United States [20], but conflicts with a study in Delhi, India, which found no significant difference among trimesters [27]. However, the latitude of Delhi is 28.6°N, and this region enjoys abundant sunlight during most of the year, in contrast to the region of the present study (36°N). This study is the first to assess vitamin D status across pregnancy trimesters in Asia at latitudes near 36°N. Although the National Health and Nutrition Examination Survey was conducted in the United States at a latitude similar to this study (36°N) [20] and reported that later trimester was independently associated with a higher 25(OH)D level—Asian pregnant women were only a small percentage of the participants and were categorized with other ethnic minorities. It is of particular note that, although the latitudes of the studied regions were similar to the latitude in this study, the vitamin D levels were higher in Western countries (the United States and the Spanish Mediterranean seacoast) than in Asian countries, including Korea. This difference could be due to other covariates such as demographics, genetic backgrounds of different ethnic groups, vitamin D supplement use, and outdoor activities [1,14]. Our results are most relevant to vitamin D studies of Asian populations in temperate climate areas.

In the present study, we compared the prevalence of vitamin D deficiency between pregnant women and healthy nonpregnant women. A high prevalence was observed in both groups (79.2% in healthy nonpregnant women and 77.3% in pregnant women). The finding that severe vitamin D deficiency was more prevalent in pregnant women (28.6%) than in nonpregnant women (7.2%) suggests that pregnancy itself could be a risk factor for vitamin D deficiency. This finding could be due to physiological changes resulting from nutrient demand and loss during pregnancy [14].

Interestingly, in addition to trimester and season as risk factors for vitamin D deficiency, we also identified a history of gynecological disease (*i.e.*, leiomyomas of the uterus or benign ovarian cysts) as a risk factor for vitamin D deficiency through multivariable logistic regression analysis (adjusted OR 3.4662; 95% CI 1.1550–10.3999; $p < 0.05$). Previous studies have suggested an association between vitamin D status and uterine diseases such as uterine myoma and endometriosis in both black and white women, although the mechanisms underlying this association remain to be clarified [28,29]. However, the present study is the first study of an Asian population to reveal an association between vitamin D deficiency and gynecological disease. Although bacterial vaginosis, which has been reported to be associated with vitamin D deficiency among pregnant women in western populations [30], was not evaluated in the present study, future research should investigate the relationship between bacterial vaginosis and vitamin D deficiency in Asian populations.

The Endocrine Society recently recommended that pregnant women consume at least 1500–2000 IU of vitamin D per day [31]. A recent randomized controlled trial showed that vitamin D supplementation for pregnant women of 4000 IU/day was both safe and the most effective level [32]. However, vitamin D supplementation is not part of most routine antenatal care programs in Korea. Although obstetricians in Korea usually recommend that pregnant women take a vitamin supplement during pregnancy, no consensus has yet been reached among physicians regarding whether the consumption of vitamin D-fortified food or specific vitamin D supplementation should be recommended. This lack of consensus is due at least in part to the lack of sufficient data on vitamin D status, vitamin D supplementation, and their associations with pregnancy-related outcomes to establish guidelines for the Korean population. The present study provides a foundation on which future research on vitamin D status and its associations with pregnancy-related outcomes in Korea can build. Vitamin D supplementation should only be recommended when many factors are taken into consideration. First, the designs and settings of the studies that inform these recommendations should be carefully considered. For instance, the current study included low-risk pregnant women and only looked at a few outcomes; moreover, the current study only enrolled participants with low vitamin D concentrations. Vitamin D expenditure should also be considered in the context of the plasma half-life of vitamin D. The details of supplementation regimens could also be important factors since different doses, boluses, and forms of supplementation could lead to varying biological effects. Moreover, geographical characteristics should also be considered because vitamin D needs can vary significantly within a country, particularly in countries that span large latitudes. During pregnancy, alterations in metabolism such as changes in vitamin D and calcium equilibrium compared with the non-pregnant state support the need for assessing vitamin D status and supplementation in the context of pregnancy. Improved assay methodologies that can detect vitamin D metabolites would also be useful for informing vitamin D supplementation needs, since most studies only report a minority of vitamin D metabolites. All these parameters should be taken into consideration in the design of future vitamin D supplementation trials.

The potential impact of vitamin D deficiency during pregnancy on maternal and neonatal health has attracted much interest in recent years. However, a causal link between vitamin D deficiency during pregnancy and adverse pregnancy-related outcomes remains to be determined using Hill's criteria [33], which may be due in part to our limited knowledge. Although one report supported a possible link between a low 25(OH)D status and poor neonatal outcomes [5], the precise mechanisms underlying this association are yet to be determined. A recent systematic review and meta-analysis found that spontaneous preterm birth and childbirth with SGA were significantly associated with 25(OH)D levels <20 ng/mL [34]. In the present study, two pregnancy outcomes (preterm delivery and childbirth with SGA) were examined, and no significant association was found between vitamin D deficiency and either pregnancy outcome. These results are comparable with those of a study of pregnant Spanish women [3]. This agreement may be due to the small numbers of adverse pregnancy outcomes in both studies and the high prevalences of vitamin D deficiency among pregnant Korean women in the groups with and without adverse pregnancy-related outcomes. However, this finding limits the comparisons that can be made, thus warranting further research in this area. Another limitation of the current study is its lack of data about UVB levels and vitamin D intake. However, the current study is also valuable because it is the first to assess potential associations between vitamin D deficiency, preterm delivery, and SGA in a temperate climate region in an ethnically homogeneous Korean population.

In conclusion, our data indicate a high prevalence of vitamin D deficiency among pregnant women in Korea. Even during the summer months, a majority of pregnant women suffered from vitamin D deficiency. Being in the first trimester of pregnancy and the winter season were both associated with an increased risk of vitamin D deficiency in pregnant Korean women. Although no significant associations between vitamin D deficiency and preterm delivery or delivery of SGA babies were observed in the present study, this work will serve as a foundation for future research on vitamin D status and/or supplementation associated with pregnancy-related outcomes among pregnant Korean women.

Acknowledgments: This study was supported by a grant of the Korean Health technology R & D Project, Ministry for Health & Welfare, Republic of Korea (HI13C0871).

Author Contributions: All authors contributed to the preparation of the manuscript. R.C., S.-Y.O., H.Y., Y.Y.C., S.W.K., J.H.C., S.K., and S.-Y.L. collected samples, obtained data, and/or analyzed data; R.C. and S.-Y.L. designed the study and S.-Y.L. secured its funding; and S.-Y.L. had full access to all data in the study and takes responsibility for the integrity of the data and the accuracy of the data analysis. All authors read and approved the final manuscript.

Conflicts of Interest: The authors declare no conflict of interest.

References

1.   Holick, M.F. Vitamin D deficiency. *New Engl. J. Med.* **2007**, *357*, 266–281.
2.   Stepman, H.C.; Vanderroost, A.; van Uytfanghe, K.; Thienpont, L.M. Candidate reference measurement procedures for serum 25-hydroxyvitamin D3 and 25-hydroxyvitamin D2 by using isotope-dilution liquid chromatography-tandem mass spectrometry. *Clin. Chem.* **2011**, *57*, 441–448.

3.   Fernandez-Alonso, A.M.; Dionis-Sanchez, E.C.; Gonzalez-Salmeron, M.D.; Perez-Lopez, F.R.; Chedraui, P. First-trimester maternal serum 25-hydroxyvitamin D(3) status and pregnancy outcome. *Int. J. Gynaecol. Obstet.* **2012**, *116*, 6–9.

4.   Thorne-Lyman, A.; Fawzi, W.W. Vitamin D during pregnancy and maternal, neonatal and infant health outcomes: A systematic review and meta-analysis. *Paediatr. Perinat. Epidemiol.* **2012**, *26* (Suppl. 1), 75–90.

5.   Aghajafari, F.; Nagulesapillai, T.; Ronksley, P.E.; Tough, S.C.; O'Beirne, M.; Rabi, D.M. Association between maternal serum 25-hydroxyvitamin D level and pregnancy and neonatal outcomes: Systematic review and meta-analysis of observational studies. *BMJ Clin. Res. Ed.* **2013**, *346*, f1169.

6.   Bener, A.; Al-Hamaq, A.O.; Saleh, N.M. Association between vitamin D insufficiency and adverse pregnancy outcome: Global comparisons. *Int. J. Womens Health* **2013**, *5*, 523–531.

7.   Bedner, M.; Lippa, K.A.; Tai, S.S. An assessment of 25-hydroxyvitamin D measurements in comparability studies conducted by the vitamin D metabolites quality assurance program. *Clin. Chim. Acta* **2013**, *426*, 6–11.

8.   Heijboer, A.C.; Blankenstein, M.A.; Kema, I.P.; Buijs, M.M. Accuracy of 6 routine 25-hydroxyvitamin D assays: Influence of vitamin d binding protein concentration. *Clin. Chem.* **2012**, *58*, 543–548.

9.   Farrell, C.J.; Herrmann, M. Determination of vitamin D and its metabolites. *Best Pract. Res. Clin. Endocrinol. Metab.* **2013**, *27*, 675–688.

10. Karras, S.N.; Shah, I.; Petroczi, A.; Goulis, D.G.; Bili, H.; Papadopoulou, F.; Harizopoulou, V.; Tarlatzis, B.C.; Naughton, D.P. An observational study reveals that neonatal vitamin D is primarily determined by maternal contributions: Implications of a new assay on the roles of vitamin d forms. *Nutr. J.* **2013**, *12*, 77.

11. Simoens, C.; Goffin, F.; Simon, P.; Barlow, P.; Antoine, J.; Foidart, J.M.; Arbyn, M. Adverse obstetrical outcomes after treatment of precancerous cervical lesions: A belgian multicentre study. *BJOG Int. J. Obstet. Gynaecol.* **2012**, *119*, 1247–1255.

12. Wildman, R.P.; Gu, D.; Reynolds, K.; Duan, X.; He, J. Appropriate body mass index and waist circumference cutoffs for categorization of overweight and central adiposity among chinese adults. *Am. J. Clin. Nutr.* **2004**, *80*, 1129–1136.

13. Institute of Medicine. *Dietary Reference Intakes for Calcium and Vitamin*; Ross, A.C., Taylor, C.L., Eds.; The National Academies Press: Washington, DC, USA, 2011.

14. Mulligan, M.L.; Felton, S.K.; Riek, A.E.; Bernal-Mizrachi, C. Implications of vitamin D deficiency in pregnancy and lactation. *Am. J. Obstet. Gynecol.* **2010**, *202*, 429.e1–429.e9.

15. Jiang, L.; Xu, J.; Pan, S.; Xie, E.; Hu, Z.; Shen, H. High prevalence of hypovitaminosis D among pregnant women in southeast China. *Acta Paediatr.* **2012**, *101*, e192–e194.

16. Shibata, M.; Suzuki, A.; Sekiya, T.; Sekiguchi, S.; Asano, S.; Udagawa, Y.; Itoh, M. High prevalence of hypovitaminosis D in pregnant Japanese women with threatened premature delivery. *J. Bone Miner. Metab.* **2011**, *29*, 615–620.

17. Song, S.J.; Zhou, L.; Si, S.; Liu, J.; Zhou, J.; Feng, K.; Wu, J.; Zhang, W. The high prevalence of vitamin D deficiency and its related maternal factors in pregnant women in Beijing. *PloS ONE* **2013**, *8*, e85081.

18. Wang, J.; Yang, F.; Mao, M.; Liu, D.H.; Yang, H.M.; Yang, S.F. High prevalence of vitamin D and calcium deficiency among pregnant women and their newborns in Chengdu, China. *World J. Pediatr. WJP* **2010**, *6*, 265–267.

19. Xiang, F.; Jiang, J.; Li, H.; Yuan, J.; Yang, R.; Wang, Q.; Zhang, Y. High prevalence of vitamin D insufficiency in pregnant women working indoors and residing in Guiyang, China. *J. Endocrinol. Investig.* **2013**, *36*, 503–507.

20. Ginde, A.A.; Sullivan, A.F.; Mansbach, J.M.; Camargo, C.A., Jr. Vitamin D insufficiency in pregnant and nonpregnant women of childbearing age in the United States. *Am. J. Obstet. Gynecol.* **2010**, *202*, 436.e1–436.e8.

21. Maghbooli, Z.; Hossein-Nezhad, A.; Shafaei, A.R.; Karimi, F.; Madani, F.S.; Larijani, B. Vitamin D status in mothers and their newborns in Iran. *BMC Pregnancy Childbirth* **2007**, *7*, 1.

22. Nicolaidou, P.; Hatzistamatiou, Z.; Papadopoulou, A.; Kaleyias, J.; Floropoulou, E.; Lagona, E.; Tsagris, V.; Costalos, C.; Antsaklis, A. Low vitamin D status in mother-newborn pairs in Greece. *Calcif. Tissue Int.* **2006**, *78*, 337–342.

23. Perez-Lopez, F.R.; Fernandez-Alonso, A.M.; Ferrando-Marco, P.; Gonzalez-Salmeron, M.D.; Dionis-Sanchez, E.C.; Fiol-Ruiz, G.; Chedraui, P. First trimester serum 25-hydroxyvitamin D status and factors related to lower levels in gravids living in the Spanish Mediterranean coast. *Reprod. Sci.* **2011**, *18*, 730–736.

24. Ustuner, I.; Keskin, H.L.; Tas, E.E.; Neselioglu, S.; Sengul, O.; Avsar, A.F. Maternal serum 25(OH) D levels in the third trimester of pregnancy during the winter season. *J. Matern. Fetal Neonatal Med.* **2011**, *24*, 1421–1426.

25. Brannon, P.M.; Picciano, M.F. Vitamin D in pregnancy and lactation in humans. *Annu. Rev. Nutr.* **2011**, *31*, 89–115.

26. Charatcharoenwitthaya, N.; Nanthakomon, T.; Somprasit, C.; Chanthasenanont, A.; Chailurkit, L.O.; Pattaraarchachai, J.; Ongphiphadhanakul, B. Maternal vitamin D status, its associated factors and the course of pregnancy in Thai women. *Clin. Endocrinol.* **2013**, *78*, 126–133.

27. Marwaha, R.K.; Tandon, N.; Chopra, S.; Agarwal, N.; Garg, M.K.; Sharma, B.; Kanwar, R.S.; Bhadra, K.; Singh, S.; Mani, K.; *et al.* Vitamin D status in pregnant indian women across trimesters and different seasons and its correlation with neonatal serum 25-hydroxyvitamin D levels. *Br. J. Nutr.* **2011**, *106*, 1383–1389.

28. Paffoni, A.; Somigliana, E.; Vigano, P.; Benaglia, L.; Cardellicchio, L.; Pagliardini, L.; Papaleo, E.; Candiani, M.; Fedele, L. Vitamin D status in women with uterine leiomyomas. *J. Clin. Endocrinol. Metab.* **2013**, *98*, E1374–E1378.

29. Sayegh, L.; Fuleihan Gel, H.; Nassar, A.H. Vitamin D in endometriosis: A causative or confounding factor? *Metab. Clin. Exp.* **2014**, *63*, 32–41.

30. Hensel, K.J.; Randis, T.M.; Gelber, S.E.; Ratner, A.J. Pregnancy-specific association of vitamin D deficiency and bacterial vaginosis. *Am. J. Obstet. Gynecol.* **2011**, *204*, 41.e1–41.e9.

31. Holick, M.F.; Binkley, N.C.; Bischoff-Ferrari, H.A.; Gordon, C.M.; Hanley, D.A.; Heaney, R.P.; Murad, M.H.; Weaver, C.M. Evaluation, treatment, and prevention of vitamin D deficiency: An endocrine society clinical practice guideline. *J. Clin. Endocrinol. Metab.* **2011**, *96*, 1911–1930.

32. Dawodu, A.; Saadi, H.F.; Bekdache, G.; Javed, Y.; Altaye, M.; Hollis, B.W. Randomized controlled trial (RCT) of vitamin D supplementation in pregnancy in a population with endemic vitamin D deficiency. *J. Clin. Endocrinol. Metab.* **2013**, *98*, 2337–2346.

33. Hill, A.B. The environment and disease: Association or causation? *Proc. R. Soc. Med.* **1965**, *58*, 295–300.

34. Wei, S.Q.; Qi, H.P.; Luo, Z.C.; Fraser, W.D. Maternal vitamin D status and adverse pregnancy outcomes: A systematic review and meta-analysis. *J. Matern. Fetal Neonatal Med.* **2013**, *26*, 889–899.

Vitamin D Status and Related Factors in Newborns in Shanghai, China

Xiaodan Yu, Weiye Wang, Zhenzhen Wei, Fengxiu Ouyang, Lisu Huang, Xia Wang, Yanjun Zhao, Huijuan Zhang and Jun Zhang

Abstract: With the increasing recognition of the importance of the non-skeletal effects of vitamin D (VitD), more and more attention has been drawn to VitD status in early life. However, the VitD status of newborns and factors that influence VitD levels in Shanghai, China, remain unclear. A total of 1030 pregnant women were selected from two hospitals in Shanghai, one of the largest cities in China located at 31 degrees north latitude. Umbilical cord serum concentrations of 25-hydroxy vitamin D [25(OH)D] were measured by LC-MS-MS, and questionnaires were used to collect information. The median cord serum 25(OH)D concentration was 22.4 ng/mL; the concentration lower than 20 ng/mL accounted for 36.3% of the participants, and the concentration lower than 30 ng/mL for 84.1%. A multivariable logistic regression model showed that the determinants of low 25(OH)D status were being born during autumn or winter months and a lack of VitD-related multivitamin supplementation. The relative risk was 1.7 for both autumn (95% CI, 1.1–2.6) and winter (95% CI, 1.1–2.5) births ($p < 0.05$). VitD-related multivitamin supplementation more than once a day during pregnancy reduced the risk of VitD deficiency [adjusted OR (aOR) = 0.6, 95% CI (0.45–1.0) for VitD supplementation] ($p < 0.05$). VitD deficiency and insufficiency are common in newborns in Shanghai, China, and are independently associated with season and VitD supplementation. Our findings may assist future efforts to correct low levels of 25(OH)D in Shanghai mothers and their newborn children.

Reprinted from *Nutrients*. Cite as: Yu, X.; Wang, W.; Wei, Z.; Ouyang, F.; Huang, L.; Wang, X.; Zhao, Y.; Zhang, H.; Zhang, J. Vitamin D Status and Related Factors in Newborns in Shanghai, China. *Nutrients* **2014**, *6*, 5600–5610.

1. Introduction

VitD deficiency during pregnancy and early childhood leads to a variety of health problems for both the mother and the child [1–3]. Although VitD status during pregnancy has important implications regarding maternal complications, including decreased weight gain [4], gestational diabetes [5], preeclampsia [6], infections [7], and caesarean section [8], it may actually have more important implications for the general health of the developing fetus and newborn child. VitD deficiency in the newborn has been linked to hypocalcaemia, low birth weight, allergies, type I diabetes, impaired development, heart failure and rickets [9–11].

243

Over the past decade, numerous studies have reported on VitD status in adults, the elderly and, increasingly, pregnant women. However, studies regarding the prevalence of VitD deficiency among newborns are limited. In China, although there have been some reports of VitD status in pregnant women, there have only been two reports of newborns' VitD status with a small sample size: one in Beijing (40 degrees north latitude) and one in Chengdu (30 degrees north latitude) [12,13]. Shanghai, one of the largest cities in China with more than 20 million people, is located in East China at 31 degrees north latitude. According to the only study on VitD levels in pregnant women in Shanghai, over 90.5% of these women had 25(OH)D levels below 30 ng/mL [14]. VitD supplementation of 10 μg/day during pregnancy, suggested by the Chinese Nutrition Medicine Association, was equal to the recommended amount for the adult. In addition, it was reported, although the data is limited, that the vast majority of Chinese women do not in reality take VitD supplementation during pregnancy [12]. To date, the VitD status of Shanghai newborns has not been reported.

To address this gap in the literature, we measured serum levels of 25(OH)D in the cord blood of 1030 healthy newborns in Shanghai to determine their VitD status. Having documented a high prevalence of VitD deficiency (defined as 20 ng/mL), we then examined factors that independently predicted VitD status at birth.

2. Experimental Methods

2.1. Study Design and Subjects

The Shanghai Allergy Cohort Study was a prospective study with a birth cohort of 1071 infants recruited between 2012 and 2013 at Xinhua Hospital and the International Peace Maternity and Child Hospital, two large tertiary hospitals in Shanghai. Prior to delivery, written informed consent was obtained from the mothers, and trained nurses conducted face-to-face interviews. At birth, study nurses collected the newborn's anthropometric details and umbilical cord blood, when available. Ethics approval was obtained by the Ethics Committees of both Xinhua Hospital affiliated to Shanghai Jiao Tong University School of Medicine and the International Maternal and Children Care Hospital.

2.2. Umbilical Cord Blood 25(OH)D

The primary outcome measurement of the present study was the cord serum level of 25(OH)D. Cord blood was available for 1071 of the newborn participants, and 1030 of those newborns' mothers completed the questionnaires. The cord blood samples were centrifuged and transferred to $-80\,^{\circ}\mathrm{C}$ freezers within 2 h. We used the sensitive liquid chromatography tandem mass spectrometry (LC-MS/MS) analytical method to detect serum 25(OH)D following the procedure reported by our previous study [15]. In this assay, the level of sensitivity for LC/MS/MS assay was 0.05 ng/mL for 25(OH)D$_2$, and 0.1 ng/mL for 25(OH)D$_3$. The serum samples (100 μL) were deproteinised and precipitated using methanol, acetonitrile, zinc sulfate, and internal standards that included deuterated 25(OH)D$_2$ and 25(OH)D$_3$ (Sigma, St. Louis, MO, USA). Chromatographic separations were obtained using an Agilent Poroshell 120 EC-C18 (50 × 2.1 mm, 2.7 μm) column with a gradient of water (containing 0.1% formic acid) and methanol as the mobile phase at a flow rate of 0.5 mL/min. Multiple reaction monitoring (MRM) of the analyses was performed under electrospray ionization (ESI) in the positive mode at m/z 401.3→383.2 and 401.3→159.1 for 25(OH)D$_3$, m/z 413.3→395.3 and 413.3→355.2 for 25(OH)D$_2$, and m/z 404.3→386.3 and 416.4.3→398.3 for d3-25(OH)D$_3$ and d3-25(OH)D$_2$, respectively. Although there is no consensus on optimal levels of 25(OH)D as measured in serum, Vit D deficiency has been historically defined and recently recommended by the Institute of Medicine (IOM) as a 25(OH)D of less than 20 ng/mL [16,17]. VitD deficiency was defined as a serum 25(OH)D concentration <20 ng/mL, and VitD insufficiency was defined as a serum 25(OH)D concentration <30 ng/mL [18,19].

2.3. Risk Factors

The questionnaire documented socioeconomic status, maternal age, weight and height of the mother prepregnancy, VitD and other multivitamin supplementations, and outdoor activity during pregnancy. Gestational age, newborn sex, month of birth, and birth weight were obtained from the participants' medical records.

2.4. Data Analysis

Serum 25(OH)D concentrations were expressed in ng/mL. We first determined the percentiles of 25(OH)D and the prevalence of VitD deficiency in the newborns (Table 1). Then, we performed a univariate analysis to examine the correlations of 25(OH)D level with different groups of related factors (Table 2) and used multivariable analysis to estimate the independent relationship between 25(OH)D deficiency and the analyzed related factors after adjusting for potential confounders (Table 3). P Values of <0.05 were considered significant. All analyses were performed using Empower(R) (www.empowerstats.com, X&Ysolutions, Inc., Boston, MA, USA) and R (http://www.R-project.org).

3. Results

Table 1 showed the quartile values of 25(OH)D (Q1 = 18.5 ng/mL, Q2 = 22.4 ng/mL, Q3 = 27.5 ng/mL), 25(OH)D$_2$ (Q1 = 3.7 ng/mL, Q2 = 4.6 ng/mL, Q3 = 5.3 ng/mL) and 25(OH)D$_3$ (Q1 = 14.1 ng/mL, Q2 = 17.9 ng/mL, Q3 = 23.0 ng/mL). Participants had a median cord blood 25(OH)D concentration of 22.4 ng/mL. The 25(OH)D$_3$ (Q2 = 17.9 ng/mL) concentration was higher than the 25(OH)D$_2$ (Q2 = 4.6 ng/mL) concentration, and the ratio of 25(OH)D$_3$:25(OH)D$_2$

was 4:1. Overall, 36.3% of Shanghai newborns had serum 25(OH)D levels <20 ng/mL and 84.1% had levels <30 ng/mL (Table 1).

Table 1. Vitamin D level and the prevalence of vitamin D deficiency in newborns ($n = 1030$).

	25(OH)D$_2$	25(OH)D$_3$	25(OH)D
Q1	3.7	14.1	18.5
Q2	4.6	17.9	22.4
Q3	5.3	23.0	27.5
Min (ng/mL)	0.1	8.3	11.5
Max (ng/mL)	11.5	45.1	51.1
Mean ± SD (ng/mL)	4.5 ± 1.2	19.0 ± 6.1	23.5 ± 6.2
The prevalence of VitD deficiency (%) [25(OH)D < 20 ng/mL]	-	-	36.3
The prevalence of VitD insufficiency (%) [25(OH)D < 30 ng/mL]	-	-	84.1

The unadjusted associations between the various characteristics and VitD status were strongest for month (season) of birth and VitD related multivitamin supplementation (all p for trend <0.001). As expected, the median serum 25(OH)D concentrations peaked in infants born during summer months and were lower for infants born in the autumn and winter. The unadjusted analyses also indicated that outdoor activity on weekdays was a potential determinant of newborn vitamin D status ($p < 0.05$) (Table 2).

Table 2. The correlations of various factors with cord blood 25(OH)D by univariate analysis ($n = 1030$).

Variable	(%)	25(OH)D (Mean ± SD) (ng/mL)	p value
Vitamin D category (ng/mL)			
<20	36.3	17.5 ± 1.8	0.0000 **
≥20	63.7	26.9 ± 5.1	
Maternal age (years)			
<30	51.0	23.3 ± 6.2	0.2914
30–34	39.5	23.5 ± 6.2	
35–39	8.5	24.4 ± 6.0	
40+	1.0	25.5 ± 6.7	
Maternal prepregnancy BMI			
<28	95.3	23.5 ± 6.2	0.2292
≥28	4.7	22.4 ± 5.4	
Maternal education			
Middle school or lower	2.8	22.7 ± 6.2	0.7719
High school	11.5	23.5 ± 7.0	

Table 2. *Cont.*

Variable	(%)	25(OH)D (Mean ± SD) (ng/mL)	p value
College or higher	85.7	23.5 ± 6.1	
Gestational age (weeks)			
<37	3.5	23.7 ± 6.2	0.1122
37–39	71.7	23.5 ± 6.2	
40+	24.8	22.8 ± 6.1	
Birth weight (g)			
<2500	2.4	24.5 ± 6.9	0.4224
≥2500	97.1	23.5 ± 6.2	
Gender			
boy	50.4	23.2 ± 6.2	0.4504
girl	49.6	23.7 ± 6.3	
Month of birth			
Summer (Jun.–Aug.)	16.7	23.3 ± 6.1	0.0009 **
Autumn (Sep.–Nov.)	46.5	22.6 ± 6.0	
Winter (Dec.–Feb.)	36.8	22.4 ± 6.3	
VitD supplementation during pregnancy			
No	78.7	23.0 ± 6.1	0.0000 **
≤6 times/week	4.1	24.7 ± 6.3	
≥1 time/day	17.2	25.3 ± 6.3	
Calcium supplementation during pregnancy			
No	18.2	22.3 ± 5.9	0.0013 **
≤6 times/week	11.7	22.6 ± 6.0	
≥1 time/day	70.1	23.9 ± 6.3	
DHA supplementation during pregnancy			
No	63.1	23.0 ± 6.0	0.0024 **
≤6 times/week	6.6	24.4 ± 6.5	
≥1 time/day	30.3	24.4 ± 6.4	
Outdoor activity in weekdays			
<0.5 h	43.6	22.9 ± 5.9	0.0267 *
≥0.5 h	56.4	23.8 ± 6.3	
Outdoor activity in weekend			
<0.5 h	48.6	23.1 ± 6.1	0.1328
≥0.5 h	51.4	23.7 ± 6.3	
Husband smoke during pregnancy			
No	99.7	23.7 ± 6.2	0.0779
Yes	0.3	22.9 ± 6.2	

$* p < 0.05, ** p < 0.001.$

After adjusting for multiple newborn and maternal characteristics, season of birth and VitD related multivitamin supplementation remained associated with newborn VitD status. Newborns born in September through February were at a higher risk of VitD deficiency. The relative risk was 1.7 (95% CI, 1.1–2.6) in both autumn and winter (95% CI, 1.1–2.5) ($p < 0.05$). VitD or DHA supplementation more than once a day during pregnancy reduced the risk of VitD deficiency [adjusted OR (aOR) = 0.6, 95% CI (0.45–1.0) for VitD supplementation, and aOR= 0.7, 95% CI (0.51–0.95) for DHA supplementation] ($p < 0.05$) (Table 3).

Table 3. Factors associated with cord serum 25(OH)D < 20 ng/mL by multivariable analysis ($n = 1030$).

Variable	Crude OR	95% CI	P-value	aOR	95% CI	P-value
Gestational age (weeks)						
<37	1.0			1.0		
37–39	1.1	(0.55, 2.2)	0.778	1.0	(0.49, 2.3)	0.903
40+	1.4	(1.1, 1.9)	0.021*	1.3	(0.96, 1.8)	0.087
Maternal age (years)						
<30	1.0			1.0		
30–34	0.99	(0.75, 1.3)	0.917	0.98	(0.74, 1.3)	0.916
35–39	0.6	(0.36, 1.0)	0.052	0.61	(0.36, 1.1)	0.078
40+	0.42	(0.088, 2.0)	0.276	0.22	(0.026, 1.8)	0.156
Maternal prepregnancy BMI						
<28	1.0			1.0		
≥28	0.77	(0.43, 1.4)	0.395	0.75	(0.4, 1.4)	0.370
Maternal education						
Middle school or lower	1.0			1.0		
High school	0.64	(0.28, 1.4)	0.280	0.8	(0.32, 2.0)	0.615
College or higher	0.59	(0.28, 1.2)	0.161	0.73	(0.32, 1.7)	0.458
Birth weight (Kg)	1.0	(1.0, 1.0)	0.551	1.0	(0.98, 1.0)	0.738
Month of birth						
Summer (Jun.–Aug.)	1.0			1.0		
Autumn (Sep.–Nov.)	1.6	(1.1, 2.3)	0.017 *	1.7	(1.1, 2.6)	0.015*
Winter(Dec.–Feb.)	1.7	(1.2, 1.4)	0.015 *	1.7	(1.1, 2.5)	0.014*
VitD supplementation during pregnancy						
No	1.0			1.0		
≤6 times/week	0.57	(0.28, 1.1)	0.115	0.78	(0.35, 1.7)	0.552
≥1 time/day	0.52	(0.35, 0.75)	<0.001 **	0.6	(0.45, 1.0)	0.045
Calcium supplementation during pregnancy						
No	1.0			1.0		
≤6 times/week	0.86	(0.54, 1.4)	0.531	1.1	(0.63, 1.8)	0.817
≥1 time/day	0.72	(0.52, 1.0)	0.050 *	0.8	(0.56, 1.2)	0.243
DHA supplementation during pregnancy						
No	1.0			1.0		
≤6 times/week	0.61	(0.35, 1.1)	0.080	0.66	(0.36, 1.2)	0.197
≥1 time/day	0.67	(0.5, 0.9)	0.007 *	0.7	(0.51, 0.95)	0.022
Outdoor activity in weekdays						
<0.5 h	1.0			1.0		
≥0.5 h	0.93	(0.72, 1.2)	0.558	0.84	(0.58, 1.2)	0.371
Outdoor activity in weekend						
<0.5 h	1.0			1.0		
≥0.5 h	1.0	(0.81, 1.4)	0.720	1.3	(0.92, 1.9)	0.128
Husband smoke during pregnancy						
No	1.0			1.0		
Yes	1.2	(0.94, 1.6)	0.139	1.2	(0.9, 1.7)	0.184

All parameter estimates were adjusted for other covariates. * $P < 0.05$.

4. Discussion

We found that 25(OH)D levels in cord blood from 1030 healthy Shanghai infants were quite low overall—almost 1/3 of the children had less than 20 ng/mL 25(OH)D in early life. Cord blood 25(OH)D level was positively correlated with summer birth and multivitamin supplementation containing VitD, two strong predictors of high VitD status.

A high prevalence of VitD insufficiency in newborns confirms that VitD insufficiency or deficiency is a major health problem in Shanghai. Our data, which showed that the median 25(OH)D level was 22.4 ng/mL with 36.3% of newborn participants having VitD deficiency and 84.1% having VitD insufficiency, was similar to that of Tao et al. [14] in a study of pregnant women in Shanghai (mean: 17.57 g/mL, deficiency: 69%, insufficiency: 91%). However, the prevalence of VitD insufficiency was much higher than that reported by a study of small sample size newborns in Beijing (insufficiency: 100%, $n = 58$) [12].

Serum 25(OH)D is the best indicator of VitD status [20]. Although a number of assays are now available for measuring 25(OH)D in the serum or plasma, recently liquid chromatography tandem mass spectrometry (LC–MS/MS) systems have been used for more rapid, specific and sensitive assessment [21] and are gaining wide-spread acceptance [22–24]. LC–MS/MS can accurately measure the different forms of VitD, including $VitD_2$ and $VitD_3$. In this study, the ratio of $25(OH)D_3:25(OH)D_2$ was 4:1, which is similar to that reported by Karras et al. (3:1) [25]. In humans, $VitD_3$ is produced from its precursor, 7-dehydrocholesterol, during exposure to ultraviolet rays contained in sunlight, or it can be consumed in the diet. The human body does not make $VitD_2$, and the typically low level of $VitD_2$ that is observed in humans is from dietary intake. Given that $VitD_2$ is the only high-dose preparation of VitD available in many countries, potential differences in the ability of assays to accurately detect $25(OH)D_2$ and $25(OH)D_3$ are of clinical importance in cases where supplementation is suggested [25].

The seasonality of serum 25(OH)D levels in older children and adults has been well documented [26–28]. In contrast, few studies have examined this issue in newborns. Our study demonstrates seasonal variation in neonatal 25(OH)D levels. We found neonatal 25(OH)D levels were highest for newborns born from June to August and then decreased during the autumn and winter, from September through February. Our data are in accordance with two previous studies in New Zealand and Norway [29,30], but showed a relative weak seasonal variation. The lack of strong seasonal correlation could be due to the fact that Shanghai is an urban city with limited opportunities for exposure to the sun, and the Chinese women have the habit of avoiding exposure (umbrellas, hats, and sunscreen). Pregnant women also tend to stop working and stay indoors. VitD supplementation is also uncommon in China.

In our study, only 21.3% of pregnant women took the VitD supplementation during their pregnancy, and they took a low dose at 200–400 IU/day.

Our study also showed that VitD related multivitamin supplementation during pregnancy was positively correlated with neonatal 25(OH)D levels. VitD fortified food is rare in China. Thus, VitD supplementation is the main source of VitD for pregnant women. DHA supplementation can also improve 25(OH)D level, possibly because VitD co-exists in DHA preparations. The Chinese Association of Obstetrics & Gynecology has not suggested any guideline for VitD supplementation for pregnant women. Accordingly, Chinese obstetricians do not pay any attention to the VitD status of pregnant women and few hospitals perform vitamin D detection. Thus, further research into VitD status and related health outcomes in China is urgently needed.

In addition, we did not find an association between VitD status and gestational age, especially in newborns born preterm. We speculate that this is because the prevalence of preterm deliveries was low (3.5%). This was a relative large cohort study of neonatal VitD levels. However, the present study has some limitations. We did not collect blood samples from the mothers. Thus, we could not measure maternal 25(OH)D levels, even though a strong positive association between maternal 25(OH)D and neonatal 25(OH)D has been well proven [31–33]. Notably, we are performing a follow-up study of the outcomes of the children in this study, including allergies and asthma.

5. Conclusions

In summary, VitD deficiency and insufficiency are common in newborns in Shanghai, China. At present, maternal VitD status is not a major concern in China. Our findings may help increase awareness of this problem and promote VitD supplementation during pregnancy to improve VitD status both in mothers and their newborn children.

Acknowledgments: This study was funded by the Chinese National Natural Science Foundation (no. 81373004) and the Foundation of Science and Technology Commission of Shanghai Municipality (no. 13430710300).

Author Contributions: This study was based on original clinical work supported by Yanjun Zhao, Lisu Huang, Xia Wang and Huijuan Zhang. This study was conceived and monitored, the data was analyzed, and the paper was written by Xiaodan Yu, Weiye Wang, Fengxiu Ouyang and Jun Zhang. The collection of data was assisted by Xiaodan Yu and Zhenzhen Wei.

Conflicts of Interest: The authors declare no conflicts of interest.

References

1. Weinert, L.S.; Silveiro, S.P. Maternal-fetal impact of vitamin D deficiency: A critical review. *Matern. Child Health J.* **2014**.

2. Wei, S.Q.; Qi, H.P.; Luo, Z.C.; Fraser, W.D. Maternal vitamin D status and adverse pregnancy outcomes: A systematic review and meta-analysis. *J. Matern. Fetal Neonatal Med.* **2013**, *26*, 889–899.

3. Camargo, C.A.; Rifas-Shiman, S.L.; Litonjua, A.A.; Rich-Edwards, J.W.; Weiss, S.T.; Gold, D.R.; Kleinman, K.; Gillman, M.W. Maternal intake of vitamin D during pregnancy and risk of recurrent wheeze in children at 3 y of age. *Am. J. Clin. Nutr.* **2007**, *85*, 788–795.

4. Johnson, D.D.; Wagner, C.L.; Hulsey, T.C.; McNeil, R.B.; Ebeling, M.; Hollis, B.W. Vitamin D deficiency and insufficiency is common during pregnancy. *Am. J. Perinatal.* **2011**, *28*, 7–12.

5. Lacroix, M; Battista, M.C.; Doyon, M.; Houde, G.; Ménard, J.; Ardilouze, J.L.; Hivert, M.F.; Perron, P. Lower vitamin D levels at first trimester are associated with higher risk of developing gestational diabetes mellitus. *Acta Diabetol.* **2014**.

6. Tabesh, M.; Salehi-Abargouei, A.; Tabesh, M.; Esmaillzadeh, A. Maternal vitamin D status and risk of pre-eclampsia: A systematic review and meta-analysis. *J. Clin. Endocrinol. Metab.* **2013**, *98*, 3165–3173.

7. Mehta, S.; Hunter, D.J.; Mugusi, F.M.; Spiegelman, D.; Manji, K.P.; Giovannucci, E.L.; Hertzmark, E.; Msamanga, G.I.; Fawzi, W.W. Perinatal outcomes, including mother-to-child transmission of HIV, and child mortality and their association with maternal vitamin D status in Tanzania. *J. Infect. Dis.* **2009**, *200*, 1022–1030.

8. Savvidou, M.D.; Makgoba, M.; Castro, P.T.; Akolekar, R.; Nicolaides, K.H. First-trimester maternal serum vitamin D and mode of delivery. *Br. J. Nutr.* **2012**, *108*, 1972–1975.

9. Kaushal, M.; Magon, N. Vitamin D in pregnancy: A metabolic outlook. *Indian J. Endocrinol. Metab.* **2013**, *17*, 76.

10. Elidrissy, A.T.H.; Munawarah, M.; Alharbi, K.M. Hypocalcemic rachitic cardiomyopathy in infants. *J. Saudi Heart Assoc.* **2013**, *25*, 25–33.

11. Miettinen, M.E.; Reinert, L.; Kinnunen, L.; Harjutsalo, V.; Koskela, P.; Surcel, H.M.; Allardt, C.; Tuomilehto, J. Serum 25-hydroxyvitamin D level during early pregnancy and type 1 diabetes risk in the offspring. *Diabetologia* **2012**, *55*, 1291–1294.

12. Song, S.J.; Si, S.; Liu, J.; Chen, X.; Zhou, L.; Jia, G.; Liu, G.; Niu, Y.; Wu, J.; Zhang, W.; Zhang, J. Vitamin D status in Chinese pregnant women and their newborns in Beijing and their relationships to birth size. *Public Health Nutr.* **2013**, *16*, 687–692.

13. Wang, J.; Yang, F.; Mao, M.; Liu, D.-H.; Yang, H.-M.; Yang, S.-F. High prevalence of vitamin D and calcium deficiency among pregnant women and their newborns in Chengdu, China. *World J. Pediatr.* **2010**, *6*, 265–267.

14. Tao, M.; Shao, H.; Gu, J.; Zhen, Z. Vitamin D status of pregnant women in Shanghai, China. *J. Matern. Fetal Neonatal Med.* **2012**, *25*, 237–239.

15. Li, L.; Zhou, H.; Yang, X.; Zhao, L.; Yu, X. Relationships between 25-hydroxyvitamin D and nocturnal enuresis in five-to seven-year-old children. *PLoS One* **2014**, *9*, e99316.

16. Ross, A.C.; Manson, J.A.E.; Abrams, S.A.; Aloia, J.F.; Brannon, P.M.; Clinton, S.K.; Durazo-Arvizu, R.A.; Christopher, G.J.; Gallo, R.L.; Christopher, S.G.; *et al.* The 2011 report on dietary reference intakes for calcium and vitamin D from the Institute of Medicine: what clinicians need to know. *J. Clin. Endocrinol. Metab.* **2011**, *96*, 53–58.

17. Holick, M.F.; Binkley, N.C.; Bischoff-Ferrari, H.A.; Gordon, C.M.; Hanley, D.A.; Hassan, M.M.; Weaver, C.M. Evaluation, treatment, and prevention of vitamin D deficiency: An Endocrine Society clinical practice guideline. *J. Clin. Endocrinol. Metab.* **2011**, *96*, 1911–1930.

18. Vieth, R. Why the minimum desirable serum 25-hydroxyvitamin D level should be 75 nmol/L (30 ng/mL). *Best Prac. Res. Clin. Endocrinol. Metab.* **2011**, *25*, 681–691.

19. Wahl, D.A.; Cooper, C.; Ebeling, P.R.; Eggersdorfer, M.; Hilger, J.; Hoffmann, K.; Josse, R.; Kanis, J.A.; Mithal, A.; Pierroz, D.D.; *et al.* A global representation of vitamin D status in healthy populations. *Arch. Osteoporos.* **2012**, *7*, 155–172.

20. Gallo, S.; Comeau, K.; Agellon, S.; Vanstone, C.; Sharma, A.; Jones, G.; L'Abbé, M.; Khamessan, A.; Weiler, H.; Rodd, C. Methodological issues in assessing plasma 25-hydroxyvitamin D concentration in newborn infants. *Bone* **2014**, *61*, 186–190.

21. Singh, R.J. Quantitation of 25-OH-vitamin D (25OHD) using liquid tandem mass spectrometry (LC-MS-MS). In *Clinical Applications of Mass Spectrometry*; Humana Press: NJ, USA, 2010; pp. 509–517.

22. Chen, H.; McCoy, L.F.; Schleicher, R.L.; Pfeiffer, C.M. Measurement of 25-hydroxyvitamin D3 (25OHD3) and 25-hydroxyvitamin D2 (25OHD2) in human serum using liquid chromatography-tandem mass spectrometry and its comparison to a radioimmunoassay method. *Clin. Chim. Acta* **2008**, *391*, 6–12.

23. Singh, R.J.; Taylor, R.L.; Reddy, G.S.; Grebe, S.K. C-3 epimers can account for a significant proportion of total circulating 25-hydroxyvitamin D in infants, complicating accurate measurement and interpretation of vitamin D status. *J. Clin. Endocrinol. Metab.* **2006**, *91*, 3055–3061.

24. Aronov, P.A.; Hall, L.M.; Dettmer, K.; Stephensen, C.B.; Hammock, B.D. Metabolic profiling of major vitamin D metabolites using Diels–Alder derivatization and ultra-performance liquid chromatography-tandem mass spectrometry. *Anal. Bioanal. Chem.* **2008**, *391*, 1917–1930.

25. Karras, S.N.; Shah, I.; Petroczi, A.; Goulis, D.G.; Bili, H.; Papadopoulou, F.; Harizopoulou, V.; Tarlatzis, B.C.; Naughton, D. An observational study reveals that neonatal vitamin D is primarily determined by maternal contributions: implications of a new assay on the roles of vitamin D forms. *Nutr. J.* **2013**, *12*, 77.

26. Klenk, J.; Rapp, K.; Denkinger, M.D.; Nagel, G.; Nikolaus, T.; Peter, R.; Koenig, W.; Böhm, B.O.; Rothenbacher, D. Seasonality of vitamin D status in older people in Southern Germany: implications for assessment. *Age Ageing* **2013**, *42*, 404–408.

27. Yu, X.D.; Zhang, J.; Yan, C.; Shen, X. Relationships between serum 25-hydroxyvitamin D and quantitative ultrasound bone mineral density in 0–6 year old children. *Bone* **2013**, *53*, 306–310.

28. Luick, B.; Bersamin, A.; Stern, J.S. Locally harvested foods support serum 25-hydroxyvitamin D sufficiency in an indigenous population of Western Alaska. *Int. J. Circumpolar Health* **2014**.

29. Camargo, C.A.; Ingham, T.; Wickens, K.; Thadhani, R.I.; Silvers, K.M.; Epton, M.J.; Town, G.I.; Espinola, J.A.; Crane, J. Vitamin D status of newborns in New Zealand. *Br. J. Nutr.* **2010**, *104*, 1051–1057.

30. Godang, K.; Frøslie, K.F.; Henriksen, T.; Qvigstad, E.; B.ollerslev, J. Seasonal variation in maternal and umbilical cord 25 (OH) vitamin D and their associations with neonatal adiposity. *Eur. J. Endocrinol.* **2014**, *170*, 609–617.

31. Parlak, M.; Kalay, S.; Kalay, Z.; Kirecci, A.; Guney, O.; Koklu, E. Severe vitamin D deficiency among pregnant women and their newborns in Turkey. *J. Matern. Fetal Neonatal Med.* **2014**.

32. El Koumi, M.A.; Ali, Y.F.; Abd, E.R.R.N. Impact of Maternal Vitamin D Status during Pregnancy on Neonatal Vitamin D Status. *Turkish J. Pediatr.* **2013**, *55*, 371–377.

33. Josefson, J.L.; Feinglass, J.; Rademaker, A.W.; Metzger, B.E.; Zeiss, D.M.; Price, H.E.; Langman, C.B. Maternal obesity and vitamin D sufficiency are associated with cord blood vitamin D insufficiency. *J. Clin. Endocrinol. Metab.* **2012**, *98*, 114–119.

Sun Exposure and Vitamin D Supplementation in Relation to Vitamin D Status of Breastfeeding Mothers and Infants in the Global Exploration of Human Milk Study

Adekunle Dawodu, Barbara Davidson, Jessica G. Woo, Yong-Mei Peng, Guillermo M. Ruiz-Palacios, Maria de Lourdes Guerrero and Ardythe L. Morrow

Abstract: Although vitamin D (vD) deficiency is common in breastfed infants and their mothers during pregnancy and lactation, a standardized global comparison is lacking. We studied the prevalence and risk factors for vD deficiency using a standardized protocol in a cohort of breastfeeding mother-infant pairs, enrolled in the Global Exploration of Human Milk Study, designed to examine longitudinally the effect of environment, diet and culture. Mothers planned to provide breast milk for at least three months post-partum and were enrolled at four weeks postpartum in Shanghai, China ($n = 112$), Cincinnati, Ohio ($n = 119$), and Mexico City, Mexico ($n = 113$). Maternal serum 25(OH)D was measured by radioimmunoassay (<50 nmol/L was categorized as deficient). Serum 25(OH)D was measured in a subset of infants (35 Shanghai, 47 Cincinnati and 45 Mexico City) seen at 26 weeks of age during fall and winter seasons. Data collected prospectively included vD supplementation, season and sun index (sun exposure × body surface area exposed while outdoors). Differences and factors associated with vD deficiency were evaluated using appropriate statistical analysis. vD deficiency in order of magnitude was identified in 62%, 52% and 17% of Mexican, Shanghai and Cincinnati mothers, respectively ($p < 0.001$). In regression analysis, vD supplementation ($p < 0.01$), obesity ($p = 0.03$), season ($p = 0.001$) and sites ($p < 0.001$) predicted maternal vD status. vD deficiency in order of magnitude was found in 62%, 28%, and 6% of Mexican, Cincinnati and Shanghai infants, respectively ($p < 0.001$). Season ($p = 0.022$), adding formula feeding ($p < 0.001$) and a higher sun index ($p = 0.085$) predicted higher infant vD status. vD deficiency appears to be a global problem in mothers and infants, though the prevalence in diverse populations may depend upon sun exposure behaviors and vD supplementation. Greater attention to maternal and infant vD status starting during pregnancy is warranted worldwide.

Reprinted from *Nutrients*. Cite as: Dawodu, A.; Davidson, B.; Woo, J.G.; Peng, Y.-M.; Ruiz-Palacios, G.M.; de Lourdes Guerrero, M.; Morrow, A.L. Sun Exposure and Vitamin D Supplementation in Relation to Vitamin D Status of Breastfeeding Mothers and Infants in the Global Exploration of Human Milk Study. *Nutrients* **2015**, *7*, 1081–1093.

1. Introduction

Vitamin D (vD) is a prohormone that is synthesized in humans following skin exposure to ultraviolet B radiation in the range of 280–320 nm. In comparison to sunlight, diet provides less than 10% of the body's vD requirement in unsupplemented individuals [1,2]. Vitamin D is necessary to maintain calcium homeostasis and bone health, and there are increasing reports of its role in innate and autoimmune functions [3]. Vitamin D deficiency is detrimental to the health of mothers and children because of increased risk of osteomalacia in adults and rickets and delayed growth in infants and children [4–6]. In addition, vD deficiency or low vD intake has been associated with increased risk of autoimmune diseases in adults and children [7,8] and lower respiratory tract infection in children [9–12].

Recently, vD deficiency has been reported to be a public health problem worldwide despite abundant sunshine in many countries and the demonstration of the efficacy of vD supplements to prevent vD deficiency [7]. A review of recent studies suggests that vD deficiency is a global problem during pregnancy [13]. The prevalence of serum 25(OH)D levels <50 nmol/L, considered vD deficiency [14], ranges between 33% in the USA [15] and 42% in Canada [16] to 75%–77% in the UK [17] and Finland [18] and from 74% to 98% in India [19], New Zealand [20] and the United Arab Emirates [21]. The high prevalence of vD deficiency in pregnancy raises concern about increased risk of low vD status in mothers and infants after birth and especially the segments that breastfeed, because of the low vD content of breast milk. Furthermore, in view of the drive to increase the prevalence and duration of exclusive breastfeeding and the reported increased risk of rickets in breastfeeding infants [5], the vD status of lactating women and their infants should be of global health concern. The reported few studies appear to indicate that vitamin D deficiency is common in breastfeeding infants, and rickets may represent the tip of the iceberg. Some authors have suggested that vD deficiency may be an under-diagnosed public health problem in breastfeeding mothers and their infants in many countries [5,9], but standardized comparisons of global prevalence are lacking. For example, the cutoff values for vD deficiency, age of study, season of study and methods of assessment of risk factors varied among the studies [9]. The objectives of this study were to compare the prevalence and risk factors for vD deficiency in a cohort of breastfeeding mothers and infants in Shanghai, China, Cincinnati, Ohio, and Mexico City, Mexico, using the same study design and serum vD level measurement in a single center. The mothers and infant dyads were enrolled in the longitudinal Global Exploration of Human Milk study, which was designed to explore the effects of different environments and diets on human milk composition, infant nutrition and health.

255

2. Methods

2.1. Subjects

One hundred and twenty mother-infant pairs were enrolled at 4 weeks postpartum in Shanghai and Cincinnati and 125 in Mexico City. The protocol of the parent study was approved by the Review Boards of Fudan Children's Hospital of Fudan University in Shanghai, China, Cincinnati Children's Hospital Medical Center in Cincinnati, Ohio, and the National Institute of Medical Sciences and Nutrition in Mexico City, Mexico. The parent study was a longitudinal international cohort study of breastfeeding mother-infant pairs designed to assess the relationship between bioactive factors in human milk and infant growth and health status over the first year of life. All of the mothers delivered singleton infants at term ($\geq$37 weeks) and planned to provide breast milk for at least 3 months postpartum. Mothers with health problems that could interfere with breastfeeding or who delivered prematurely (<37 weeks) were excluded from the study. Healthy mothers were recruited from those who delivered at International Peace Maternity and Child Health Hospital in Shanghai, China, The Christ Hospital in Cincinnati, Ohio, and Gea Gonzalez Hospital in Mexico City, Mexico, between March, 2007, and September, 2008.

The primary outcome of this study is the prevalence and risk factors for vD deficiency (measured by serum 25(OH)D concentration) in mothers at 4 weeks postpartum in Mexico City, latitude 19$°$ N, (n = 113), Shanghai, latitude 31$°$ N, (n = 112), and Cincinnati, latitude 39$°$ N, (n = 119) by season. We also studied a subset of 35 Shanghai, 47 Cincinnati and 45 Mexican infants who were assessed during fall and winter seasons at 26 weeks of life at the 3 sites, because they had serum available for 25(OH)D measurement. Cincinnati infants were multi-racial (white (80%), black (10%) and other racial groups (10%)).

2.2. Design

A registered nurse visited family homes at 2 weeks postpartum to enroll the mothers after consent had been obtained. For the parent study, postpartum visits took place at 4 weeks, 13 weeks, 26 weeks, 52 weeks and 108 weeks to complete demographic data and follow-up questionnaires. The data collected prospectively for the purpose of this study included socio-demographics, maternal vD supplementation intake reported during the interview and sunlight exposure behaviors in mothers and infants. Maternal report of vD supplementation to the infant was incomplete in all 3 sites, and therefore, comparisons of vD supplementation of infants at the 3 sites was not available. Infant milk source during the follow-up was documented using standardized questionnaires during weekly phone follow-up interviews. It was, therefore, possible to determine the prevalence of formula usage, which could impact infant's vD intake and, thus, vD status.

Sun exposure behavior was assessed by recording the duration of direct sun exposure (h/week) in the week prior to the interview. Body surface area (BSA) exposure while outdoors was based on a modified questionnaire [22] for assessing sun exposure to sunlight in adults and infants using a mode of outdoor clothing. For example, exposure of head and neck is assigned an area of 5% for the mother and 14% for the infant. The total percentage of BSA exposed to sunlight was calculated as the sum of the percentage BSA exposed while outdoors associated with all of the subject's responses. A sun exposure index was calculated by multiplying the percentage of BSA exposed by the hours of exposure to sunlight per week. This index has been shown to correlate with vD status in adults and children [23–25].

Blood samples were drawn by venipuncture from the mothers and the infants, and the date of blood collection was recorded. The serum samples were frozen at −80 °C and shipped to the Cincinnati vD research lab from Shanghai and Mexico City sites for evaluation of vD status of mothers and infants. Serum concentrations of 25(OH)D were measured by radioimmunoassay (DiaSorin, Stillwater, MN, USA) in nmol/L, as previously described [22]. The intra- and inter-assay coefficients of variation for 25(OH)D concentration measurement were 4% and 11%, respectively. Serum 25(OH)D concentration <50 nmol/L was defined as deficient [14]; values of 30 to <50 nmol/L were categorized as moderate deficiency, and values <30 nmol/L, consistent with increased risk of rickets or osteomalacia, were categorized as severe deficiency [26,27]. Blood samples were available to measure serum intact parathyroid hormone (PTH) using the immunoradiometric assay (DiaSorin) method in Shanghai and Cincinnati mothers. The normal adult range in the laboratory using this assay is 13–54 pg/mL.

2.3. Statistical Analysis

The primary variables for this study were maternal serum 25(OH)D concentrations at 4 weeks postpartum at the 3 sites and the infant serum 25(OH)D concentrations at 26 weeks postpartum. Analysis of variance was used to compare mothers by site and within each season for serum 25(OH)D concentrations and sun exposure index. Infant serum 25(OH)D concentrations during fall and winter seasons at 26 weeks of age by site was compared using ANOVA.

We also compared selected maternal socio-demographic factors, prevalence of vD supplementation and sun exposure behaviors by sites using nonparametric statistical tests. Multivariate multiple regression models with the vD status of the mothers at 4 weeks postpartum and the infants at 26 weeks of age during the fall/winter season as the outcome variable were constructed to control for other potential confounding variables.

3. Results

3.1. Maternal Results

Table 1 shows the comparison of the maternal baseline characteristics by site. Cincinnati mothers were older ($p < 0.001$), included mothers with higher prevalence of obesity ($p = 0.0001$), four-year college education ($p = 0.0001$) and vD supplementation rate ($p = 0.0001$). The mean sun index was negligible in Shanghai (10.0) and Mexican mothers (0.87) compared with Cincinnati mothers (239.0), $p < 0.001$.

At four weeks postpartum, maternal mean serum 25(OH)D concentrations differed ($p < 0.001$) by site (Figure 1). The mean values of 48.6 nmol/L in Shanghai and 48.2 nmol/L in Mexico City were lower than the value of 70.2 nmol/L in Cincinnati. Vitamin D deficiency (serum 25(OH)D <50 nmol/L) in order of magnitude was found in 62%, 52% and 17% of Mexican, Shanghai and Cincinnati mothers, respectively ($p < 0.001$).

Table 1. Maternal demography, vitamin D (vD) supplementation and sun index by city.

	Shanghai Latitude 31° N	Cincinnati Latitude 39° N	Mexico City Latitude 19° N	p-Value
Age (mean (SD))	29.3 (3.7)	31.5 (5.2)	24.4 (5.6)	0.001
Obese (BMI >30) (n (%))	1 (0.8)	33 (28.0)	5 (4.5)	0.0001
Education (n (%)), completed 4-y college	69 (57.5)	82 (68.3)	5 (4.2)	0.0001
vD supplementation (n (%))	22 (18.3)	94 (87.0)	44 (35.2)	0.0001
Sun index (mean (SD))	10 (24)	239 (301)	0.87 (1.1)	0.001

p-values by Fisher's or the Kruskal–Wallis test.

Figure 2 displays the maternal serum 25(OH)D concentrations and sun indices by sites and season. The sun index varies by season among Cincinnati mothers, but there was lack of seasonal variation among Shanghai and Mexican mothers. Maternal vD status as measured by serum 25(OH)D concentrations showed seasonal variation, with the highest values among Cincinnati mothers within each season.

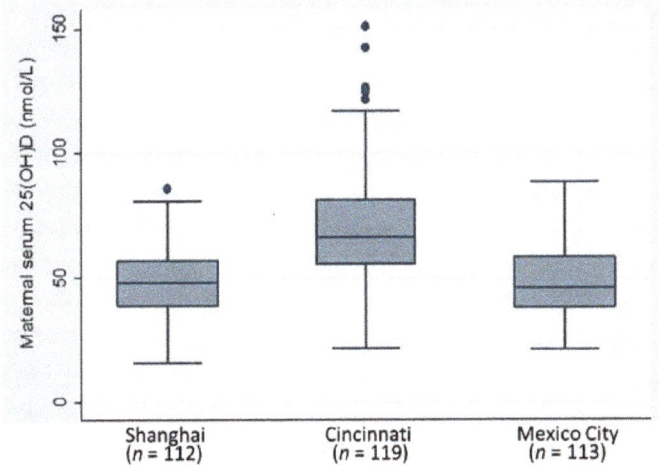

Figure 1. Maternal serum 25(OH)D concentrations, $p = 0.001$ by ANOVA.

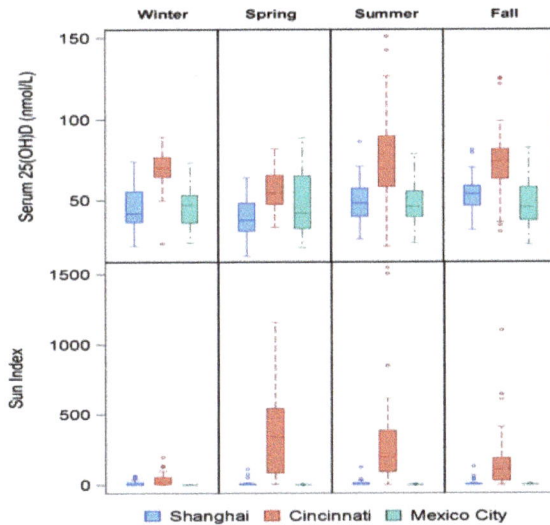

Figure 2. Maternal vD status and sun index by season and site, $p < 0.001$ by ANOVA, comparing mothers by site within each season for vitamin D and sun exposure index.

3.2. Infant Results

Comparing infants seen during the fall/winter seasons at 26 weeks of age at the three sites, the mean serum 25(OH)D concentrations were lower in Mexico City (44.0 nmol/L) and Cincinnati (68.3 nmol/L) than Shanghai (95.3 nmol/L), $p < 0.001$ (Figure 3). Vitamin D deficiency in order of magnitude was found in 62%,

28% and 6% of Mexican, Cincinnati and Shanghai infants, respectively ($p < 0.001$). Sunlight exposures during the fall/winter seasons were different by sites and were higher in Shanghai infants at 26 weeks than in Cincinnati and Mexican infants. The duration of sun exposure in hours per week (median, IQR) were 3.0 (1.1, 4.4) vs. 2.0 (0.5, 5.3) vs. 1.0 (0.3, 1.7) in Shanghai, Cincinnati and Mexican infants, respectively. The median (IQR) percent of BSAs exposed were 26 (14, 26) vs. 14 (7, 26) vs. 19 (14, 24) in Shanghai, Cincinnati and Mexican infants, respectively. Median (IQR) sun index (BSA × duration of sun exposure) values were 55 (22,104) vs. 27 (3.8, 65) vs. 21 (7.1, 29.1) in Shanghai, Cincinnati and Mexican infants, respectively. In spring/summer seasons, the infant sun index was higher in the Cincinnati cohort followed by Shanghai and lowest in the Mexico City cohort, but we did not have enough blood for infant serum 25(OH)D measurement in the Shanghai and Mexico City cohorts. Serum 25(OH)D in infants are associated with their sun index, including all infants measured in the fall/winter season ($r = 0.39$, $p < 0.001$) across the three sites. This is also true for infants in the Cincinnati site in the fall/winter season ($r = 0.37$, $p = 0.01$), but not for the other two sites independently.

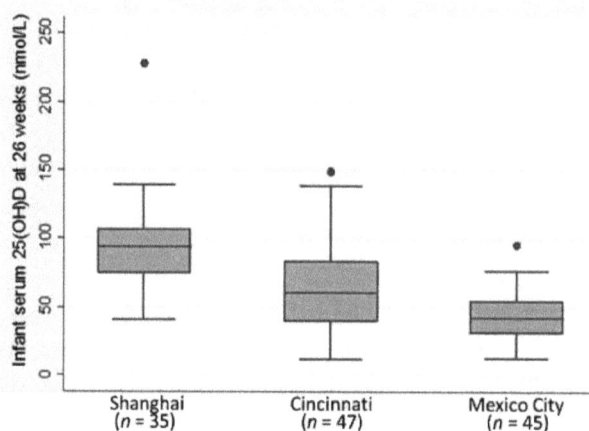

Figure 3. Infant serum 25(OH)D concentrations in fall/winter seasons at 26 weeks of age, $p < 0.001$ by ANOVA.

3.3. Categories of vD Deficiency in Mothers and Infants

The different categories of low vD status, moderate (serum 25(OH)D 30 to <50 nmol/L) and severe (serum 25(OH)D <30 nmol/L) deficiency, in mothers and infants differed by site and are shown in Table 2. Overall, less than 4% of the mothers were severely deficient, and the percent of mothers with severe deficiency was over two-fold higher in Mexican mothers than Shanghai and Cincinnati mothers. About half of the Shanghai and Mexican mothers had moderate deficiency compared with 14% of Cincinnati mothers. Overall, 12.5% of the infants evaluated during the fall/winter season at 26 weeks of age were severely deficient. In contrast to maternal findings, the percent of infants with severe and moderate deficiencies were lower in Shanghai compared with Cincinnati and Mexico City cohorts.

Table 2. Categories of vitamin D status in mothers and infants.

	All	Shanghai	Cincinnati	Mexico City
Categories				
Mothers * at 4 weeks postpartum	344	112	119	113
n (%) <30 nmol/L	13 (3.8)	3 (2.7)	3 (2.5)	7 (6.2)
n (%) 30 to <50 nmol/L	135 (39.2)	55 (49.1)	17 (14.3)	63 (55.8)
n (%) ≥50 nmol/L	196 (57.0)	54 (48.2)	99 (83.2)	43 (38.0)
Infants * at 26 weeks of age	128	36	47	45
n (%) <30 nmol/L	16 (12.5)	0 (0)	6 (12.8)	10 (22.2)
n (%) 30 to <50 nmol/L	27 (21.0)	2 (5.6)	7 (14.9)	18 (40.0)
n (%) ≥50 nmol/L	85 (66.4)	34 (94.4)	34 (72.3)	17 (37.8)

* $p \leq 0.001$ by Fisher's exact test comparing categories of vD status by site.

3.4. Factors Independently Associated with vD Status in Mothers and Infants in Regression Analysis

In the mothers, regression analysis with serum 25(OH)D concentration as the primary outcome showed that vD supplement intake (β ± SE, 5.5 ± 2.2, $p = 0.01$) and summer/fall season (β ± SE, 7.3 ± 1.8, $p < 0.001$) were associated with higher maternal serum 25(OH)D concentrations, while obesity (β ± SE, −6.7 ± 3.1, $p = 0.03$) and sites (Shanghai (β ± SE, −19.9 ± 2.8, $p < 0.001$) and Mexico City (β ± SE, −20.8 ± 6, $p < 0.001$)) were associated with low maternal serum 25(OH)D concentrations. Factors evaluated in the model were obesity or prepregnancy, BMI, age, education, season, vD supplementation, sun index and sites. In the Cincinnati cohort only was there a higher sun index, a significant predictor of maternal vD status. In regression analysis, formula feeding ($p = 0.001$), season ($p = 0.022$), sun index ($p = 0.085$) and sites ($p \leq 0.001$) were independent predictors of higher serum 25(OH)D concentration status in the infants at 26 weeks of age. Factors evaluated in the model were sun index log, percent formula fed, mother's serum 25(OH)D level, maternal vitamin D deficiency and sites.

3.5. Maternal Serum 25(OH)D Concentrations and PTH Relationship in Cincinnati and Shanghai

There was a negative correlation between serum 25(OD) concentrations and PTH concentrations ($r = -0.2$, $p = 0.002$) (Figure 4) in mothers at four weeks postpartum based on the data from Shanghai and Cincinnati. Blood samples were insufficient to measure PTH concentrations in mothers from Mexico City.

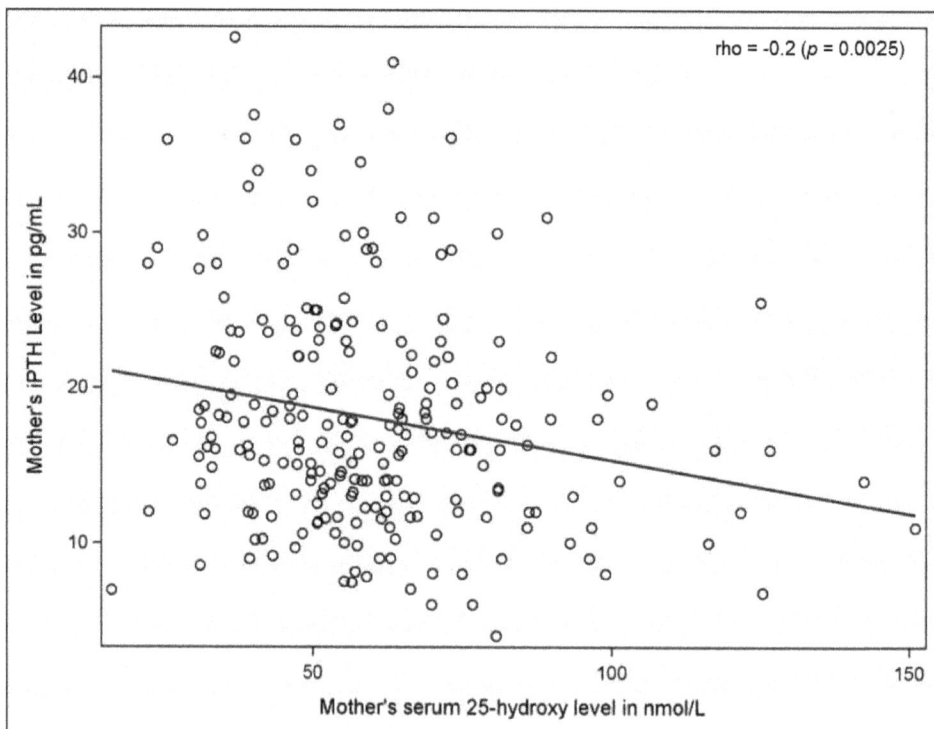

Figure 4. Correlation between parathyroid hormone (PTH) (pg/mL) and 25(OH)D (nmol/L) levels at four weeks post-partum in Shanghai and Cincinnati mothers. Analyzed together, serum 25(OH)D and PTH were negatively correlated.

4. Discussion

In this prospective study of urban population in North America, Latin America and China using the same study design, we found vD deficiency to be common in breastfeeding mothers from Shanghai and Mexico City and less common in mothers in Cincinnati. The mean serum 25(OH)D concentration in lactating mothers in Mexico City (48.2 nmol/L) and in Shanghai (48.6 nmol/L) was lower than the recommended target value of >50 nmol/L [27]. At four weeks postpartum, over 60% of the mothers in Mexico City and half of the mothers in Shanghai were vD deficient ()serum 25(OH)D concentration <50 nmol/L) compared with 17% of mothers in Cincinnati. Most of the vD deficient mothers had moderate vD deficiency (serum 25(OH)D levels of 30 to <50 nmol/L) while 2% of the mothers in Shanghai and Cincinnati and 6.2% of Mexican mothers had severe deficiency (serum 25(OH)D levels <30 nmol/L), which is associated with increased risk of osteomalacia. As expected, there was an inverse relationship between 25(OH)D levels and serum PTH levels, indicating an inadequate vD status in the mothers, which is associated with elevated levels of serum PTH. The degree of severe vD deficiency is significantly lower than previously reported from other countries. Based on previous studies, 61% of breastfeeding mothers from the United Arab Emirates [28], 48% of mothers in India [29] and 46% of breastfeeding mothers from Turkey [30] had severe deficiency (serum 25(OH)D concentration <25 nmol/L), which is associated with increased risk of osteomalacia [27]. Such a low vD status would also predispose breastfeeding infants without vD supplementation to vD deficiency. It thus appears that moderate to severe vD deficiency in early postpartum in breastfeeding mothers is a common problem in many countries and may be under recognized.

In this study, the higher vD status in mothers from Cincinnati was associated with higher sun index and vD supplementation intake compared with mothers in Shanghai and Mexico City. It is of note that the restricted exposure to sunlight during postpartum among Shanghai and Mexican mothers is related to cultural practices in which mothers are restricted from outdoor activities and are cared for by family members. This practice of restricting mothers from outdoor exposure in the immediate postpartum convalescent period (known as "doing the month") in China has been associated with increased risk of low vD status and rickets in some rural Chinese communities [31]. Recognition of the possible impact of these cultural practices on vD nutrition in postpartum mothers should heighten attention to the need for vD supplementation in such settings. In all of the cohorts from the three sites, vD intake, obesity and season were independent predictors of maternal vD status in multivariate regression analysis. In individual site analysis, high maternal sun index (>500) was associated with high maternal vD status only in the Cincinnati cohort, which attained such a high index. Therefore, differences in the prevalence of these potential risk factors among populations will impact maternal global prevalence, as well as the degree of maternal vD deficiency. For example, in the study from the United Arab Emirates, where severe vD deficiency is more common than in this study, it was found that mothers were more severely sunshine deprived during lactation and had a lower rate of vD supplement intake [28,32].

The vitamin D status of breastfeeding infants who were seen at 26 weeks of age during the fall and winter seasons were lower in the Mexican infants (mean serum 25(OH)D 44 nmol/L) and Cincinnati infants (68.3 nmol/L) than in Shanghai infants (95.3 nmol/L). Vitamin D deficiency, defined as serum 25(OH)D <50 nmol/L, was ten-fold higher in Mexican infants and almost five-fold higher in Cincinnati infants than in Shanghai (62% *vs.* 28% *vs.* 6%, respectively). In addition, severe deficiency (serum 25(OH)D <30 nmol/L) was over two-fold higher in Mexican than in Shanghai and Cincinnati infants. This degree of severe deficiency could theoretically predispose Mexican infants to increased risk of rickets [26,27].

Other recent studies indicate that the prevalence of serum 25(OH)D <30 nmol/L is high and variable worldwide in breastfeeding infants, and lack of sun exposure and vD supplementation have been suggested as contributing factors [9]. Twenty-seven percent of breastfeeding infants in Ioannina in Greece [33], 43%–48% of breastfed infants from New Delhi, India [29,34], and 82% of exclusively breastfed infants in Al Ain, the United Arab Emirates [28], had serum 25(OH)D <25 nmol/L at 3–6 months of age. It therefore appears that moderate to severe vD deficiency is common in sunshine-deprived and unsupplemented breastfed infants, and reports of clinical rickets may not represent the true picture of low vitamin D status in breastfed infants.

Although the mothers and infants in Shanghai were sunshine deprived in the immediate postpartum period, it is of interest that the infants had a higher sun index than the Cincinnati and Mexican infants during the fall/winter season at 26 weeks of age. Clinical experience also suggested that most (80%) of breastfeeding infants in Shanghai would be on vD supplements, because it is encouraged by care providers [35]. Higher sun index, intake from formula feeding and possible high vD supplementation probably contributed to the higher vD status in Shanghai infants. Using available data from the cohorts from the three sites in the regression analysis, a higher sun index and formula feeding, which increased infant vD intake, were predictors of higher infant vD status at 26 weeks of age. In a previous report, which focused on the Cincinnati site, a shorter duration of exclusive breastfeeding was also predictive of vD sufficiency [22].

The strength of the study is that we had data to examine the effect of sun exposure and vD supplement intake on maternal vD status at three international sites using the measurement of 25(OH)D levels in a single center. Our study also had a number of limitations. The measurement of 25(OH)D was at only one time point, and we did not have data to compare mother-infant pairs over time. There was lack of information on the vD status of the infants between birth and 26 weeks of age, which could have provided better longitudinal data on the relationship between feeding pattern and serum 25(OH)D concentration in the infant. We did not have blood samples in the infants for comparison of 25(OH)D concentrations during all four seasons across the three sites. We did not evaluate the role of skin pigmentation, which could contribute to vitamin synthesis and serum 25(OH)D levels, especially in Cincinnati cohorts. Additionally, an important limitation was lack of data on the rate of vD supplement intake in the infants at two of the three sites.

The reported vD supplementation rate in infants in the Cincinnati cohort was only 19%. Other studies from the U.S. have also reported a low vD supplementation rate of 5%–19% in breastfeeding infants [36,37], while two recent studies from Canada found high vD supplementation rates of 80%–98% [38] and 88%–98% in breastfed infants [39]. Advice on vD supplement use from healthcare providers was a positive predictor of supplementation in the Canadian [38,39] and one U.S. [37] study. In general, breastfed infants rely on transplacental transfer of vD, skin synthesis of vD or vD supplementation. However, due to concern about skin cancer, professional organizations recommend that infants avoid sun exposure [40]. Therefore, if breast milk is a major source of feeding in a setting of low maternal vD status and limited sun exposure, awareness among healthcare providers and caregivers of the need for vD supplement intake should be heightened to prevent vD deficiency in breastfeeding infants.

5. Conclusions

Vitamin D deficiency is detrimental to the health of mother and infant. From this comparative study using the same study design, it is possible that vD deficiency may be a global health problem in the breastfeeding mother-infant dyad and is related to sun exposure behaviors and vD supplement use between populations. Greater attention to maternal and infant vD status, preferably starting during pregnancy, is warranted worldwide.

Acknowledgments: This study was supported, in part, by Mead Johnson Pediatric Nutrition Institute, Inc., and NIH HD13021.

Author Contributions: Adekunle Dawodu, Jessica G. Woo, Ardythe L. Morrow, Barbara Davidson, Yong-Mei Peng, Guillermo M. Ruiz-Palacios and Maria de Lourdes Guerrero contributed to the design of the study. Ardythe L. Morrow and Jessica G. Woo provided statistical analysis of the data. Adekunle Dawodu, Ardythe L. Morrow and Jessica G. Woo participated in the initial draft of the manuscript. All the authors contributed to the review and content of the manuscript and have given approval to the final version of the paper.

Conflicts of Interest: The authors declare no conflict of interest.

References

1. Holick, M.F. Mccollum award lecture, 1994: Vitamin D—New horizons for the 21st century. *Am. J. Clin. Nutr.* **1994**, *60*, 619–630.
2. Macdonald, H.M.; Mavroeidi, A.; Fraser, W.D.; Darling, A.L.; Black, A.J.; Aucott, L.; O'Neill, F.; Hart, K.; Berry, J.L.; Lanham-New, S.A.; *et al.* Sunlight and dietary contributions to the seasonal vitamin d status of cohorts of healthy postmenopausal women living at northerly latitudes: A major cause for concern? *Osteoporos. Int.* **2011**, *22*, 2461–2472.
3. Bikle, D. Nonclassic actions of vitamin D. *J. Clin. Endocrinol. Metab.* **2009**, *94*, 26–34.
4. Holick, M.F. Vitamin d: Importance in the prevention of cancers, type 1 diabetes, heart disease, and osteoporosis. *Am. J. Clin. Nutr.* **2004**, *79*, 362–371.
5. Dawodu, A.; Wagner, C.L. Mother-child vitamin D deficiency: An international perspective. *Arch. Dis. Child.* **2007**, *92*, 737–740.
6. Thacher, T.D.; Fischer, P.R.; Strand, M.A.; Pettifor, J.M. Nutritional rickets around the world: Causes and future directions. *Ann. Trop. Paediatr.* **2006**, *26*, 1–16.
7. Holick, M.F. Vitamin d deficiency. *N. Engl. J. Med.* **2007**, *357*, 266–281.
8. Hypponen, E.; Laara, E.; Reunanen, A.; Jarvelin, M.R.; Virtanen, S.M. Intake of vitamin d and risk of type 1 diabetes: A birth-cohort study. *Lancet* **2001**, *358*, 1500–1503.

9. Dawodu, A.; Wagner, C.L. Prevention of vitamin d deficiency in mothers and infants worldwide—A paradigm shift. *Paediatr. Int. Child Health* **2012**, *32*, 3–13.

10. Wayse, V.; Yousafzai, A.; Mogale, K.; Filteau, S. Association of subclinical vitamin d deficiency with severe acute lower respiratory infection in Indian children under 5 y. *Eur. J. Clin. Nutr.* **2004**, *58*, 563–567.

11. McNally, J.D.; Leis, K.; Matheson, L.A.; Karuananyake, C.; Sankaran, K.; Rosenberg, A.M. Vitamin D deficiency in young children with severe acute lower respiratory infection. *Pediatr. Pulmonol.* **2009**, *44*, 981–988.

12. Roth, D.E.; Shah, R.; Black, R.E.; Baqui, A.H. Vitamin d status and acute lower respiratory infection in early childhood in sylhet, Bangladesh. *Acta Paediatr.* **2010**, *99*, 389–393.

13. Dawodu, A.; Akinbi, H. Vitamin d nutrition in pregnancy: Current opinion. *Int. J. Women's Health* **2013**, *5*, 333–343.

14. Holick, M.F.; Binkley, N.C.; Bischoff-Ferrari, H.A.; Gordon, C.M.; Hanley, D.A.; Heaney, R.P.; Murad, M.H.; Weaver, C.M. Evaluation, treatment, and prevention of vitamin d deficiency: An endocrine society clinical practice guideline. *J. Clin. Endocrinol. MeTable* **2011**, *96*, 1911–1930.

15. Ginde, A.A.; Sullivan, A.F.; Mansbach, J.M.; Camargo, C.A., Jr. Vitamin d insufficiency in pregnant and nonpregnant women of childbearing age in the united states. *Am. J. Obstet. Gynecol.* **2010**, *202*, e431–e438.

16. Newhook, L.A.; Sloka, S.; Grant, M.; Randell, E.; Kovacs, C.S.; Twells, L.K. Vitamin D insufficiency common in newborns, children and pregnant women living in newfoundland and labrador, canada. *Matern. Child Nutr.* **2009**, *5*, 186–191.

17. Holmes, V.A.; Barnes, M.S.; Alexander, H.D.; McFaul, P.; Wallace, J.M. Vitamin d deficiency and insufficiency in pregnant women: A longitudinal study. *Br. J. Nutr.* **2009**, *102*, 876–881.

18. Viljakainen, H.T.; Saarnio, E.; Hytinantti, T.; Miettinen, M.; Surcel, H.; Makitie, O.; Andersson, S.; Laitinen, K.; Lamberg-Allardt, C. Maternal vitamin d status determines bone variables in the newborn. *J. Clin. Endocrinol. MeTable* **2010**, *95*, 1749–1757.

19. Sahu, M.; Bhatia, V.; Aggarwal, A.; Rawat, V.; Saxena, P.; Pandey, A.; Das, V. Vitamin D deficiency in rural girls and pregnant women despite abundant sunshine in northern India. *Clin. Endocrinol. (Oxf.)* **2009**, *70*, 680–684.

20. Judkins, A.; Eagleton, C. Vitamin d deficiency in pregnant New Zealand women. *N. Z. Med. J.* **2006**, *119*, U2144.

21. Dawodu, A.; Saadi, H.F.; Bekdache, G.; Javed, Y.; Altaye, M.; Hollis, B.W. Randomized controlled trial (rct) of vitamin d supplementation in pregnancy in a population with endemic vitamin D deficiency. *J. Clin. Endocrinol. MeTable* **2013**, *98*, 2337–2346.

22. Dawodu, A.; Zalla, L.; Woo, J.G.; Herbers, P.M.; Davidson, B.S.; Heubi, J.E.; Morrow, A.L. Heightened attention to supplementation is needed to improve the vitamin d status of breastfeeding mothers and infants when sunshine exposure is restricted. *Matern. Child Nutr.* **2014**, *10*, 383–397.

23. Specker, B.L.; Valanis, B.; Hertzberg, V.; Edwards, N.; Tsang, R.C. Sunshine exposure and serum 25-hydroxyvitamin d concentrations in exclusively breast-fed infants. *J. Pediatr.* **1985**, *107*, 372–376.

24. Dawodu, A.; Absood, G.; Patel, M.; Agarwal, M.; Ezimokhai, M.; Abdulrazzaq, Y.; Khalayli, G. Biosocial factors affecting vitamin d status of women of childbearing age in the united arab emirates. *J. Biosoc. Sci.* **1998**, *30*, 431–437.

25. Barger-Lux, M.J.; Heaney, R.P. Effects of above average summer sun exposure on serum 25-hydroxyvitamin d and calcium absorption. *J. Clin. Endocrinol. MeTable* **2002**, *87*, 4952–4956.

26. Dawodu, A.; Agarwal, M.; Sankarankutty, M.; Hardy, D.; Kochiyil, J.; Badrinath, P. Higher prevalence of vitamin d deficiency in mothers of rachitic than nonrachitic children. *J. Pediatr.* **2005**, *147*, 109–111.

27. Institute of Medicine. *Dietary Reference Intakes for Calcium and Vitamin D*; The National Academies Press: Washington, DC, USA, 2011.

28. Dawodu, A.; Agarwal, M.; Hossain, M.; Kochiyil, J.; Zayed, R. Hypovitaminosis d and vitamin d deficiency in exclusively breast-feeding infants and their mothers in summer: A justification for vitamin D supplementation of breast-feeding infants. *J. Pediatr.* **2003**, *142*, 169–173.

29. Seth, A.; Marwaha, R.K.; Singla, B.; Aneja, S.; Mehrotra, P.; Sastry, A.; Khurana, M.L.; Mani, K.; Sharma, B.; Tandon, N. Vitamin D nutritional status of exclusively breast fed infants and their mothers. *J. Pediatr. Endocrinol. MeTable* **2009**, *22*, 241–246.

30. Andiran, N.; Yordam, N.; Ozon, A. Risk factors for vitamin d deficiency in breast-fed newborns and their mothers. *Nutrition* **2002**, *18*, 47–50.

31. Strand, M.A.; Perry, J.; Guo, J.; Zhao, J.; Janes, C. Doing the month: Rickets and post-partum convalescence in rural China. *Midwifery* **2009**, *25*, 588–596.

32. Saadi, H.F.; Dawodu, A.; Afandi, B.O.; Zayed, R.; Benedict, S.; Nagelkerke, N. Efficacy of daily and monthly high-dose calciferol in vitamin D-deficient nulliparous and lactating women. *Am. J. Clin. Nutr.* **2007**, *85*, 1565–1571.

33. Challa, A.; Ntourntoufi, A.; Cholevas, V.; Bitsori, M.; Galanakis, E.; Andronikou, S. Breastfeeding and vitamin d status in Greece during the first 6 months of life. *Eur. J. Pediatr.* **2005**, *164*, 724–729.

34. Jain, V.; Gupta, N.; Kalaivani, M.; Jain, A.; Sinha, A.; Agarwal, R. Vitamin D deficiency in healthy breastfed term infants at 3 months & their mothers in india: Seasonal variation & determinants. *Indian J. Med. Res.* **2011**, *133*, 267–273.

35. Peng, Y.M.; Children's Hospital of Fudan University, Shanghai, China. *Personal Observation*, 2014.

36. Davenport, M.L.; Uckun, A.; Calikoglu, A.S. Pediatrician patterns of prescribing vitamin supplementation for infants: Do they contribute to rickets? *Pediatrics* **2004**, *113*, 179–180.

37. Taylor, J.A.; Geyer, L.J.; Feldman, K.W. Use of supplemental vitamin D among infants breastfed for prolonged periods. *Pediatrics* **2010**, *125*, 105–111.

38. Crocker, B.; Green, T.J.; Barr, S.I.; Beckingham, B.; Bhagat, R.; Dabrowska, B.; Douthwaite, R.; Evanson, C.; Friesen, R.; Hydamaka, K.; *et al.* Very high vitamin d supplementation rates among infants aged 2 months in vancouver and richmond, british columbia, canada. *BMC Public Health* **2011**, *11*, 905.

39. Gallo, S.; Jean-Philippe, S.; Rodd, C.; Weiler, H.A. Vitamin d supplementation of Canadian infants: Practices of montreal mothers. *Appl. Physiol. Nutr. Metab.* **2010**, *35*, 303–309.

40. American Academy of Pediatrics. Committee on Enrivonmental Health. Ultraviolet light: A hazard to children. *Pediatrics* **1999**, *104*, 328–333.

MDPI AG

St. Alban-Anlage 66

4052 Basel, Switzerland

Tel. +41 61 683 77 34

Fax +41 61 302 89 18

http://www.mdpi.com

Nutrients Editorial Office

E-mail: nutrients@mdpi.com

http://www.mdpi.com/journal/nutrients